Progress in Behaviour Therapy

Chief Editor: J.C. Brengelmann

Editors: J.T. Quinn P.J. Graham
J.J.M. Harbison H. McAllister

With 75 Figures

Springer-Verlag
Berlin · Heidelberg · New York 1975

J.C. Brengelmann
Max-Planck-Institut für Psychiatrie,
Kraepelinstraße 10, 8000 München 40, Germany

J.T. Quinn, P.J. Graham, J.J.M. Harbison, H. McAllister
Departments of Mental Health, Psychology, and Social Studies,
Queen's University of Belfast, Belfast BT 7 INN, Ireland

ISBN-13:978-3-642-66106-8 e-ISBN-13:978-3-642-66104-4
DOI: 10.1007/978-3-642-66104-4

Library of Congress Cataloging in Publication Data: Progress in Behaviour Therapy. Selections from the proceedings of the second meeting of the European Association for Behaviour Therapy and Modification and of the fourth annual meeting of the Behavioural Engineering Association, held at Wexford, Ire. Bibliography: p. Includes index. 1. Behaviour therapy – Congresses. I. Brengelmann, Johannes C. II. European Association for Behaviour Therapy and Modification. III. Behavioural Engineering Association. RC489.B4P69 616.8'914 75-5542.

Softcover reprint of the hardcover 1st edition 1975

Preface

This book contains a selection of the proceedings of the Second Meeting of the European Association for Behaviour Therapy and Modification, and of the Fourth Annual Meeting of the Behavioural Engineering Association. The conference, held at Wexford, Ireland, was attended by 320 delegates from most European countries and North America.

In the foreword to the proceedings of the previous European Conference Brengelmann and Tunner commented upon the extension of the basis of behaviour therapy. They pointed out that behaviour therapy had developed from the position in the early days, when treatments were derived by almost literal translation of learning principles to the clinic, to the more modern position where therapies were developed from considerations of the results from all experimental disciplines devoted to the study of both human and animal behaviour. Even a superficial consideration of the breadth of the topics represented in this volume will indicate that this trend has continued.

There has been in recent years some emphasis upon the value of integrating therapies derived from experimental procedures with clinical skills not far removed from those generally assumed to be possessed by psychotherapists and others with more traditional clinical experience. The interest in such approaches as those of Masters and Johnston, the use of group methods, interest in marital interaction – all these chronicle the penetration of behavioural therapy into areas previously regarded as the domain of the psychotherapist. Indeed, it is not surprising that some behaviour therapists now wish to be known as behavioural psychotherapists. This trend is also represented in the present volume.

It would, however, be a pity if, in an attempt to make up for possible past neglect of clinical skills by behaviour therapists, we were to blur the central stigmata of our discipline—an insistence that the development of the subject should continue to bear a close relationship to, and to look for, many of its therapeutic innovations from experimental psychology in the laboratory. It is therefore a matter of some satisfaction to the organisers of this conference that, while interest in clinical skills and the breadth of the topics involving behaviour therapy continue to grow, we have been able to attract papers relating to methodology, measurement, and even experimental animal psychology.

This volume is the first of a series on behaviour therapy that will appear at irregular intervals.

Our special thanks go to the publishers, Springer-Verlag, for all their help in producing this volume.

München, May 1975

J.T. QUINN
P.J. GRAHAM
J.J.M. HARBISON
H. McALLISTER
J.C. BRENGELMANN

Table of Contents

List of Contributors

Ashcroft, J.B., Moss Side Hospital, School Lane, Maghull, Liverpool, Lancs L31 1BD

Bancroft, J., Warneford Hospital, Oxford OX3 7JX

Becker-Carus, Ch., Abteilung Psychologie, Max-Planck-Institut für Psychiatrie, 8 München 40, Kraepelinstraße 10

Birbaumer, N., Psychologisches Institut der Universität München, Klinische Abteilung, 8 München 40, Kaulbachstraße 93

Brengelmann, J.C., Abteilung Psychologie, Max-Planck-Institut für Psychiatrie, 8 München 40, Kraepelinstraße 10

Brown, P.T., Central Hospital, Psychology Department, Hatton, Warwick

Chriswell, F., Department of Psychiatry, University of California, San Francisco, California

Crombach, C., Abteilungen für Psychiatrie und Psychologie, Max-Planck-Institut für Psychiatrie, 8 München 40, Kraepelinstraße 10

Crowe, M.J., Institute of Psychiatry, De Crespigny Park, London SE5 8AF

Dellam, A.M.P., Whitchurch Hospital, Whitchurch, Cardiff

Eaves, D., Department of Psychiatry, The University of Liverpool, Liverpool

Evans, P.D., Department of Psychology, The North East London Polytechnics, London

Ferstl, R., Abteilung Psychologie, Max-Planck-Institut für Psychiatrie, 8 München 40, Kraepelinstraße 10

Gerlinghoff, M., Abteilung Psychiatrie, Max-Planck-Institut für Psychiatrie, 8 München 40, Kraepelinstraße 10

Gottwald, P., Abteilung Psychologie, Max-Planck-Institut für Psychiatrie, 8 München 40, Kraepelinstraße 10

Graham, P. Joan, Department of Social Studies, Queen's University of Belfast, Belfast

Halliday, M., Dingleton Hospital, Melrose, Roxburghshire, Scotland

Harbison, J.J.M., Department of Mental Health, Queen's University of Belfast, Belfast

Heyse, H., Abteilung Psychiatrie, Max-Planck-Institut für Psychiatrie, 8 München 40, Kraepelinstraße 10

Hopkins, H.G., Dingleton Hospital, Melrose, Roxburghshire, Scotland

Innerhofer, P., Abteilung Psychologie, Max-Planck-Institut für Psychiatrie, 8 München 40, Kraepelinstraße 10

Jacob, R.G., St. Göran's Children's Hospital and the Department of Education, Stockholm

Jeffree, D., Hester Adrian Research Centre for the Study of Learning Processes in the Mentally Handicapped, University of Manchester, Manchester

Johnson, G., Department of Mental Hygiene, The Langley Porter Neuropsychiatric Institute, 401 Parnassus Avenue, San Francisco, California 94122

Jongmans, H., Psychologisch Laboratorium, University of Amsterdam, Weesperplein 8, Amsterdam

Kenyon, P.M., Central Hospital, Warwick, and Department of Psychology, University of Birmingham

Kolaszynska-Carr, A., Central Hospital, Warwick, and Department of Psychology, University of Birmingham

Kraemer, S., Abteilung Psychologie, Max-Planck-Institut für Psychiatrie, 8 München 40, Kraepelinstraße 10

Longabaugh, R., Department of Psychiatry, University of California, San Francisco, California

Mai, N., Abteilung Psychologie, Max-Planck-Institut für Psychiatrie, 8 München 40, Kraepelinstraße 10

Marks, I., Institute of Psychiatry, Maucsley Hospital, De Crespigny Park, London SE5 8AF

McAllister, H., Department of Psychology, Queen's University, Belfast

McAuley, R., Department of Mental Health, Queen's University, Belfast

Mittler, P., Hester Adrian Research Centre for the Study of Learning Processes in the Mentally Handicapped, University of Manchester

Morgan, R.T.T., University of Leicester, School of Social Work, Leicester

Nias, D.K.B., Shirley House, Upper Beeding, Steyning, Sussex

Nolan, P.J., Social Work Department, Rainhill Hospital, Prescot, Lancs

Nordlung, O., St. Göran's Children's Hospital and the Department of Education, Stockholm

Oelkers, C., Abteilung Psychologie, Max-Planck-Institut für Psychiatrie, 8 München 40, Kraepelinstraße 10

O'Gorman, E., Department of Mental Health, Queen's University, Belfast

Olley, M., Department of Mental Health, Queen's University, Belfast

Ott, H., Kinderabteilung, Max-Planck-Institut für Psychiatrie, 8 München 40, Kraepelinstraße 10

Peck, D.F., Department of Psychiatry, Edinburgh University, Edinburgh, Scotland

Peikert, V., Abteilungen für Psychiatrie und Psychologie, Max-Planck-Institut für Psychiatrie, 8 München 40, Kraepelinstraße 10

Phillips, J.P.N., Senior Lecturer, Department of Psychology, The University, Hull

Quinn, J.T., Department of Mental Health, Queen's University, Belfast

Ramsay, R.W., Psychologisch Laboratorium, University of Amsterdam, Weesperplein 8, Amsterdam

Raskin, M., Department of Psychiatry, University of California, San Francisco, California

Redlin, W., Psychologisches Institut der Universität München, Klinische Abteilung, 8 München 40, Kaulbachstraße 93

Revenstorff, D., Abteilung Psychologie, Max-Planck-Institut für Psychiatrie, 8 München 40, Kraepelinstraße 10

Rondestvedt, J., Department of Psychiatry, University of California, San Francisco, California

Schultze, B., Dingleton Hospital, Melrose, Roxburghshire, Scotland

Schwarz, D., Abteilung Psychiatrie, Max-Planck-Institut für Psychiatrie, 8 München 40, Kraepelinstraße 10

Schwieler, G.H., St. Göran's Children's Hospital and the Department of Education, Stockholm

Sedlmayr, E., Abteilung Psychologie, Max-Planck-Institut für Psychiatrie, 8 München 40, Kraepelinstraße 10

Stoffelmayer, B.E., Klinikum Höhenried, 8131 Höhenried

Surtees, P., Department Mental Health, University of Aberdeen

Thornton, E.W., Department of Psychology, University of Liverpool, Liverpool

Tunner, W., Psychologisches Institut der Universität München, Klinische Abteilung, 8 München 40, Kaulbachstraße 93

Ullrich, R., Abteilungen für Psychiatrie und Psychologie, Max-Planck-Institut für Psychiatrie, 8 München 40, Kraepelinstraße 10

Ullrich-de Muynck, R., Abteilungen für Psychiatrie und Psychologie, Max-Planck-Institut für Psychiatrie, 8 München 40, Kraepelinstraße 10

Walker, L.G., Department Mental Health, University of Aberdeen

Wilhelm, H., Abteilung Psychologie, Max-Planck-Institut für Psychiatrie, 8 München 40, Kraepelinstraße 10

Williams, C., Lea Hospital, Bromsgrave

Wheldall, K., Hester Adrian Research Centre for the Study of Learning Processes in the Mentally Handicapped, University of Manchester, Manchester

I. Behaviour Modification with Children

Mannerisms, Mutilation and Management

C. WILLIAMS and P. SURTEES

> A changing sensory environment seems essential for human beings. Without it the brain ceases to function in an adequate way and abnormalities of behaviour develop.
>
> HERON, 1957

The general conclusions to be drawn from work on experimentally induced sensory deprivation appear to suggest that an environment offering little or no stimulus change is an aversive state, and, as such, would tend to result in behaviours that serve to avoid such a state (SCHULTZ, 1965).

Apart from the deliberate restriction of sensory input as used in laboratory studies, there can also be naturally occurring sensory deprivation conditions of which probably the best exemplars are those conditions resulting from either:

1. congenital defects of the sense organs

or

2. environments severely restricted in stimulus change.

In 1941 GREGG, an Australian ophthalmologist, first reported an association between the infection of the mother with rubella virus, especially during the first trimester, and the subsequent congenital defects of the foetus. Cataracts, malformation of the heart and deafness are the most noticeable defects produced by congenital rubella, and they form the common symptom triad of the rubella syndrome. Defects of the nervous system, intellectual retardation and behavioural anomalies are now also recognized as belonging to this syndrome (CHESS et al., 1971). Hence, any individual suffering from such a syndrome can be viewed as a natural analogue of the experimental subject in a sensory deprivation study.

The first part of this paper describes work currently being carried out on such a group of children and presents some of the results of the effects of stimulation on the baseline repertoires of individuals from such a group when studied under stimulus controlled conditions.

The second naturally occurring sensory deprivation condition we identify is that present in many wards in hospitals for the severely subnormal where staff shortages produce conditions in which many individuals receive only minimal stimulation and where attention from staff is largely contingent on disruptive behaviour.

In the second part of this paper we present an experimental study on such a patient whose limited behavioural repertoire included bouts of very severe self-mutilation by repeated head-banging.

I. Study 1

In an earlier report (WILLIAMS, 1972) it was noted that observation of a group of retarded rubella syndrome children would show that much of their activity involves the performance of repetitive and stereotyped movement patterns involving rocking, arm-flapping, head-banging, finger-waving and eye-poking. A continuous taped commentary of samples of behaviour of an eight year old SSN rubella syndrome child indicated that the child spent some 40% of the total observation time eye-poking - that is, inserting the first finger of his right hand into his right eye socket and moving the eyeball itself up and down. Clearly eye-poking has reinforcing consequences, but without direct evidence it is difficult to identify precisely what these are. The child is probably experiencing similar visual phenomena to those experienced by sighted persons pressing on closed eyelids by pressure stimulation of the optic nerve endings. Since the optic defect of rubella children is largely restricted to the lens there is little reason to suppose that the retina, the optic nerve and the visual cortex are not at least physiologically reactive.

In this same subject, rocking occupied a further 25% of his free operant repertoire. He was free from any form of stereotyped self-stimulatory activity during only 11% of the observation period. However, when tactile stimulation was applied by using a vibration tube worn against his back, the percentage of time spent without stereotypy increased significantly to 26% ($p = .001$). Thus, the provision of a continuous tactile stimulation decreased self-stimulation markedly.

A further finding from preliminary observations of this group was that some of them, instead of physically poking their eyes, would wave their fingers back and forth in front of their eyes, especially in areas of particularly bright light. A common feature among this group was that some remnant of vision was present and that the lens was sufficiently transparent to allow at least light-dark discrimination.

The present study grew in part from that described above in an attempt to modify the tactile stimulus presentation so that it was subject-operated and hence analogous to a standard operant manipulandum through providing tactile feedback as a result of bar pressing.

Three major hypotheses were to be tested:

1. that rubella children who showed finger-waving in their free operant repertoire would be able to discriminate light stimuli and that they would approach such stimuli. In other words, given partial sight, but deafness, light stimuli would reinforce approach behaviour;
2. that the provision of subject-operated stimuli would compete with self-stimulation;

   and
3. that tactile stimulation would serve to reinforce bar-pressing activity.

The studies described below were done using two additional experimental subjects. Preliminary results are presented to show how such subjects can be investigated under control conditions and the contribution they can make to a theoretical formulation of stereotypy and self-mutilation.

II. Subjects

Subject 1, whose study has provided the results for testing the first hypothesis, is a 4 1/2-year-old female whose mother contracted rubella at 6 weeks of pregnancy. She has the classical rubella symptom triad though her sensory defect is not total in that the cataracts have been needled and she is now light sensitive. She is also reactive to sounds above 80 decibels at all frequencies. She can walk and feed herself with a spoon. She has a Maxfield-Buchholtz adapted Vineland SQ of 43 and is currently on no regular medication. Baseline frequency counts of her behaviour in the observation area indicated a mean percentage of 55% visually oriented mannerisms (finger-wave and eye-poke).

Subject 2, used for testing the second and third hypotheses, is a young man of 8 1/2 years, diagnosed as rubella syndrome, whose mother was affected at 3 weeks of pregnancy. He presently feeds himself but is not toilet trained. There is no speech present. He has only minimal light-dark discrimination following cataract needling. His Maxfield-Buchholtz adapted Vineland SQ is 38, and he is receiving 20 mg of Pemoline t.d.s. His free operant repertoire consists largely of finger-sucking, arm-flapping and eye-poking.

III. Apparatus

1. The observation area used for these studies was specially constructed inside a larger room. It consists of four 6' high wood walls enclosing a 9' x 9' floor area. This floor area is marked off in 16 equal squares, each one numbered.

2. A stimulus box was made measuring 60 cm by 45 cm by 30 cm. The top has a sloping panel of translucent plastic mounted in a sponge rubber frame and is pressure sensitive. Pressing on the panel operates a micro-switch which activates a vibration unit mounted beneath the panel. The sensitivity of the micro-switch was adjusted to be sensitive to the lightest possible touch but to switch off when released.

   A 150 watt electric light bulb giving a white light was fixed inside the box. Operation of either the vibration or light circuit is controlled by the experimenter, who uses over-ride switches.

IV. Method

Each child was observed from a vantage point outside the marked floor area using a time sampling technique. The observer wore a hearing aid ear piece through which was fed an auditory signal every ten seconds at which time the observer would write down in code those behaviours exhibited by the child. The coding of behaviours was determined previously using two independent observers, and the reliability of the procedure was established. This observation procedure was continued for 50 observations per experimental condition, the number of conditions for any one session being determined by the particular experimental design in use at the time. All observations were taken in dimmed light to enhance the light-dark contrast.

V. Results

1. The data from the study using subject 1 are presented in a classical graph form (Fig. 1).

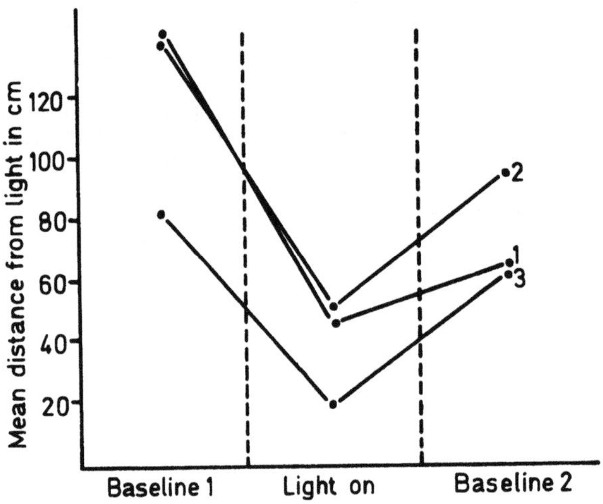

Fig. 1. Relationship between spatial position and sensory input

They indicate a clear situational preference in that in all three sessions she moved towards the box whenever the light came on and moved away when the light was switched off. The first hypothesis is therefore supported, and evidence for positive phototropism is provided.

2. The data from subject 2 are presented in the form of cumulative curves (Fig. 2) showing the results of two similar sessions run on different days. Each session consists of an ABA design - each part of which consists of 50 ten-second time samples of behaviour.

   The curves are drawn by recording observations of stereotypy along the abscissa and absence of stereotypy along the ordinate (the term 'gaze' has been adopted as the code for absence of stereotypy, though it is clear no gazing as such is possible).

It can be seen from the cumulative curves that:

1. in both sessions the baseline free operant rate of gaze is about 25% of the time;
2. when vibration-contingent panel-pressing is made available on a CRF schedule, the subject makes use of such a contingency indicating the reinforcing consequences of vibration (each hatch mark indicates a panel press response of sufficient strength to activate the vibrator);
3. the percentage gaze under the CRF-VIB condition is 100 %, indicating a total suppression' of stereotypy;

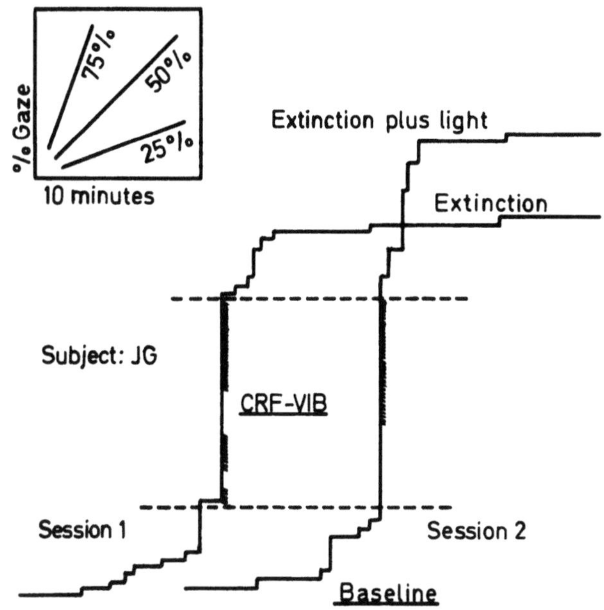

Fig. 2. Cumulative curves of 'gaze' against stereotypy under various conditions of contingent sensory reinforcement

4. extinction is very rapid, and response contingent vibration produces no long-term behavioural effect when the contingencies are removed;
5. in the extinction period of session 2 the box light was left on, and the extinction of the 'gaze-suppression' effect was delayed until the light was switched off.

VI. Summary of Results

These data support the three experimental hypotheses in that in rubella syndrome subjects, sensory stimulation reinforces approach behaviour, and tactile stimulation from a subject-operated manipulandum competes with self-generated stimulation, thereby reducing markedly stereotyped mannerisms.

VII. Discussion

Drawing on theoretical and experimental data published by other workers on various aspects of non-specific sensory stimulation, the present authors have noted particularly the following:

1. a hypothesis suggesting the existence of a mechanism in the brain mediating behavioural functions having to do with levels of alertness (MALMO, 1959);
2. that visual stimulation will reinforce operant behaviour in visually deprived animals (FOX, 1972; SACKETT et al., 1963; WENDT et al., 1963);
3. a reported relationship between stimulus intensity and hedonic tone (BERLYNE, 1969);

4. a relationship between high levels of arousal as indexed by EEG and the occurrence of stereotypy in autistic children (HUTT and HUTT, 1968);

5. a statement by the HUTTs that 'whilst the autists' stereotyped behaviours occur significantly more frequently with increase in environmental complexity, those of the defectives seem to occur predominantly in the absence of stimulation;

6. heart rate data from a group of children diagnosed as autistic, indicating the possibility of a pathology in arousal control in such children (MacCULLOCH and WILLIAMS, 1971; MacCULLOCH and SAMBROOKS, 1972).

From such studies plus those extensively reviewed by BERLYNE (1967), the authors have interpreted the present findings firstly using the arousal model shown in Fig. 3.

The proposed arousal-stereotypy relationship is seen as producing a U-shaped curve relating the two variables. As arousal level decreases through 'boredom' for normal subjects to conditions of environmental deprivation in 'retardates', the amount of stereotypy increases, and, conversely, as arousal level increases through 'stress' with normal subjects to over-arousal with 'autistics' then similarly, stereotypy again increases. The model implies that an optimal level of arousal could exist where stereotypy is at a minimum and that any divergence from this optimal level could serve as a drive cue in the Hullian sense to initiate stereotyped behaviour whose function was related to arousal regulation.

There is, however, a growing dissatisfaction amongst certain theorists over the use of such 'internal' concepts as arousal (SKINNER, 1969; BLACKMAN and THOMAS, 1971). As a result, the present authors felt that a more parsimonious model for our data should relate, not to 'events taking place somewhere else, at some other level of observation, described in different terms and measured, if at all, in different dimensions' (SKINNER, 1950), but to observable environmental events.

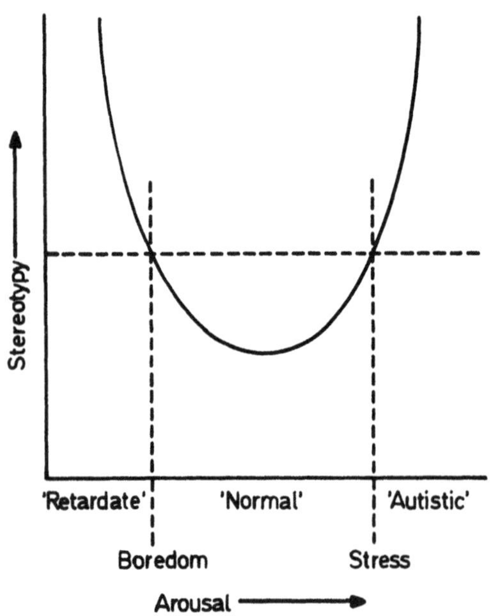

Fig. 3. Hypothetical relationship between stereotypy and arousal level

Accordingly the U-shaped model was used to plot the two variables stereotypy and stimulus level such that both extremes of stimulation, over-stimulation and under-stimulation, are directly related to increase in stereotypy (Fig. 4).

We feel that our present data fit well with the model when considering the retarded individual and the congenitally sensory-deprived individual at the lower end of the stimulus level continuum. There is, however, little data to support the placing of the autistic group at the higher end of such a continuum; the justification for doing so will depend upon demonstrating a behavioural counterpart to the concept of hyperarousal. The physiological model (MacCULLOCH and SAMBROOKS, 1972) provides a mechanism whereby one could suppose that the stimulus input in autistics is over-amplified by the ascending reticular activating system of the mid-brain which would support, in theory, such a placement on the model. Until further evidence is available we present this solely as a very tentative suggestion.

We would now like to introduce the second part of the study by reiterating a number of points:

1. Under conditions of sensory deprivation individuals are reinforced by events that provide non-specific stimulation.
2. Present staff shortages on hospital wards ensure that a state of social deprivation exists for many patients.
3. Staff attention is a reinforcing event and can serve to strengthen behaviour patterns upon which it is contingent (GARDNER, 1971).

Given these factors we propose a model for the genesis of self-mutilation from initial self-stimulatory behaviours resulting from deprivation, developing to severe self-mutilation by a process of shaping, unwittingly carried out by staff, who intervene progressively later in the chain of mutilation responses. Since the opportunity for acquiring incompatible behaviours in some cases is lacking, we feel that

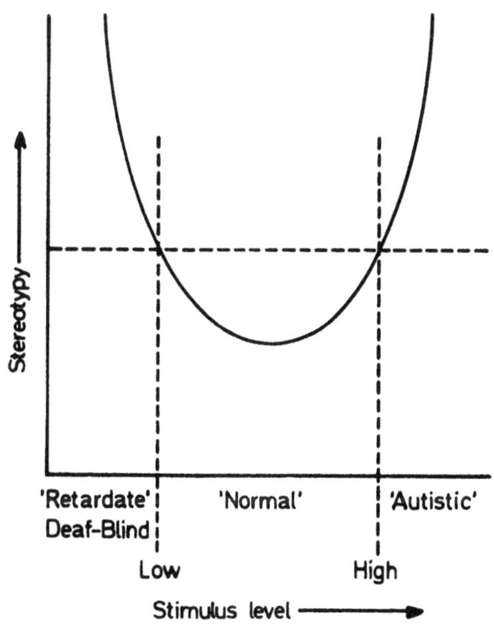

Fig. 4. Hypothetical relationship between stereotypy and stimulus level

self-mutilation can be viewed as an operant that becomes maintained by the resultant staff attention which such behaviour elicits. As such it was considered that an operant approach to the treatment of self-mutilation should be attempted in one particularly severe case.

The subject for this study was a 24-year-old female, institutionalised at the age of 6 years, when her parents felt they could no longer control her behaviour. Her early admission notes describe her as an "idiot" showing persistent head banging and biting. She is totally blind and has no executive speech. She can now feed herself but is not toilet trained. Her present drug regime consists of Phenobarbitone 60 mg t.d.s. and Pericyazine 30 mg t.d.s. Her head-banging is at present so severe that throughout the day she is seated on her ward with her hands in restraints to prevent the self-injury that would occur should she be released. This regime has been in existence for 15 years prior to the present study.

Most of the self-injurious behaviour consists of raising her left wrist and repeatedly striking her forehead with blows of increasing strength until it becomes necessary to intervene with attention to prevent serious damage. The result of this behaviour is that she has produced a number of prominent swellings on her head which need repeated nursing attention to prevent infection.

The problem as we saw it was, therefore, chronic, incompatible with ultimate rehabilitation and resistant to current treatment practices.

The following is an account of the procedures we adopted in an attempt to modify this behaviour.

VIII. Experimental and Treatment Procedures

Baseline Measures

In view of the problem of allowing the head-banging to occur when unrestrained, the subject's forehead was protected with cotton wool and crepe bandage to prevent serious injury. This procedure would clearly alter quite drastically the stimulus situation under which the response was occurring. The authors, however, did not feel justified in allowing such injury to occur solely in order to establish 'good' baseline data.

This baseline period was essentially a series of extinction trials and appears as such in the graph of the cumulative curves (Fig. 5). The curve is made up of the total pre-treatment observation time of 110 three-minute periods taken over one month in 40 minute sessions. A steady state of head-banging of approximately 12 responses per minute was recorded up to the eighteenth three-minute observation period, when they ceased completely. This extinction was specific to the experimental room, as would be predicted (LOVAAS and SIMMONS, 1969), and did not generalise to the ward where she would again be placed in the restraints. Clearly extinction is not an adequate procedure.

The second experimental study involved the presentation of response contingent negative reinforcement. A shock box designed to give a two millisecond pulse at 90 volts^{+} across two electrodes placed on the calf

$^{+}$ The maximum current possible from any of the shock boxes used in this study was measured at 8 milliamps through a direct short of nil resistance.

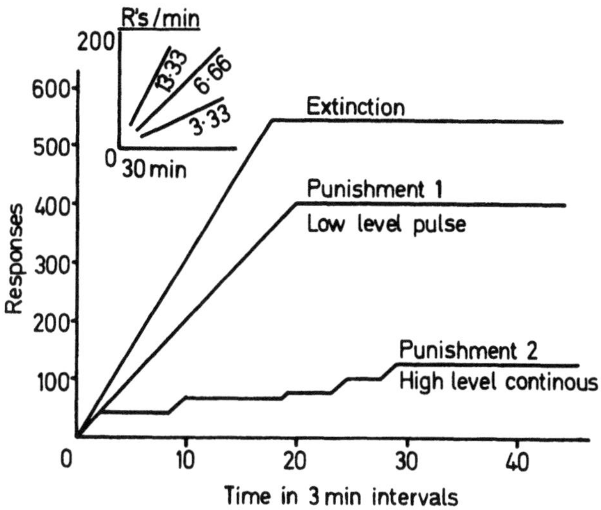

Fig. 5. Cumulative curves of head-banging responses under three treatment conditions

of the left leg was used to present the aversive stimulation. The target response was defined as any hand-to-forehead contact that was similar to the early steps in the self-injury chain of behaviour.

The results of this period are shown as punishment 1 in Fig. 5 and indicate the cessation of head-banging responses after 400 shock contingent trials (it should be noted that this represents a total shock time of only 0.8 seconds). Not only was the response rate markedly reduced but the force with which the hand was moved to the forehead also diminished until during the final punishment trials what had been previously a severe head-bang became a light touch to the head.

The third experimental study involved the presentation of a relatively higher level of continuous shock at 125 volts. On each trial the shock was terminated upon cessation of head-banging. The effect of this procedure was to produce a markedly accelerated cessation curve, shown in the graph as punishment 2. This decrement in self-injury responses was produced even though it may have been predicted that an adaptation effect should have occurred following the previous use of low level shock (AZRIN and HOLZ, 1966).

In view of the situational specificity of the punishment procedures, we felt that a direct suppression of the self-injury responses by using high shock level was grossly unsatisfactory, particularly in this case where self-injury constituted the major component of the subject's behavioural repertoire. We therefore decided to teach a response incompatible with self-injury. Since previous attempts using food as a reinforcer on a DRO schedule had not proved very successful in producing a lasting effect, it was decided to attempt such training using escape-avoidance conditioning. The incompatible response to be trained was defined as having both hands holding a toy doll. The subject had been tested with the doll during the initial observation periods but with no effect on the self-injury frequency. The avoidance response of doll holding was shaped by using escape training in a procedure similar to that described by WHALEY and MALOTT (1971, pp. 377-383). A loud buzzer was used as the CS, having been paired with shock as the UCS. The electrodes on these trials were attached to the subject's left arm where it was felt that the point of punishment would be more clearly associated with the self-injury behaviour.

The subject's right hand was placed on the doll whilst her left arm was raised by the second experimenter to the position adopted prior to each self-injury response. Both buzzer and shock were then switched on and the subject's left hand was taken down from its position and held to the doll when both buzzer and shock would be terminated. No protective head covering was used during these escape training trials.

During the first 15 minutes, 35 such training trials were completed, followed by 15 minutes of unrestrained doll holding, after which a further shaped escape trial was performed. Again, unrestrained doll holding occured, this time for a period of 45 minutes, after which time the first signalled avoidance responses were made when the subject raised her left hand to strike her forehead, the buzzer was sounded and she replaced her hand to the doll without shock being delivered. The doll holding continued for the remainder of the session. The progress of this phase of the treatment is shown in Fig. 6.

During the follow-up sessions the subject, when given the doll, ceased head-banging and actively resisted when the experimenters attempted to get her to raise her left hand to her head. The follow-up sessions were conducted over a further period of 1 hour 45 minutes observation time.

Since it was now felt that the self-injury response had been brought under control in the laboratory, it was decided to repeat additional shaped escape training trials in more realistic situations:

1. seated in the ward day room,
2. seated in the ward dormitory,
3. seated at the meal table,
4. lying on her bed at night.

In all of these situations the shaped escape procedure was used, and in a total training time of 2 hours, 14 shaped escape trials were used and 10 spontaneous avoidance responses occurred. Following these training trials it was possible to exchange the doll for a number of other toys with similar effects, and observation for a whole day using only the buzzer as a CS indicated a successful suppression of her previous self-injury.

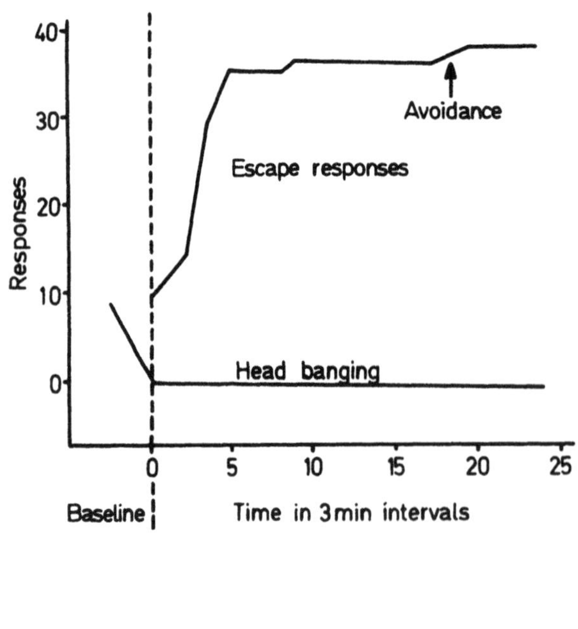

Fig. 6. Cumulative curve of head-banging responses and escape-avoidance responses during escape-avoidance training

Subsequent follow-up, however, has indicated that the suppression effect has not been permanent and that arm restraints have been re-introduced by the nursing staff.

We would like to suggest a number of reasons for this failure to control self-injury except under specific stimulus conditions.

1. Not only was the buzzer acting as a CS for avoidance learning, but the experimenters themselves also acquired CS properties associated with the sounds specific to the training procedures.
2. The nursing staff on the ward were unable to continue with the procedures necessary to maintain the avoidance response by virtue of the constraints of ward shortage and lack of available time for special treatment of an individual.
3. As a result of foregoing factors, the subject acquired a discriminated avoidance response, only restraining from self-injury when the experimenters were present. The staff were, therefore, obliged to react to her head-banging by attention to prevent injury and subsequently by arm restraints for more permanent control.

IX. Conclusion

Self-injury behaviour can be controlled effectively using an escape-avoidance training procedure. This procedure, however, is only recommended with extreme caution since, unless the established avoidance response can be maintained by, and in the presence of the permanent care staff of the ward, the self-injury responses will be reinstated. It is our belief that unless an incompatible response that is to some extent self-maintaining can be taught to such individuals, it will remain very difficult to deal with severe cases of self-injury, particularly when those individuals' behavioural repertoires are as limited as was the repertoire of the individual described in this paper.

References

AZRIN, N.H., HOLZ, W.C.: Punishment. In: HONIG, W.K. (Ed.): Operant Behaviour: Areas of Reserach and Application. New York: Appleton-Century-Crofts 1966.

BERLYNE, D.E.: Arousal and reinforcement. In: LEVINE, D. (Ed.): Nebraska Symposium on Motivation. Nebraska: University of Nebraska Press 1967.

BERLYNE, D.E.: Arousal, reward and learning. Ann. N.Y. Acad. Sci. 159, 1059-1070 (1969).

BLACKMAN, D.E., THOMAS, G.V.: Critical notice: reinforcement and information. Brit. J. Psychol. 62, 403-407 (1971).

CHESS, S., KORN, S.J., FERNANDEZ, P.B.: Psychiatric Disorders of children with Congenital Rubella. London: Butterworths 1971.

FOX, S.S.: Self-maintained sensory input and sensory deprivation in monkeys: a behavioural and neuropharmacological study. J. comp. physiol. Psychol. 55, 438-444 (1972).

GARDNER, W.I.: Behaviour Modification in Mental Retardation. London: University of London Press 1971.

GREGG, N.M.: Congenital cataract following German measles in mother. Trans. ophthal. Soc. Aust. 3, 35-46 (1941).

HERON.W.: The pathology of boredom. Scientific American 196, 52-56 (1957).

HUTT, S.J., HUTT, C.: Stereotypy, arousal and autism. Hum. Develop. 11, 277-286 (1968).

LOVAAS, O.I., SIMMONS, J.Q.: Manipulation of self-destruction in three retarded children. J. appl. behav. Anal. 2, 143-157 (1969).

MacCULLOCH, M.J., SAMBROOKS, J.E.: An aetiological theory of infantile autism. Paper presented at the Second European Conference of Behaviour Modification, Wexford/Ireland 1972.

MacCULLOCH, M.J., WILLIAMS, C.: On the nature of infantile autism. Acta psychiat. scand. 47, 295-314 (1971).

MALMO, R.B.: Activation: a neuropsychological dimension. Psychol. Rev. 66, 367-386 (1959).

SACKETT, G.P., KEITH-LEE, P., TREAT, R.: Food versus perceptual complexity as rewards for rats previously subjected to sensory deprivation. Science 141, 518-520 (1963).

SCHULTZ, D.P.: Sensory Restriction: Effects on Behaviour. New York: Academic Press 1965.

SKINNER, B.F.: Are theories of learning necessary? Psychol. Rev. 57, 193-216 (1950).

SKINNER, B.F.: Contingencies of Reinforcement. New York: Appleton-Century-Crofts 1969.

WENDT, R.H., LINDSLEY, D.F., ROSS ADEY, W., FOX, S.S.: Self-maintained visual stimulation in monkeys after long-term visual deprivation. Science 139, 336-338 (1963).

WHALEY, D.L., MALOTT, R.W.: Elementary Principles of Behaviour. New York: Appleton-Century-Crofts 1971.

WILLIAMS, C.: A functional analysis of stereotypy in the rubella child. Conf. report No. 62, The Southern Regional Association for the Blind 1972.

Acquisition of the Two-Word "Pivot-Open" Structure in Subnormal Children: A Case Study+

K. WHELDALL, D. JEFFREE and P. MITTLER

I. Summary

The aim of this project was to test the hypothesis that early two-word utterances of the 'pivot-open' type could be taught to young, severely subnormal children. The subjects were two four-year-old mongol boys, equated developmentally, who were judged to be using only single word utterances at the beginning of the study. The design involved both between-subject and within-subject control procedures.

Both the children were initially taught the appropriate use of ten nouns and one participle, these words being taken mostly from their existing repertoires. Play for the experimental child was then structured to encourage 'pivot-open' utterances, based on a combination of five of the original ten nouns plus the pivot 'gone'. The control child had virtually the same conditions except that his play was relatively unstructured in that no 'pivot-open' models were given. When criterion level was reached for the experimental child using the first five nouns, he was exposed to the second five nouns to test for generalization. It was shown that generalization did occur. The control child, who had not produced any 'pivot-open' constructions, was then switched to the experimental condition and quickly learnt both to imitate and generalize the 'pivot-open' construction.

A follow-up study revealed considerable transfer to the classroom situation.

II. Introduction

Normal children, after passing through a one-word labelling stage, begin to structure two-word, pivot-open type sentences at around 18 months without having had any specific training. These take the form, for example, of utterances like "allgone boy", "allgone sock", "allgone vitamins", as cited by McNEILL (1966).

The appearance of a child's earliest two-word utterances represents a landmark of considerable importance in the language and cognitive development of a young child. The child equipped with even a small number of two-word utterances can begin to express increasingly complex intentions and meanings (e.g. 'no dinner'; 'my car'; 'more

+ The research reported in this paper was supported by S.S.R.C. Grant 840/1.

dinner'). He has progressed from the stage of labelling, using mainly nouns, to his first statements of situations and relationships. The ability to combine two words marks not only the beginning of his use of grammar and syntax, but also enables him to express a far wider range of ideas.

Nevertheless, despite the importance of this behaviour, it has to be admitted that we know relatively little about the way in which normal children progress from the one-word to the two-word stage. Linguists have described these utterances in terms of a 'pivot-open' distinction (BRAINE, 1963). Pivots (P) are words which occur with high frequency on which a much larger number of 'open' (O) class words are hung. MILLER and ERVIN (1964) have also referred to pivots as operators. Thus, 'allgone' might be a pivot preceding open class words such as 'dinner', 'potty', 'Daddy' etc; similarly '<u>no</u> bye bye'; '<u>no</u> dinner', etc. The pivot can also follow the open word, as in 'sock <u>gone</u>' 'car <u>gone</u>' etc. (McNEILL, 1966 gives a representative list from three studies of early child grammars). SLOBIN (1972), reporting the results of several projects on early language development, points out that the child's speech is more differentiated than the surface form of his utterances might suggest, and interpretation must depend on non-linguistic factors. Lois BLOOM (1972) reports that one of the children she studied said "Mummy sock" on two distinct occasions - when picking up her mother's sock and while being dressed by her mother. Both context and gesture are used to disambiguate such sentences. To avoid misunderstanding it must be pointed out that not every two-word utterance is of this type. Some seem to be acquired and used as invariant units (e.g. 'here y'are').

Research into the development of two-word utterances in subnormal children is overdue, as subnormal children appear to encounter special difficulties at this stage. Several studies have pointed to the subnormal child's tendency to get stuck at the one-word labelling stage. It appears that teachers and parents may unwittingly reinforce one-word utterances. JEFFREE and CASHDAN (1971) found that mothers of severely subnormal children fired innumerable questions at them simply in order to get them to talk at all. Such questions which took the form of "Wat is that?" tended to constrain replies to single-word responses or required only yes or no answers.

There has been a recent surge of interest in the use of operant techniques to initiate or improve the use of expressive language in retardates. BRICKER and BRICKER (1970) reported a systematic programme, progressing from imitation of gesture to appropriate labelling responses. They suggest that the next stage in such a programme might be an attempt to train the use of 'pivot-open' sentences (BRICKER, 1972). The problem is whether the same techniques are equally appropriate to what is essentially the learning of a very different kind of response. In acquiring an initial vocabulary, responses to <u>objects</u> are demanded, whereas pivot-open utterances are responses to <u>events</u>. Furthermore, the objective is not merely to train the child to use a specific response to a secific event, but to allow generalization of the structure of these responses to similar situations.

In order to do this, the vocabulary used should already be familiar to the child and related to his own interests; also the meaning conveyed by the combination of words should be a translation of an active experience with which he is already familiar.

In light of these considerations, the aim of the present study was to see if it was feasible to facilitate the acquisition of pivot-open utterances in young mongol children, who were at the single-word labelling stage. This modification of behaviour was to be achieved without severe control of the reinforcement contingencies.

III. Method

In view of the exploratory nature of the procedures, it was decided to use only two subjects within a controlled experimental design.

Two mongol boys were selected from the same class at the same Special School for the severely subnormal. Both were of the same chronological age (4 years) and developmental stage as determined by several measures, including those of WOODWARD (1966) and KIRK et al. (1968). They were both near the end of the sensori-motor stage of development; their language development was between 18 months and 2 years, their motor-development and stage of play between 2 and 3 years (on the scale devised by KIRK et al.). (See Table 1).

Table 1. Developmental Level of Subjects

	Experimental child	Control child
CA	4.3	4.0
sensori-motor stage	V	V-V1
language age	18m.+	18m.+
motor-development	2-3 yrs	2-3 yrs
play	2-3 yrs	2-3 yrs

Both were clearly at the one-word naming stage and used a similar number of single words (about 30) as well as a few word strings used as invariant units. This was established after eleven mornings of classroom observation during which a neutral observer noted down everything the two children said. The home background was probably not so closely matched, one child being a second generation immigrant.

The design consisted of a combination of between-subject and within-subject control procedures. The control subject subsequently functioned in the experimental condition also.

1. Equating on Single Words

An examination of the observed verbal behaviour revealed that thirteen words were common to the vocabularies of both children; of these, four (book, ball, bus, baby) were selected as suitable open class words. In addition to this, to make up a total of ten such words, three more were selected from each child's vocabulary (pen, bag, soap; shoe, car, cup).

Both children were taught to recognise and use all these words appropriately. In addition they were taught to use the selected pivot word 'gone' as one-word utterance in the context of one of the experimenters hiding from the children. 'Gone' was selected as the experimental pivot, as it had not been produced by either child and because it is frequently reported as a pivot which is learned early in the child's language development.

In the preliminary sessions, when these single words were being taught, the boys were encouraged to compete for social approval dependent upon the requisite verbal performance. One of the experimenters played with the children whilst the other took careful note of everything the children said and of the context in which it was said. We paid particular attention to discriminating between

a) direct imitation of the target word,

b) spontaneous, appropriate use of the target word.

The demonstration of 'goneness' consisted of the 'recorder' hiding or leaving the room whilst the 'teacher' gave the appropriate cue ("gone") and either demanded an imitation, or gave no cues and tried to induce a spontaneous appropriate response (by, for example, looking surprised or expectant).

2. Directive Play

Five of the target words were then chosen (ball, bus, baby, pen, car) balanced for familiarity for both subjects. The experimental subject was then started on a program of directive play sessions in which he was reinforced (by social reinforcement and the use of specially designed toys) first for imitating and later for spontaneously producing pivot-open utterances upon presentation of the appropriate stimuli.

The control subject was given an equal number of non-directive play sessions closely paralleling the experimental situation, except that only single-word models, and no models of the pivot-open utterance, were provided and 'gone' was only demonstrated as in the previous sessions.

The same procedure was adopted for these sessions as in the initial sessions except that the children were taught separately and were now using only five words (plus 'gone'), instead of ten. Thus, for the control child the sessions were merely a continuation of the previous ones, whilst the experimental child's sessions were modified so that the pivot-open constructions were demonstrated and like utterances demanded in return. Social reinforcement was continued in the form of smiles and praise, being allowed to play a favourite game, applause etc., as the situation demanded. Primary reinforcement (with sweets) was used at the beginning of the experiment but discontinued as it proved distracting; the children, not surprisingly, started saying "sweet", almost to the exclusion of everything else.

3. Generalization

To test whether generalization of the concept had occurred, we then introcuded the second group of five words, previously learned. Over the next ten sessions no model utterances using these words, ('book gone', 'cup gone' etc.) were produced in front of the child, although the previous models, 'ball gone' etc. were still occasionally used.

4. Transfer to the Classroom

One morning's classroom observation was then carried out with each child by an independent observer and compared with the eleven observation mornings prior to the experiment. These speech samples were analysed for number of nouns, number of verbs, number of two- and three-word utterances and number of words used.

5. Change in Experimental Conditions

From this point the experimental child was dropped from the main body of the experiment, and the control child was now treated as a new experimental subject. As before, a model was given for five pivot-open utterances and an opportunity to generalize five more when no model was given.

IV. Apparatus

The Pivot-Open Practice Instrument (POP-IN) proved to be of considerable value for establishing and reinforcing appropriate responses. It consisted of a large posting box into which model objects (book, baby, ball etc.) could be dropped and then made to reappear by the child pulling a lever after having made the appropriate utterance (see Fig. 1). That is to say he was only allowed to pull the lever and make the toy shoot out of the pop-in after making the appropriate response. Dropping the toy into the box ('ball gone') was important as a demonstration of the event that the response is describing. In addition, expanded polystirene cubes, displaying pictures of five target words and one blank panel, were used to cue in the correct response. Thus, the panel showing a picture of a bus was shown to the child and then flipped over to the blank panel, while providing the verbal model 'bus gone'. The children also played with model toys and hid them under flower pots and put them away in a case. Picture books, as well as model objects, were used in all the sessions.

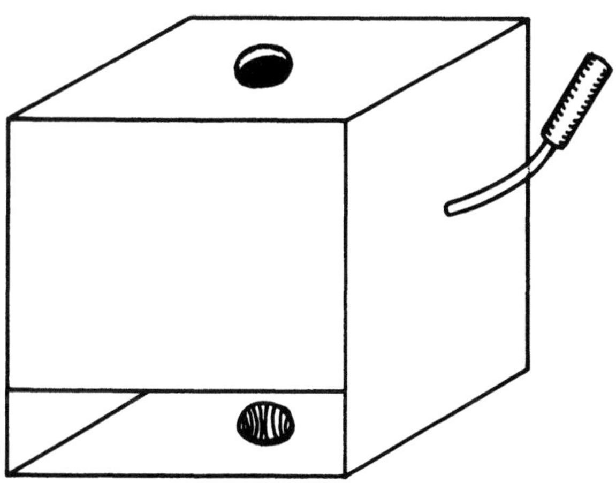

Fig. 1. The Pivot-Open Practise Instrument (POP-IN)

V. Results

Results are summarized graphically in Fig. 2.

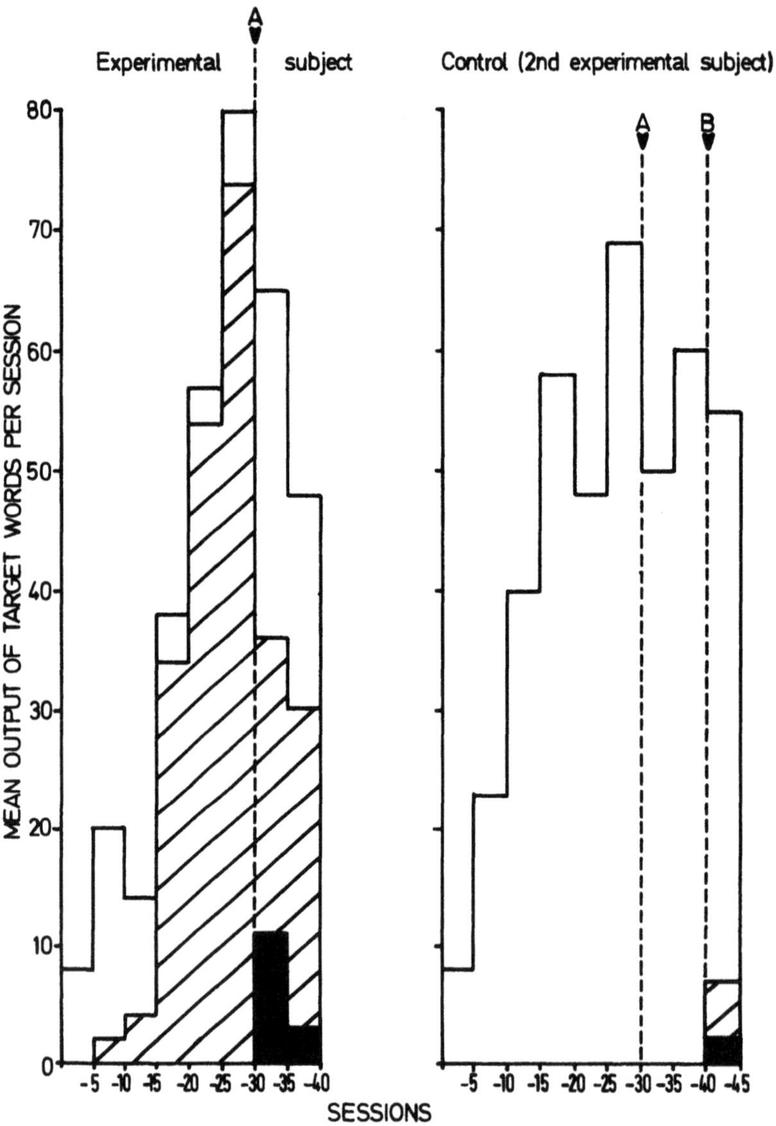

Fig. 2. Graph to show the relative number of spontaneously produced and appropriately used target words, pivot-open utterances and "transferred" pivot-open utterances for the experimental and control subjects (averaged over 5 session periods). □ = target words. ▨ = target words structured into pivot-open utterances. ■ = "new" target words structured into "transferred" pivot-open utterances. A = introduction of "new" words for generalisation. B = point where control subject swichet to experimental condition

1. Directive Play

After thirteen quarter-hour sessions of initial training, both children were spontaneously naming and identifying the ten target words and imitating the word 'gone'. Over a period of thirty sessions the experimental subject progressed from a baseline where he was using no pivot-open utterances, through an intermediate stage where he was using mainly directly imitated utterances, to a final stage of appropriate spontaneous utterances virtually to the exclusion of everything else. In the control condition the number of appropriate, spontaneous single-word utterances rose dramatically to an average of sixty per session, but no pivot-open utterances were elicited. The number of target words spoken by both children in the last five sessions of directive play was about four times as great as during the first five sessions. They were both successfully co-operating and increasing their verbal output. For the experimental subject, 90% of these target words were structured into two-word sentences and 65.5% were both spontaneous and appropriate. No such two-word sentences were used by the control subject, but 79% of the target words used in these last five sessions were spontaneous and appropriate.

2. Generalization

Over a period of ten sessions the experimental subject spontaneously generated thirty-six sentences which he had not previously heard; for example, when cup (one of the second set of five objects) was posted in the POP-IN he said, 'cup gone', not having previously heard these words put together.

The new experimental subject learned both the spontaneous use of the pivot-open construction and its generalization to new words in five sessions, at the end of which he had spontaneously used 18 such constructions which he had previously heard, and generated six constructions with new words. Unfortunately, the sessions had to be terminated at this point due to absences.

3. Transfer to Classroom

Data summarizing pre- and two post-test measures are summarized in Table 2.

a) Pre-test

Before the facilitation sessions neither subject was very talkative in the classroom situation. Their average output per morning was about eight words, and over eleven sessions the experimental and control subjects had uttered 85 and 91 recognisable words respectively. Their language was mainly confined to labelling except for two or three two-word utterances used as invariant units.

b) Post-test 1

After thirty sessions in which the experimental subject had learned the pivot-open construction and the control subject had only rehearsed the vocabulary, a second speech sample was analysed for each child. This sample was taken on one morning only. Both children showed great improvement in repertoire.

Table 2. Summary of Changes in Language Behaviour Before, During and After Pivot-Open Training

	Experimental			Control (Experimental 2)		
	Pre-test[a]	Post-test (1)	Post-test (2)	Pre-test[a]	Post-test (1)	Post-test (2)
No. of recognisable words	85	164	277	91	158	140
No. of different word types	30	69	90	33	71	45
% verbs	20	33	32	18	22	18
% nouns	40	25	18	64	32	33
2-word phrases	2	25	42	3	25	3
Different types	-	13	31	-	16	2
3-word phrases	-	14	31	-	10	1
Different types	1	11	12	-	4	1
4-word phrases	-	-	2	-	-	1
Different types	-	-	2	-	-	-

[a] Total over 11 sessions

The experimental subject was heard to utter 164 recognisable words (as compared with an average of 8), and he now used 69 different words. He now used 25 two-word phrases of 13 different types and 14 three-word phrases of 11 types. Seven of these seemed to be structured, e.g. 'Give us it' and 'I've got it'.

The control subject, however, was also using more mature language. He uttered 158 recognisable words, of 71 types. He used 25 two-word phrases of 16 different types and 10 three-word phrases of 4 different types. Four of these were structured, e.g. 'Get a chair'.

c) Post-test 2

After a period of 3 months, another sample of one morning's language for each child was analysed. The first experimental subject now had a total of 277 words and 90 were of different types. He also used 42 two-word utterances and these were of 31 different types. He used 31 three-word utterances of 12 different types and two four-word utterances, e.g. 'I want it out'.

The language behaviour of the second experimental subject appears to have partially extinguished over this period. Out of a total of 140 words he used 45 types. He used only three two-word phrases which were only of two types and which were used as invariant units, e.g. 'Do it' and 'Oh dear', and one three word phrase. He also structured one four-word phrase (let me have ball).

VI. Discussion

The main conclusion which can be drawn from this study is that young mongol children can be taught to generalize the structure of a two-word sentence through the imitation of several examples with appropriate contextual play. The control child who was given all the appropriate contextual play and the necessary vocabulary in isolation did not succeed in putting the words together until provided with the model, but was then successful.

The quality and quantity of language used by both children in the classroom improved greatly during the experimental period, and both started to structure their utterances in this setting, in particular with respect to the number of verbs used. Both children used only six verbs originally, but the experimental subject later used nearly four times and the control subject three times as many. This suggests some generalized effect of the program, the increased use of the verbs being a sign of linguistic maturity (MEIN, 1961). Although it is likely that the daily language sessions were a major factor in this improvement, this cannot be conclusively demonstrated in the absence of a third control subject receiving no treatment.

Because both subjects improved, it might be said that the improvement was due to maturation, helped by a generally reinforcing program, but the fact that the second subject's performance later declined suggests that this was not the case. It should also be said, that, at the stage of the first post-test, the experimental subject's classroom language was more mature than that of his control, insofar as the percentage of verbs to nouns was higher. However, the control subject did generate spontaneous, appropriate pivot-open constructions as soon as he became the second experimental subject. This is of interest when one considers his classroom language three months later, when he was again using single words almost exclusively. It is only possible to speculate on the reason for this apparent extinction. It must be mentioned that the subject had changed schools just prior to his experimental program. Another factor is that he had eight times as many unstructured play sessions (40) as structured ones (5), so that the use of single words had been consistently reinforced over a long period. He did not readily accept the new structured regime and objected vociferously when it was introduced.

It should be noted that none of the phrases taught in the experimental sessions with the pivot 'gone' was used by either child more than once in the classroom, possibly because there appeared to be nothing in the classroom situation to prompt this particular construction. It is felt that a more useful pivot might have been chosen which verbally conveyed the child's requirements. It is perhaps more functionally useful in a competitive classroom situation to be able to say 'Gimme ball' than the purely descriptive 'Ball gone'. The early appearance in the children's vocabulary of the word 'mine' seems to suggest the need for an acquisitive expression.

References

BLOOM, L.: Semantic features in language development. In: SCHIEFELBUSCH, R.L. (Ed.): Language of the Mentally Retarded. Baltimore: University Park Press 1972.

BRAINE, M.D.S.: The ontogeny of English phrase structure, the first phase. Language 59, 1-13 (1963).

BRICKER, W.A., BRICKER, D.D.: A program of language training for the severely handicapped child. Exceptional Children 37, 101-112 (1970).
BRICKER, W.A.: A systematic approach to language training. In: SCHIEFELBUSCH, R.L. (Ed.): Language of the Mentally Retarded. Baltimore: University Park Press (1972).
JEFFREE, D., CASHDAN, A.: Severely subnormal children and their parents; an experiment in language improvement. Brit. J. educ. Psychol. 41, 184-194 (1971).
McNEILL, D.: Developmental psycholinguistics. In: SMITH, F., MILLER, G.A. (Eds.): The Genesis of Language. Cambridge/Mass.: M.I.T. Press 1966.
MEIN, R.: A study of the oral vocabularies of severely subnormal patients. II Grammatical analysis of speech samples, J. ment. Defic. Res. 5, 52-59 (1961).
MILLER, W.R., ERVIN, S.M.: The development of grammar in child language. In: BELLUGI, A., BROWN, R. (Eds.): The Acquisition of Language. Monographs of the Society for Research in Child Development, Vol. 29, 1, p. 9-33 (1964).
SLOBIN, D.: Seven questions about language development. In: DODWELL, P.C. (Ed.): New Horizons in Psychology, Vol. 2, Harmondsworth: Penguin (1972).
WOODWARD, M.: Notes on techniques devised for the assessment of severely subnormal and young normal children on the basis of Piaget's observations and interpretations of sensori-motor development. Unpublished paper 1966.
KIRK, S.A., KARNES, M.B., KIRK, W.D.: You and Your Retarded Child, 2nd Ed. Palo Alto/California: Pacific Books 1968.

Comparison Among Therapists Attempting Language Training and Generalization of Punishment Effects in the Behaviour Modification of a Schizophrenic Child

P. GOTTWALD, W. REDLIN, H. OTT, P. INNERHOFER and H. WILHELM

A number of experiments have demonstrated the possibility of changing the bizarre behaviour of "psychotic" children through operant conditioning and building up a repertoire of simple and basic self-help, social and sometimes even language skills (cf. LOVAAS, 1967, 1971). Our interest in behaviour therapy with schizophrenic and autistic children has centred around programs of language acquisition. In addition, the elimination of undesirable behaviour and the development of social skills have been attempted in a number of children.

In the present case study we set for ourselves three goals:

1. to gain some experience with an evaluation technique known as "multiple baseline" (cf. BAER et al., 1968);
2. to compare the results obtained by different therapists working with similar techniques and material and to test for generalization of the effects of punishing undesirable behaviour and
3. to test the results of programs for the acquisition of 'abstract speech', in this case the use of prepositions and pronouns.

Case History. Our patient, Lotte A., was admitted to the child psychiatry ward of the Max-Planck-Institute for Psychiatry+, when she was 13 years old. She stayed for one-and-a-half years.

Family History. Lotte's mother was diagnosed as schizophrenic several weeks after Lotte was born; she was hospitalized repeatedly and is now in a state mental hospital. A brother of Lotte's mother also suffered from schizophrenia.

The child's development was overshadowed by the psychosis of her mother over the first two years. Her intellectual development was retarded, emotionally she remained withdrawn and aloof. There were, however, no signs of neurological impairment. According to her father, Lotte's development up to the age of 10 was slow but steady; after this age, it not only appeared arrested but gradually deteriorated.

Clinical Tests. Except for some indication of abnormal EEG activity, no signs of organic brain damage were found.

Informal Behaviour Observation. On our ward Lotte appeared small and underweight for her age; her facial expression and body movements were

+ We thank Dr. GERTRUD BLEEK, Head of the Department of Child Psychiatry at the Max-Planck-Institute for Psychiatry, and her staff for support of our study and considerable patience while the collection of observation data took place.

somewhat rigid. She did not, in general, answer questions. Occasionally she would demand certain toys or activities in a highly stereotyped manner. If the attending adult did not comply, Lotte would work herself into a state of great arousal, shouting her request over and over again until she was nearly exhausted.

When left alone, she did not play appropriately with toys, but handled them in a stereotyped manner, sniffed them and then dropped them. She would sit motionless for long periods of time staring into a corner or drumming extremely complex rhythms at an astonishing speed with both hand. Sometimes she would also begin a stereotypic kind of singsong which she repeated endlessly. There were phases during which she showed all the signs of extreme anxiety - she expressed fear of objects which were not present, such as cars, so that she was thought to be hallucinating. Her use of language was highly stereotyped and inappropriate. She spoke grammatically incorrectly, never saying "I". At times she uttered sentences completely out of context, which she seemed to have taken from overheard conversations, a phenomenon termed "phonographism" by TRAMER (1964) and thought of as characteristic for childhood psychosis. Echolalic speech was very common.

Psychological Test Performance. In the Stanford-Binet Test Lotte answered only a limited number of questions at the level of 3 to 5 years. She did not solve any of the problems from the Leiter International Performance Scale. Her language competence seemed to be that of a 3-year-old child.

Diagnosis. Childhood schizophrenia.

Therapy Programs

Table 1 summarizes the programs that were initiated by the different therapists.

I. Comparison between Therapists A and B and the Generalization of Punishment Effects

The therapeutic goal was

1. to establish a training situation in which to teach the child to label objects correctly and to point to a given object on request, and
2. to decrease inappropriate and bizarre behaviour. Finally, a program to develop some understanding of abstract speech (prepositions) was attempted.

The two therapists worked daily, 5 days a week, alternating between lunchtime and afternoon snacktime. Each session lasted 40 min; small portions of meals were used as positive reinforcers. The sessions took place in a well lit room, 4 x 4m, which contained only a table and 3 chairs and could be observed through a one-way window.

The following behaviour of the child was recorded:

a) "psychotic" behaviour: drumming, singing, psychotic talk, short cries;
b) normal social behaviour: eye-to-eye contact and body contact with the therapist, smiling.

Table 1. Therapy Programs

<table>
<tr><th colspan="2">Therapist</th><th>March</th><th>April</th><th>May</th><th>June</th><th>July-November</th></tr>
<tr><td rowspan="2">A</td><td>Task</td><td>Labelling Objects</td><td colspan="2">P r e p o s i t i o n s
in front of ¦ in front of/ behind</td><td rowspan="2"></td><td rowspan="2"></td></tr>
<tr><td>Contin-gencies</td><td colspan="3">Reinforcement of desired behaviour
Punishment of Motor Stereotypes ¦ Punishment of psychotic talk (May)</td></tr>
<tr><td rowspan="2">B</td><td>Task</td><td>Labelling Objects</td><td colspan="2">P r e p o s i t i o n s
under ¦ under/ on top of</td><td rowspan="2"></td><td rowspan="2"></td></tr>
<tr><td>Contin-gencies</td><td colspan="3">Reinforcement of desired behaviour
Punishment of psychotic talk ¦ Punishment of psychotic talk</td></tr>
<tr><td rowspan="3">C/D</td><td>Task</td><td>Social Interactions</td><td>Social Interactions Games</td><td>Social Interactions</td><td colspan="2">Social Interactions
Language Training
Pronouns</td></tr>
<tr><td>Contin-gencies</td><td>Reinforcement of desired behaviour</td><td>Time-contingent reinforcement</td><td>Reinforcement of desired behaviour</td><td colspan="2">Reinforcement of correct responses</td></tr>
<tr><td></td><td colspan="4">Extinction for psychotic behaviour</td><td></td></tr>
<tr><td colspan="2">Psychotic drugs</td><td colspan="4"></td><td>Melleril R 150 mg/d
Neurocil R 25 mg/d .</td></tr>
</table>

Therapeutic Contingencies included 'primary' reinforcement of correct responses in the labelling task, social reinforcement when the child returned to her seat at the table, and ignoring of drumming, singing and stereotyped requests (see above). Punishment for 'drumming' and 'psychotic talk' was administered according to the plan outlined in the table. Painful electric stimulation with a portable device served as an aversive event.

Prompting and Fading of Prompts. Manual prompting was used in the labelling task and verbal prompting during preposition training. All prompts were gradually faded out.

Results:

1. Labelling of objects; Therapists A and B, Sessions 1-10

Fig. 1a and b shows 3 parameters of the training in labelling: 'correct labelling', 'correct indicating' and '% noncompliance'.

While the first two parameters showed some fluctuation, the high proportion of correct responses seems to indicate that 'correct labelling' was not newly acquired, but rather under reinforcement control (see also decrease in % noncompliance). As can be seen there was a high frequency of 'drumming', 'singing' and 'psychotic talk' during sessions 8-10.

2. Labelling of objects; Ther. A, punishment of 'drumming', Sessions 11-15

In session 11, Therapist A punished 'drumming' three times during the first few minutes. The behaviour did not recur during the remainder

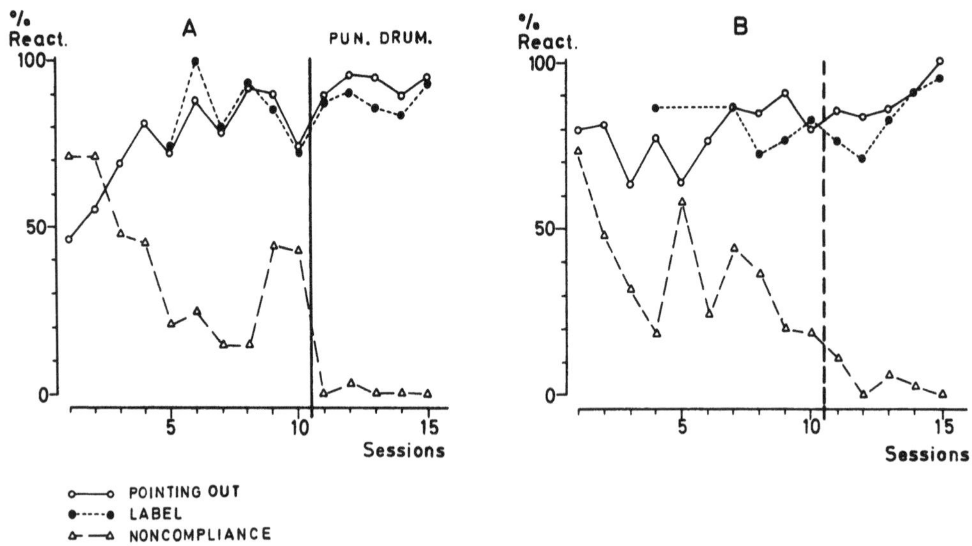

Fig. 1. Labelling and pointing to labelled objects, with therapists A and B. Per cent values of the parameters 'correct labelling', 'correct indicating' and 'noncompliance' are shown. During sessions 11-15, therapist A punished 'psychotic drumming' (motor stereotype)

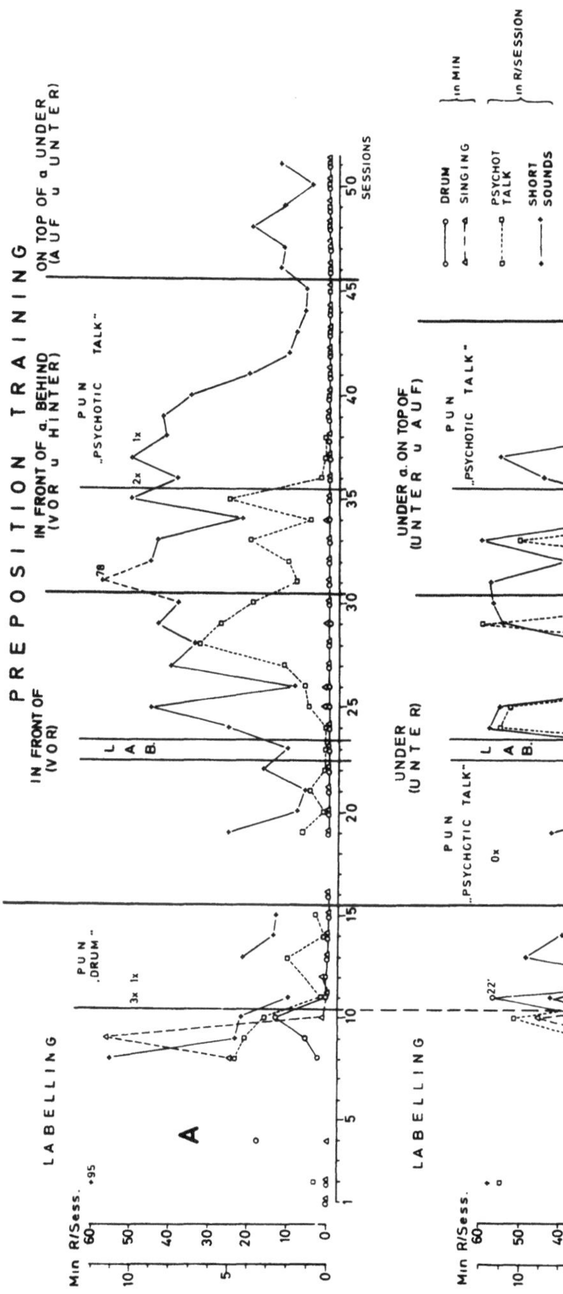

Fig. 2. Duration and frequency of psychotic behaviour over 40 sessions, therapists A and B. Total duration of 'drumming' and 'singing' is shown (left ordinate) while frequency of 'psychotic talk' and 'short cries' is given (right ordinate). Note the marked change following punishment of psychotic behaviour

of the session. After one incidence of punishment in session 12, neither 'drumming' nor 'singing' was observed during the remaining sessions. This effect generalized to the sessions with Ther. B. In the therapeutic setting of Ther. C. (see below), 'drumming' was also absent after the initiation of punishment by Ther. A. Under extinction, neither 'drumming' nor 'singing' recurred (see Fig. for details).

3. Preposition training; Ther. B, punishment of 'psychotic talk, Sessions 16-22

These sessions always took place in the same room and at the same time of day. Each therapist worked with two objects. Ther. A used a ball and a book, Ther. B, a doll and a pillow. The task was (1) to label correctly a given arrangement, e.g. the pillow is under the doll, the ball is behind the book, and (2) to arrange these objects correctly upon request. Fig. 3 shows the course of the learning parameters in these sessions. From the data it can be concluded that Lotte used only one preposition correctly, namely 'under'. Later it was shown that this correct performance was actually an artifact. The effective suppression of 'psychotic talk' through punishment by Ther. B did not generalize to Ther. A, as can be seen from Fig. 2. Under extinction (sessions 23-35), psychotic talk occurred again immediately (see Fig. 2 for details).

PREPOSITION TRAINING

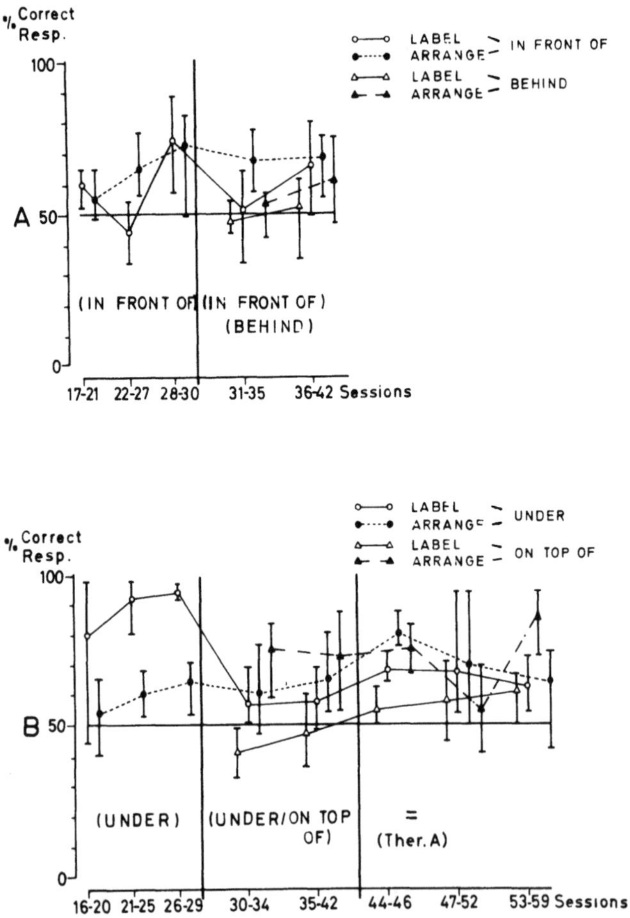

Fig. 3. Training for abstract speech (therapists A and B): Prepositions. Per cent correct response during 'labelling' and 'arranging' a given situation (e.g. book behind ball, pillow on top of doll) is shown. Data were pooled for blocks of sessions, and the range is indicated

4. Preposition training; Ther. A and B, punishment of 'psychotic talk', Sessions 36-43

When both therapists punished 'psychotic talk' (only Ther. A had to administer three shocks), 'psychotic talk' remained suppressed; the observed decrease in the frequency of 'short cries' following punishment of 'psychotic talk' is not easily interpreted. Whether it is due to the punishment or to a reduction in the demands put upon the child during training or whether it is due to habituation to the situation plus demands is by no means clear. The learning parameters in the preposition training were not affected.

5. Special preposition training; Ther. A, Sessions 43-51

When two different objects were used to be put 'on top of' or 'below' the table, the child's performance was correct. Therefore, the size of otherwise identical blocks was used as a prompting stimulus and then slowly faded out in subsequent sessions. Correct performance was maintained down to the pair of blocks with sides of 24 and 22 cm respectively. When blocks of equal size (23/23 cm) were used, the performance broke down immediately and completely.

This result attests to the considerable discriminatory powers of the child, as well as to the fact that correct performance in preposition training must have been caused by involuntary prompts, of an as yet unspecified nature, given by the therapist.

6. Social behaviour during Sessions 1-43

Neither body contact nor smiling showed clear trends or a dependency with regard to any of the conditions mentioned above. Eye-to-eye contact increased over sessions (trend analysis using the Cox-Stuart method was significant ($p < .005$) for both therapists). Closer inspection of the individual graphs in Fig. 4 seems to warrant the hypothesis that introduction of novel tasks or new contingencies led to an increase and subsequent decrease of eye-to-eye contact with both therapists.

II. Training in Social Interactions and Further Training in Abstract Speech (Pronouns); Ther. C.

In previous sessions carried out by Ther. C, the therapeutic goal was to increase the number of social interactions initiated by the child. While primary reinforcement was also given, this whole setting was less rigidly organized than the settings created by the other therapists, and more meaningful materials (e.g. toys, clothes, plates, spoons, cups, dishes, cutlery) were used. In the sessions to be reported here, utterances containing pronouns (like my, your, her and his) were systematically used. The child had to answer specific questions, e.g. "whose shirt is white?", as well as to follow commands requiring use of pronouns, e.g. "give her your doll", "give him my doll".

1. Observations and Results

Per cent correct responses were recorded. Also, every sentence uttered by the child was rated and given grades (1-4) depending upon grammatical

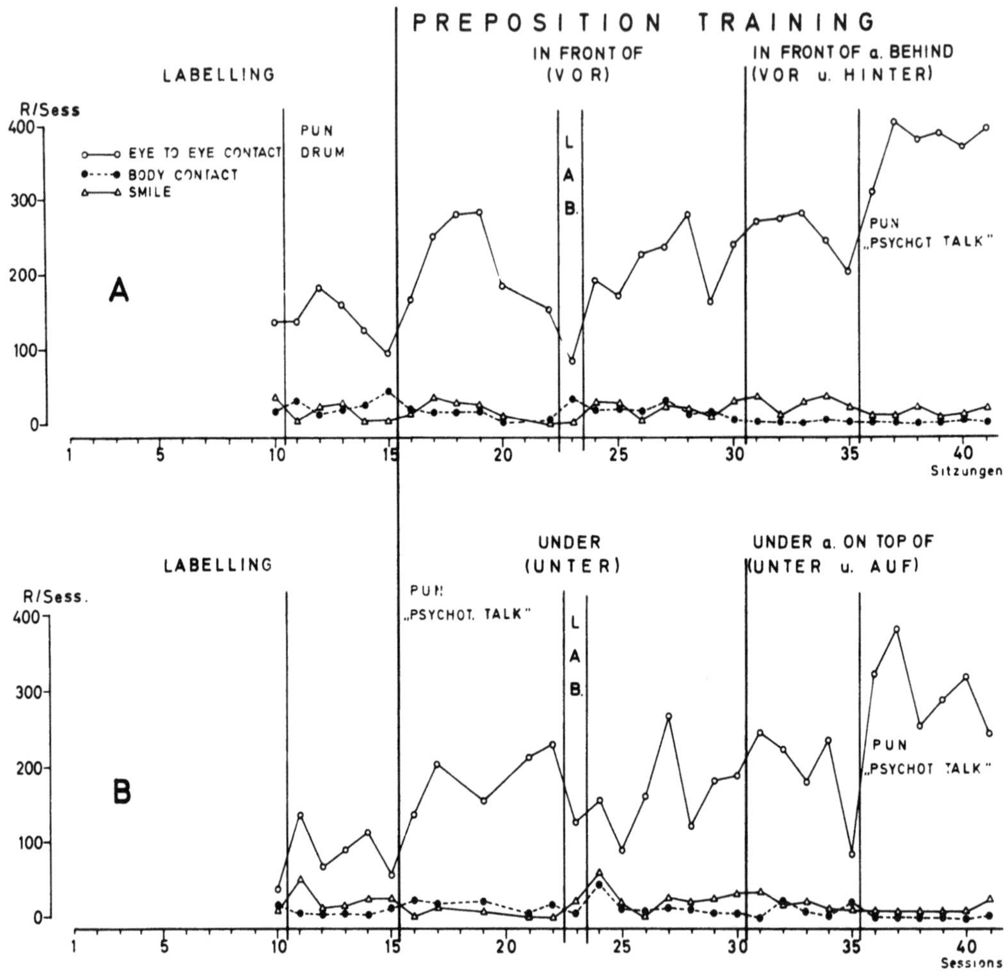

Fig. 4. Frequency of social behaviour during preposition training. Amount of 'eye-to-eye contact with the therapist', 'body contact' and 'smiling' are shown over 40 sessions. There is an overall increase in eye-to-eye contact, and in addition, a superimposed cyclic pattern of increase and decrease in novel situations in the amount of eye-to-eye contact

correctness. While there was no significant imrovement in these grades despite considerable prompting, correct use of pronouns my and your was achieved. Fig. 5 shows a temporary decline in the correct performance of 'my' and 'your' when 'his' and 'her' were introduced; the latter two pronouns were never mastered.

In Fig. 6, the frequency of eye-to-eye contact is again shown to rise and fall with any change in the situation, whether it be a new therapist or a novel therapeutic situation.

Fig. 7 shows how the child's verbal behaviour, e.g. the frequency of requests, thanking the therapist, proposing a game, and nonverbal behaviour, e.g. smiling and motionless staring, varied with the conditions of reinforcement in an ABA design. During A, reinforcement was

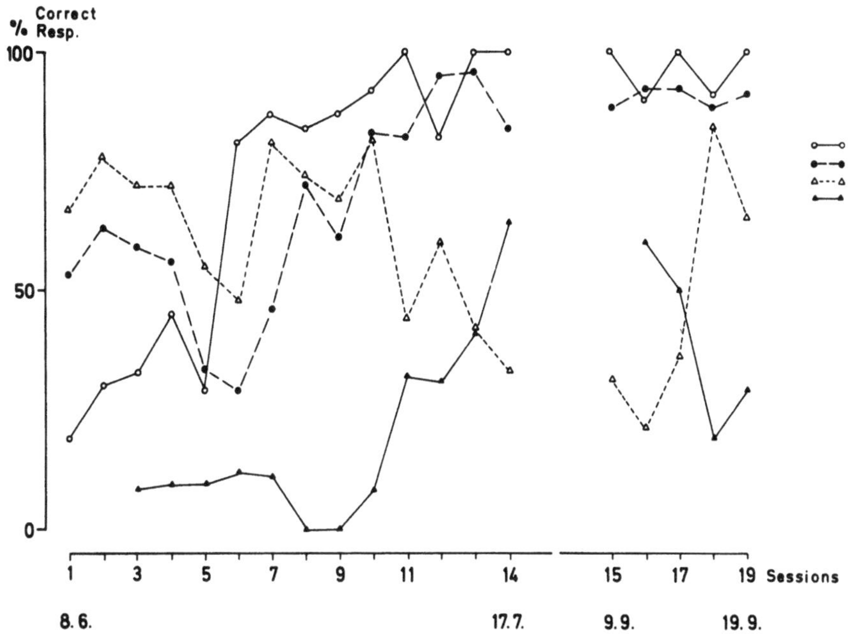

Fig. 5. Training for abstract speech: pronouns. Per cent correct performance using 'my' and 'your' falls after introduction of the new pronouns 'her' and 'his'. While 'my' and 'your' recover, 'hers' and 'his' do not reach criterium. Sessions 15-19: Follow-up after 2 months

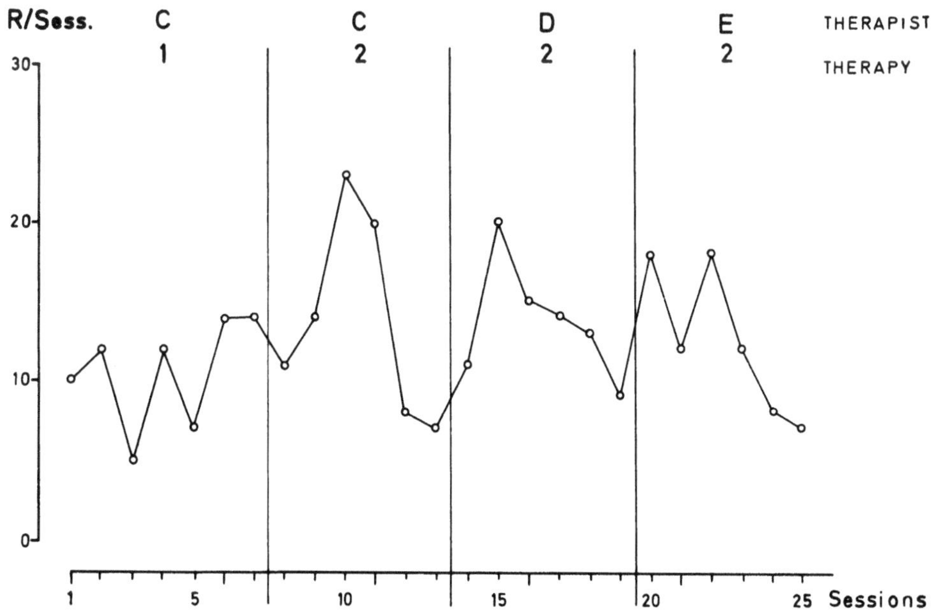

Fig. 6. Frequency of eye-to-eye contact with therapists C, D and E, in situations 1 and 2. Note the same pattern of change in frequency as is seen in Fig. 4

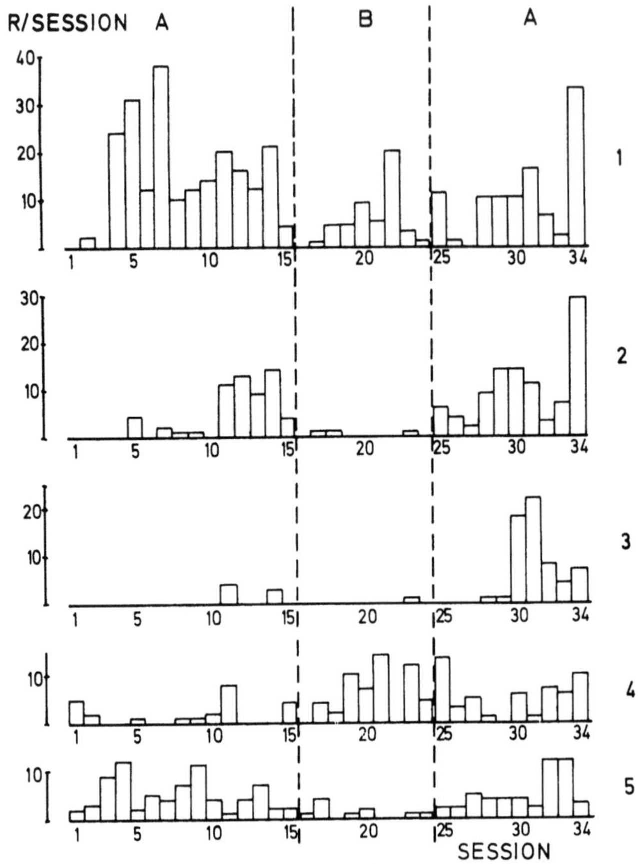

Fig. 7. Frequency of occurrence of five types of behaciour in an ABA design, with time-contingent instead of response-contingent reinforcement in B (1: made a request, 2: thanked the therapist, 3: proposed a game, 4: smiled, 5: stared motionless). During B, the child's mood seems better, while performance deteriorates

contingent upon appropriate verbal behaviour, while during B, reinforcement was time-contingent.

2. Discussion

The extent to which all therapists gained control over the deviant behaviour of the child confirms the results of earlier work in this field (RISLEY and WOLF, 1967; LOVAAS, 1967, 1971) on the effectiveness of response-contingent reinforcement of desirable behaviour and the possibility of suppressing psychotic behaviour through punishment. The results of abstract speech training are in accordance with the results in some of the cases described by LOVAAS et al. (1972). The observation of "overselectivity" in a complex stimulus situation (visual prompts in preposition training) confirms a result that was demonstrated by LOVAAS and co-workers (1971).

Attempts at a functional analysis of psychotic behaviour were successful insofar as they allowed a subdivision of the general class of psychotic behaviour into 'drumming' and 'singing' on the one hand and 'psychotic talk' and 'short cries' on the other. 'Novelty of situation', regardless of whether this was a change in situation or of therapists, materials or contingencies, seemed to be the independent variable influencing eye-to-eye contact with the experimenter. Considering the amount of time and energy spent to obtain these results, one might tend to regard them as rather trivial. However, evidence that supports the usefulness of learning principles for the prediction and control of psychotic behaviour seems important enough both theoretically and practically to justify this effort. If one is accustomed to the confusion in the literature on childhood psychosis, any step, however small, in the direction of a functional analysis is likely to be regarded as useful. There seems to be, at present, no other way open for the scientific study of severely disturbed children (cf. GOTTWALD, 1971).

There has been some controversy regarding the use of punishment in cases of childhood schizophrenia. Punishment has been used mainly to suppress self-destructive or other dangerous behaviour (LOVAAS, 1967; RISLEY, 1968; BIRNBRAUER, 1968). However, slapping has also been advocated by LOVAAS and his co-workers (1972) in cases of self-stimulation and other bizarre behaviour which may occur during therapy sessions. In discussing possible indications for punishment of these children, therapeutic goals and values and undesirable side effects, as well as problems in generalization, have to be taken into account.

Undesirable side effects of punishment have not been reported to date (cf. RISLEY, 1968; LOVAAS, 1972). In our study, evidence to the contrary has not been forthcoming. Nevertheless, the small number of cases does not allow any conclusion to be drawn. The limited generalization of the effects of punishment, which is also evident in BIRNBRAUER's study (1968), would necessitate punishment in many situations before success would be achieved. BUCHER and KING (1971) reported poor generalization but noted that fewer and fewer punishments were necessary to keep destructive activity suppressed as therapist and child moved from one situation to another. If, on the other hand, an increase in psychotic behaviour is due to demands put upon the child, e.g. starting to learn abstract speech, punishment of that behaviour seems unwarranted. It is our contention that in this case the therapeutic procedures of goals should be changed, e.g. from language training to the development of social skills. Although the present experiment was not primarily conceived as an attempt at therapy for a schizophrenic child, but rather as an attempt at a functional analysis of abnormal behaviour, we had hoped for some longer-lasting therapeutic effect. We are, to put it mildly, far from happy with the discrepancy between effort and final success, which is rather dramatic when one keeps in mind the fact that the child had to be admitted to a state mental hospital. Our failure in this respect is not, however, a valid argument against the usefulness of behaviour therapy for these children. Goals of scientific inquiry and therapeutic objectives do not easily merge in the present stage of research into childhood schizophrenia. It is to be hoped that behaviour therapy will contribute to bridging this gap.

3. Summary

Within a case study of a 12-year-old girl with the diagnosis of childhood schizophrenia dating back to the second year of life, a number of behaviour modification experiments were performed, using multiple baseline procedures, and evaluating for generalization effects between therapists and settings. Observation of psychotic behaviour (motor stereotypes, bizarre talk) and appropriate behaviour during (a) speech training, (b) an attempt at building social behaviour and (c) a combination of both, demonstrated the effectiveness of food-reinforcement in shaping desired behaviour, and of punishment in the suppression of psychotic behaviour. The general improvement in the child's behaviour within training sessions did not generalize to the daily living setting of a small group of disturbed children on a children's psychiatric ward. Since language training was only partially effective in the present case (correct use of pronouns, but not of prepositions) despite prolonged and intense efforts, focusing therapeutic attempts on training in socialization is proposed as the main therapeutic goal for such children. The use of punishment in the suppression of behaviour which is undesirable in learning situations appears debatable.

References

BAER, D.M., WOLF, M.M., RISLEY, T.R.: Some current dimensions of applied behaviour analysis. J. appl. behav. Anal. 1a, 91-97 (1968).
BIRNBRAUER, J.S.: Generalization of punishment effects - a case study. J. appl. behv. Anal. 1, 201-211 (1968).
BUCHER, B., KING, L.W.: Generalization of punishment effects in the deviant behaviour of a psychotic child. Behav. Ther. 2, 68-77 (1971).
GOTTWALD, P.: Imitation and matching-to-sample training in the behaviour therapy with autistic children: Therapeutic and classificatory objectives. In: Proceedings of the Second Congress of the International Association for the Scientific Study of Mental Deficiency (D.A.A. PRIMROSE, Ed.), 461-467. Warsaw: Polish Medical Publishers 1971.
LOVAAS, O.I.: A behaviour therapy approach to the treatment of childhood schizophrenia. In: Minnesota Symposiom on Child Psychology. University of Minnesota Press 1967.
LOVAAS, O.I.: Considerations in the development of a behavioural treatment program for psychotic children. In: CHURCHILL, ALPERN, DeMYER (Eds): Infantile Autism, 124-144. Springfield/Ill.: Ch.C. Thomas 1971.
LOVAAS, O.I., SCHREIBMAN, L., KOEGEL, R., REHM, R.: Selective responding by autistic children to multiple sensory input. J. Abnorm. soc. Psychol. 77, 211-222 (1971).
LOVAAS, O.I., KOEGEL, R., SIMMONS, J.Q., STEVENS, J.: Some generalizations and follow-up measures on autistic children in behaviour therapy. J. appl. behav. Anal., in press (1972).
RISLEY, T.R., WOLF, M.M.: Establishing functional speech in echolalic children. Behav. Res. Ther. 5, 73-88 (1967).
RISLEY, T.R.: The effects and side effects of punishing the autistic behaviours of a deviant child. J. appl. behav. Anal. 1, 21-34 (1968).
TRAMER, M.: Lehrbuch der allgemeinen Kinderpsychiatrie. Basel/Stuttgart: B. Schwabe 1964.

Treatment of Anorexia in Early Infancy - Some Behavioural Approaches+

R. G. JACOB++, O. NORDLUND and G.H. SCHWIELER+++

Treatment procedures of anorectic infants from the ages of one to six years have been reported (HEWITT and ALDRICH, 1946; WRIGHT, 1971), but no studies have been published with infants of less than one year. Many of the first interactions between mother and infant are concerned with feeding, and anorexia may be one of the first problems a mother encounters with her child.

Anorexia is often a natural concomitant of transient illnesses such as upper respiratory tract infection, but usually the anorexia is also transient. However, if the mother becomes alarmed by the child's low intake and tries to force-feed the child, a vicious circle might be started in which the forcing leads to aversion to food or the feeding situation; this, in turn, tends to reduce voluntary food intake still further, thus perpetuating the anorexia (see Fig. 1).

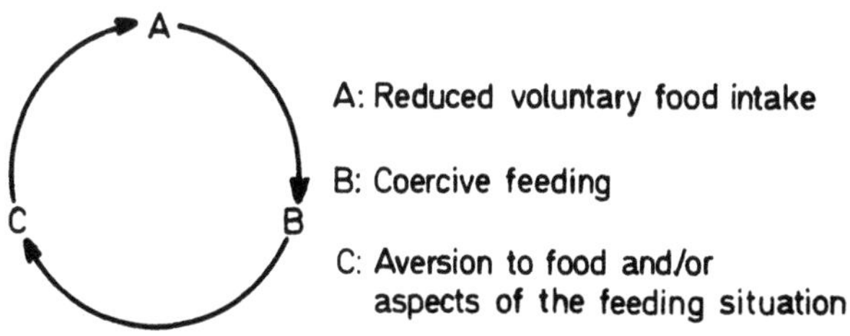

Fig. 1. A cybernetic model of the etiology of chronic anorexia in infants.

This vicious circle might be entered also at the other two critical points mentioned, i.e. forcing of food by the mother and aversion to food or the feeding situation, respectively. Thus, if the mother for some reason other than those mentioned above, e.g. strict adherence to a regular feeding schedule taught in some maternity wards (ALDRICH,

---

+ Reprints can be obtained from: O. NORDLUND, Department of Education, Fiskartorpsvägen 160 B, Fack, 10405 Stockholm 50, Sweden or from R.G. JACOB, M.D., Psychology Department, State University of New York, Stony Brook, New York, 11790.

++ R.G. JACOB is currently at the State University of New York at Stony Brook. Support during the writing of this study was provided by the Sixteen Gemzéus Fund and Anders Otto Svärd Fund.

+++ The authors thank K.D. O'LEARY, Ph.D., Psychology Department, SUNY, Stony Brook, for helpful suggestions in the writing of this paper.

1942), or a desire to have the infant look "better nourished", starts using coercive feeding methods, anorexia may develop. Aversion can be produced in a number of ways. GUNTHER (1961) describes the development of a feeding inhibition subsequent to the baby's nostrils being blocked by its upper lip or the mother's breast during the feeding situation. The results from repeated "taste aversion" experiments with animals reviewed by ROZIN and KALAT (1971) suggest that aversion to food may also arise if food intake is followed by nausea.

Infants with chronic anorexia are sometimes treated by supplementing the deficit associated with each meal through a nasogastric tube. This procedure might be effective in prolonging the course of the anorexia, since utilization of food supplements via a nasogastric tube makes normal consumatory behaviour unnecessary. Consequently, normal eating behaviour is no longer differentially reinforced. Utilizing the principle of least effort, the child would not be expected to increase his normal eating behaviour, since he is satiated via the nasogastric tube with less effort. It is consistent with this interpretation that SHARE et al. (1952) produced a depression of oral intake in dogs by giving food through a gastic fistula for 4 hours after the oral feeding each day.

The above speculations regarding the etiology of chronic anorexia in infancy provide us with some guidelines as to what treatment procedures might be useful:

I. Breaking the "anorexia loop"

   A. Increasing voluntary food intake

      1. Social reinforcement (e.g. smile or eye contact contingent on feeding)

      2. Modelling (e.g. having the child observe the parents or other children eating)

      3. Deprivation of food and/or fluid

   B. Reducing maternal coercion during feeding

      1. Instructions and counselling

      2. Videotape feedback to the mother of her feeding the child

      3. Emphasis on self-feeding

      4. Having someone other than the mother feed the child

   C. Reducing aversion to food or feeding situation

      1. Trying different kinds of food

      2. <u>In vivo</u> desensitization (e.g. nipples with hole increasing in size, playing with food, introduction of small amounts of formula into mouth between meals, rocking or singing to the child while feeding)

II. Differentially reinforcing oral food intake in cases where supplemental nourishment is given by nasogastric tube

   A. Removing the nasogastric tube

   B. Giving food intragastrically (i.e. through the tube) contingent on sucking

The authors have applied some of these methods to three cases of chronic anorexia. The first case was a 1-year-old girl, who had been given food supplements by nasogastric tube from 2 months of age. The second case was a 4-month-old child with a history of being supplemented in the same manner from 2 months of age. The third case was a 2-month-old boy with multiple congenital malformations, including tracheomalacia, who had been tube-fed since birth.

In all three cases, improvement was seen only after a deprivational state, defined as food intake of a magnitude markedly less than would be considered appropriate according to child nutritional rules, was allowed to occur. Procedures which had this effect were simply removing the nasogastric tube in cases 2 and 3, and in case 1·having the child (now 18 months old) feed itself instead of being fed.

Fig. 2 shows the improvement in case 3 after the tube was withdrawn at C. As can be seen, food intake was considerably below the required 600 ml at the beginning of this phase. (Before that, at B, a treatment according to II:2 was tried, i.e. giving formula by the gastric tube contingent on sucking. However, the procedure was not carried out correctly, since formula was also supplemented noncontingently after the child had stopped sucking; thus we may call this treatment a "pseudo-treatment".) This case subsequently maintained an adequate oral food intake throughout the one month follow-up period. Case 1 had a relapse after 4 months. Since case 2 was referred to another hospital, the food intake could not be assessed for more than one day after the removal of the tube.

In cases 1 and 2 procedures to reduce aversion to food or the feeding situation were applied before deprivation, since these children showed "distress" reactions, such as fussing and turning away the head, to aspects of the feeding situation (e.g. being seated in feeding position) or to the food itself. More specifically, in case 1 a roll of gauze bandage soaked with increasing amounts of juice was given to the child to bite on, and she was also given a tray containing a layer of

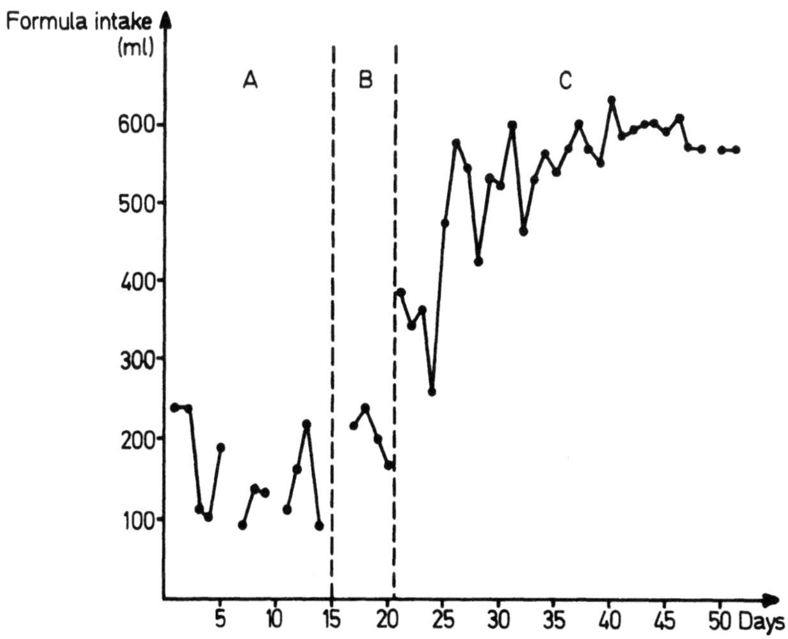

Fig. 2. Total formula intake during baseline (A), "pseudo-treatment" (B), removal of nasogastric tube (C)

her usual formula to play with. In case 2, small amounts of formula were put into the mouth with a pipette at regular intervals between meals for one day, and thereafter a hierarchy consisting of nipples with holes increasing in size was used in the feeding situation. Both children were supplemented by a gastric tube at the time these procedures were implemented. Food intake did not increase during these in vivo desensitization treatments, but negative emotional reactions seemed to diminish, according to global judgements. In case 1 we also tried to alter the coercive feeding technique used by the mother by discussions and videotape feedback, but we could not by these methods, bring about the desired change.

According to our experiences with these cases, deprivation seems to be a necessary condition for improvement, but we do not know whether it would have been a sufficient condition, since other treatments preceded the final deprivational procedures in all three cases. However, deprivation is not without danger, since it does not seem to be known for how long it can be carried on in infants without harm being done, or before demotivating "inanition factors" (BOLLES, 1967) come into play. A child with congenital heart disease and anorexia, treated with deprivation by the last author, became weaker after one day, further increasing the anorexia. In such cases the physical working capacity of the infant is probably below that needed for adequate feeding, so that trying to "cure" the anorexia is contraindicated.

We now routinely use "feeding upon demand" as the first treatment of early stages of anorexia in infants without organic disease. The child is fed only as long as it seems to be "willing" to take food, regardless of intake, thus frequently inducing a deprivational state. If the intake during the meal is low, a new opportunity for feeding is given after about one hour, or when the child shows signs of hunger, such as crying. This treatment stands in marked contrast to the feeding via a nasogastric tube for supplementation where consumatory behaviour is not reinforced.

References

ALDRICH, C.A.: Ancient processes in a scientific age, feeding aspects. Amer. J. Dis. Child. 64, 714-722 (1942).

BOLLES, R.C.: Theory of Motivation. New York: Harper and Row (1967).

GUNTHER, M.: Infant behaviour at the breast. In: B.M. FOSS (Ed.): Determinants of Infant Behaviour. London: Methuen 1961.

HEWITT, E.S., ALDRICH, C.A.: Poor eating habits of the run-about child: the role of physiologic anorexia. J. Pediat. 28, 595-596 (1946).

ROZIN, P., KALAT, J.A.: Specific hungers and poison avoidance as adaptive specializations of learning. Psychol. Rev. 78, 459-486 (1971).

SHARE, I., MARYNIUK, E., GROSSMAN, M.I.: Effects of prolonged intragastric feeding on oral food intake in dogs. Amer. J. Physiol. 169, 229-235 (1952).

WRIGHT, L.: Conditioning of consumatory responses in young children. J. clin. Psychol. 27, 416-419 (1971).

Problems in the Conditioning Treatment of Enuresis

R.T.T. MORGAN

The treatment of enuresis has for a long time, and I think with some justification, been regarded as a field in which behaviour therapy has most reliably achieved good results. Treatment is, however, beset by some major problems, partly of the type in which the prerequisite cooperation between the child patient and his familiy on the one hand, and the clinic on the other, may break down, and partly of the type in which a treatment response is not established with acceptable efficiency, stability or permanence. Our project was concerned with practical problems, occurring in a field setting.

The research was conducted in a special investigation clinic for the treatment of childhood enuresis and encopresis, which is situated in north London. Patients at the clinic are aged from 4 to 15 years, and would normally attend at monthly or forthnightly intervals, their progress being reviewed on each occasion by any one of three therapists. The clinic is one in which enuresis is treated wherever possible by conditioning techniques using the enuresis alarm. Supplementary forms of treatment are drug therapies, using normally either Tyrimide or Tofranil, very occasionally an amphetamine, or merely the maintenance of a record of wet and dry nights.

The median treatment duration at the clinic is 17.6 weeks. This may seem a somewhat high median compared with various reports in the literature, but the distribution from which it is derived includes patients whose treatment was interrupted for one reason or another, and some patients whose treatment lasted for 2 years or more. We have not, as is done in many studies, excluded as "failures" any patients remaining in treatment for more than some arbitrarily defined period. As can be seen from the figure, our modal duration of treatment is from 6 to 10 weeks.

The basic series studied comprised all cases of nocturnal enuresis referred to the clinic during 1969. After various exclusions, this series numbered 229 cases. By no means all of these patients, however, can be regarded as having achieved a successful therapeutic outcome.

Five basic pitfalls could be identified. The first was failure even to reach the stage of receiving a first appointment at the clinic, because the parents failed to reply to a letter sent on referral, requesting the name and address of the familiy general practitioner so that his permission for treatment could be obtained; 7% of all referrals fell by the wayside at this early stage. The next loss occurred when 17% of referred patients failed to arrive for their initial appointment at the clinic and did not subsequently request a further appointment. These "non-attenders" accounted for 18% of all cases given first appointments.

Of the 174 children who actually entered treatment, 32% dropped out again before achieving our initial cure criterion of 14 consecutive dry nights. These "terminators" account for another 22% of our referrals. 108 patients achieved discharge, a further 16 being still attendance at the time of data collection. On follow-up by reply-paid letter (follow-up information being obtained on all but two of these patients), we found that 26 of the discharged patients had relapsed to such an extent that retreatment became necessary. This represents a relapse rate of 24%.

We considered 32 patients to form a category of unacceptably slow responders. These children had all been in treatment for a period of 32 weeks or more, which constitutes the slowest quartile of the distribution of treatment durations. Naturally, any criterion of slow response is a little arbitrary, but we considered 32 weeks to be generous, since in the literature 3 months, 90 days or 50 alarm triggerings have variously been regarded as cut-off points for therapeutic failure.

The remaining proportion of all referrals, who may justifiably be regarded as therapeutic successes, treated with acceptable efficiency and without known relapse, is approximately one in four. This is markedly lower than the proportion of cases failing to enter or not completing treatment, but it should perhaps be emphasized that we are discussing total referrals rather than treated cases.

We selected for study the four problems of non-attendance, termination, slow response and relapse.

Comparing 38 non-attenders with the 174 children entering treatment, we found that the non-attenders had spent a significantly longer period on the waiting list for treatment. In a different series of non-attenders, it also emerged that these patients had significantly fewer wet nights per week at the time of the first appointment than did those who arrived at the clinic. It may therefore be that non-attenders are those in whom the motivation for treatment has declined since referral as a result of a reduction of enuresis while on the waiting list. Our patients await treatment for a median period of 15 weeks, and we have found a 9.7% "waiting list remission rate" during this period.

Referral source also emerged as a factor relevant to non-attendance: non-attenders were significantly more likely to have been referred by health visitors, and less likely to have been referred by their G.P.s. Referral arising from discussion between parent and doctor at a routine school medical examination did not discriminate between attenders and non-attenders. Possibly, the likelihood of entering treatment bears a positive relation to the degree of active "advice seeking" by the parents. Self-referrals probably form a unique category of cases in which the parents directly arrange the professional facilities they require, and are probably quite likely to reject them again later; self-referrals are evenly spread between the two groups.

By means of domiciliary visits, we found the major parental explanations of non-attendance, in order of frequency, to be: child now dry; left district; forgot appointment (but did not request a further appointment); and maternal illness.

Problem number two was termination. We defined termination as three consecutive appointment failures or notification of withdrawal from treatment. Comparing 50 terminators with 108 successfully discharged cases, we found that the child with a positive family history of enuresis was especially prone to termination. It is conceivable that a positive family history is associated with a certain acceptance of enuresis and poor toleration of the demands of treatment. We did find that terminators gave significantly more instances of poor cooperation with treatment than did other patients and that they were less consistent in attending the clinic before dropping out. Terminators did, however, remain in treatment for a period comparable to the normal duration of successful treatment; we found from a different series, however, that only 19% of our terminators had dropped out on becoming dry, merely failing to report this fact to the clinic. Termination, therefore, does not seem to occur when a patient is progressing well, but to represent an amalgam of inappropriate familial attitudes and poor therapeutic response.

The first 10 appointments emerged as the "failure zone" for termination, which we found to occur most rapidly in small or very large families, occurring latest in four-child families.

A major therapeutic problem which we found significantly associated with both termination and slow response to treatment was failure to awake to the auditory stimulus of an enuresis alarm, indicating the need for further research on effective alarm stimuli. On comparing three subjectively very different alarms in use at our clinic, we did not find any significant differences in therapeutic efficiency.

Regarding the problem of relapse, we found none of 40 patient, background and treatment variables to differentiate relapsing from nonrelapsing patients, although in terms of the rapidity of relapse, we did find that older children relapsed earlier. Relapse would seem to be a function of treatment rather than of its recipient.

Over the past few years, we have been evaluating the uses of an "overlearning procedure" in reducing the relapse rate. The overlearning regime is introduced once the child has achieved the initial cure criterion of 14 consecutive dry nights. He is required to drink up to 2 pints of fluid in the last hour before retiring, while continuing to use the enuresis alarm. Overlearning is continued until the cure criterion is regained, unless an unacceptably severe recurrence of wetting should occur. Normally, we consider a recurrence of more than 50% of nights wet as unacceptable, although this is not a rigid rule. The rationale of overlearning is that, where a child's learned control of nocturnal micturition cannot cope with this extra fluid, wetting will recommence and this will permit a continuation of the conditioning process, with the establishment of the desired "margin of error".

We have found that overlearning reduces the relapse rate from 35% to 13%; this reduction is significant. In a larger-scale replication study involving 344 cases, we found that overlearning reduced the relapse rate from 29% to 10%; this reduction is also highly significant. In view of these results, I would recommend the routine incorporation of overlearning in the conditioning treatment of enuresis.

In conclusion, it may be stated that anxiety and attitudinal factors may be considered of relevance to therapeutic outcome, that overlearnir appears to produce a dramatic reduction in the relapse rate, and that insufficient or inappropriate alarm stimuli seem to be a major factor in therapeutic failure. It is noteworthy that some common prognostic assumptions were not supported in this study. The outcome of treatment, for instance, seems little affected by the age and sex of the patient, the severity of enuresis, the diagnosis of primary or secondary enuresis, or the presence of diurnal eliminative disorders.

References

YOUNG, G.C., MORGAN, R.T.T.: Analysis of factors associated with the extinction of a conditioned response. Behav. Res. Ther., in press (1972a).

YOUNG, G.C., MORGAN, R.T.T.: Non-attending enuretic children. Community Medicine 127, 158-159 (1972b).

YOUNG, G.C., MORGAN, R.T.T.: Overlearning in the conditioning treatment of enuresis. Behav. Res. Ther. 10, 147-151 (1972c).

YOUNG, G.C., MORGAN, R.T.T.: Overlearning in the conditioning treatment of enuresis; a long-term follow-up study. Behav. Res. Ther., in press (1972d).

YOUNG, G.C., MORGAN, R.T.T.: Patient termination in the treatment of childhood enuresis. To be published (1972e).

YOUNG, G.C., MORGAN, R.T.T.: Reasons for appointment failure among enuretic patients. Community Medicine, in press (1972f).

YOUNG, G.C., MORGAN, R.T.T.: Speed of response to the treatment of enuresis. To be published (1972g).

YOUNG, G.C., MORGAN, R.T.T.: Stimulus intensity factors in conditioning treatment of enuresis. Behav. Res. Ther., in press (1972h).

II. Behavioural Approaches to Neurotic Disorders

Are Phobics Ill?: Subject Sampling and the Validity of Treatment Analogues of Phobic Anxiety States

H. McALLISTER and M. OLLEY

I. Summary

The development of behavioural methods of treating anxiety has led to the use of volunteer subjects in analogue studies for investigating appropriate procedures. In this study a group of volunteer subjects with specific phobias is compared with phobic patients and a normal control group. Psychometric results indicate significant differences between the volunteers and patients, although the two groups shared a common disabling symptom. Such differences raise the problem of how analogue studies should be interpreted and indicate the need for caution in the extrapolation of analogue study results to the clinical situation.

II. Introduction

Anxiety has been for many years a major factor in attempting to evaluate a person's psychiatric status because of its central involvement in psychopathology. Reliance has been placed on either the subjective report of the individual on his condition, on observations of his overt behaviour, or on the use of physiological techniques to monitor his autonomic reactivity. The monitoring of physiological activity as an assessment procedure was based on the view that autonomic reactivity provides a useful index of the person's moment-to-moment emotional state, or of his anxiety level and hence of his current psychiatric status.

However, no one of these methods alone has proved satisfactory, and a new orientation in this area of research has developed. The view has evolved that the stress reaction is most usefully seen as the simultaneous occurrence of psychological or attitudinal, behavioural or motor, and physiological responses, however imperfectly coupled these may be (LACEY, 1967; LANG, 1969). A multidimensional approach to the measurement of anxiety is now deemed essential, and several studies have looked at these three aspects of their subjects' activity that is, the subjects' self-report, ratings of his overt behaviour and measures of his autonomic reactivity.

With the growth of behavioural methods for treatment of psychiatric disorder, much effort has gone into developing techniques for modifying anxiety responses. Phobic anxiety has been an attractive area of investigation because by definition, if not in fact, those suffering from this condition manifest their anxiety or fear in a manner which permits fairly precise delineation. However, when we turn to the literature we find that most of the best controlled studies have used volunteer subjects and not psychiatric patients for the investigation of treatment procedures. Until comparatively recently such treatment usually involved the technique of systematic desensitization. PAUL (1969) summarized almost all controlled investigations of systematic desensitization between 1961 and 1969. Between the years 1963 and 1968 he cites 14 studies dealing with individual treatment; of these, 10 used screened volunteer students as subjects, and one used distressed students. Again, 10 studies of group treatment published between 1961 and 1967 are summarized. Here, 4 used volunteer students, one used 'distressed' volunteers and another, 'distressed' students. Volunteers who replied to newspaper appeals and students were used by BANDURA et al. (1969) in comparing the relative efficacy of desensitization and modelling techniques, while BARLOW et al. (1970) compared 'shaping' procedures with desensitization, using college girls as subjects.

Immediate questions arise. For example, can we extrapolate the findings of these studies to the clinic? Do volunteer phobics and phobic patients belong to the population? Can treatment procedures be evolved through the exclusive use of volunteer non-psychiatric subjects, or are additional links required between the analogue study and application to clinical treatment?

We wish to make a distinction between those in the normal population with phobias, who on encountering their phobic situation will demonstrate marked avoidance behaviour and anxiety, and those with phobias who seek psychiatric help and therefore might be designated as 'ill'. We are questioning models of phobic anxiety and the treatment of phobias that employ non-patient volunteers.

In an extensive investigation of phobic anxiety states we have adopted the multidimensional approach to the measurement of anxiety. One object of this investigation has been the endeavour to delineate the extent to which volunteer phobics may differ from those who seek psychiatric help. Both groups will exhibit avoidance behaviour if confronted with specific stimulus situations, and both can be looked at from the three facets of the stress reaction mentioned. Thus with the preceding questions in mind, we compared psychiatric patients diagnosed as having phobic anxiety states with two control groups. One of these is a volunteer group comparable to those reported in the literature and the other is a normal group matched with the patients. This paper reports only the results of the subjects' self-assessment by means of an extensive battery of psychometric tests.

III. Methods

1. Subjects

Phobic patients: N = 22: 5m, 17f. Age range: 18 years 7 months to 59 years 9 months; $\bar{m}$ = 33 years 5 months. All had phobic anxiety as the major presenting symptom and had been referred to the Department of Mental Health, Queen's University of Belfast, for treatment. All were treated on an out-patient basis and maintained, if necessary, on a minor tranquillizer, i.e. 5 mg Diazepam t.i.d.

Normal controls: N = 18: 3m, 15f. Age range: 19 years 5 months to 57 years 4 months, $\bar{m}$ = 32 years 5 months. These 18 subjects were independently matched with 18 patients as to age, sex, and Mill Hill

Vocabulary Score. None had a history of psychiatric illness, defined as not having attended a psychiatric hospital. They were chosen from extramural classes of Queen's University and from the Hospital Nursing Reserve of the Belfast City Hospital.

Volunteer phobic controls: N = 19: 3m, 16 f. Age range: 21 years 5 months to 43 years 10 months, $\bar{m}$ = 28 years 7 months. No attempt was made to match this group with either the patients or the normal control group. Instead, these subjects were actively sought among the friends and relatives of our colleagues. All exhibited anxiety and avoidance behaviour when in their feared situation. None had considered having psychiatric treatment for their phobias nor did they take drugs to alleviate their anxiety.

2. The Psychometric Tests

All subjects completed the following tests when first entering the study: Fear Survey Schedule III (FSS III) (WOLPE and LANGE, 1964); The Middlesex Hospital Questionnaire (MHQ) yielding scores on Anxiety symptoms (A), Phobic symptoms (P), Obsessional symptoms (O), Somatic symptoms (S), Depressive symptoms (D) and Hysterical symptoms (H), (CROWN and CRIPS, 1966); The Eysenck Personality Inventory (EPI) measuring Extraversion (E), Neuroticism (N), and Lie (L), (EYSENCK and EYSENCK, 1964); The Manifest Anxiety Scale (MAS) measuring Anxiety (A), Defensiveness (K), and Lie (L), (TAYLOR, 1953); The Self-Description Questionnaire, (HOQ) (CAINE and HOPE, 1967); and The Mill Hill Vocabulary Scale (MHV) (RAVEN, 1958).

3. Results

Analyses of the psychometric data using the univariate Student's 't' test are shown in Table 1.

Here we can see that the phobic patients differ significantly on almost all measures from both the normal controls and the volunteer phobic subjects. The only significant difference between the two control groups is in the Mill Hill Vocabulary Score, with the volunteer phobic subjects forming the more verbally competent group, probably due to the nature of their selection. Note that even the total score of the FSS III, a measure of common fears, yields no significant difference between the two control groups.

A more satisfactory mode of analysis for such data is provided by using multivariate techniques. A discriminant function analysis produces the results shown in Tables 2 and 3.

Table 2 shows that we could very clearly discriminate using the tests involved between all three of our groups. No control subject was 'misclassified' as a phobic patient while only two phobic patients (9.1%) were 'misclassified', one as a normal control and the other as a volunteer phobic. Likewise three volunteers were mistakenly classified as normal controls while only one normal control was misjudged, as a phobic volunteer. Thus only 6 subjects out of a total of 59 (10.2%) were misclassified, and no "non-psychiatric" subject was mistaken for a patient.

The discrimination outlined in Table 2 was made using the derived values shown in Table 3. These show that discrimination between the phobic patients and the two control groups is made mainly by Function A and is heavily dependent upon the symptom ratings emerging from the MHQ.

Table 1. Means, standard deviations and student's 't' test differences for three groups of subjects

		Phobic Pts N = 22			Vol. Phobics N = 19			Normal Contrls N = 18			Phobic Pts N = 18			
		't' tests f. independent samples						't' tests f. matched pairs						
		m.	s.d.	p.	m.	s.d.	p.	m.	s.d.	p.	m.	s.d.		
	Age in months	401.0	138.6		336.6	74.7		388.7	139.4		401.6	134.5	Age in months	
	M.H. Vocab.	52.1	9.2	xxx	66.2	7.1	xxx	54.2	8.9		53.0	9.7	M.H. Vocab.	
EPI	Extraversion	21.5	7.1		25.0	6.3		24.8	7.6		20.6	7.1	Extraversion	EPI
	Neuroticism	32.7	8.3	xxx	20.3	6.0		18.2	9.1	xxx	34.6	7.0	Neuroticism	
	Lie	4.9	2.4		3.7	2.5		5.3	3.7		4.6	2.2	Lie	
	HOQ	22.0	5.6		24.0	6.8		23.7	6.1		21.9	5.7	HOQ	
MHQ symp-toms	Anxiety	11.6	3.2	xxx	5.5	3.1		5.8	3.3	xxx	12.2	2.5	Anxiety	MHQ symp-toms
	Phobic	8.4	3.7	xxx	4.1	2.0		3.9	2.5	xxx	8.5	3.6	Phobic	
	Obsessional	9.3	3.3	xx	6.1	3.1		5.9	3.4	xx	9.6	3.5	Obsessional	
	Somatic	7.3	3.3	xxx	2.5	2.1		2.9	2.6	xxx	7.6	3.3	Somatic	
	Depressive	6.2	3.0	xxx	3.2	1.4		3.9	2.5	x	6.5	3.0	Depressive	
	Hysterical	6.3	3.4		4.6	3.5		5.1	3.0		7.0	3.2	Hysterical	
	MHQ Total	49.0	13.8	xxx	25.9	8.5		27.6	10.1	xxx	51.4	12.9	MHQ Total	
MAS	Anxiety	28.4	10.4	xxx	14.3	7.4		15.4	9.1	xxx	31.1	8.7	Anxiety	
	K	11.8	4.5		14.2	3.2		14.7	4.1		11.6	4.8	K	
	Lie	5.3	2.5	x	3.6	1.7		5.1	2.7		5.3	2.4	Lie	
	FSS III	103.2	34.3	xx	73.5	31.7		67.9	37.9	xx	110.8	27.9	FSS III	

x p .05; xx p .01; xxx p .001

Table 2. Discriminatory analysis - 'hits and misses table'

Forecast Group	Actual Group		
	Phobics	Controls	Volunteers
Phobics	20	0	0
Controls	1	17	3
Volunteers	1	1	16

Table 3. Scaled Eigenvectors: Contribution of Each Variable to the Discriminant

Variable		Factor A	Factor B
% Trace		80.94	19.06
EPI	(E	0.244	0.262
	(N	-0.217	0.841
	(L	0.291	-0.111
	HOQ	0.107	0.253
MHQ	(A	-0.621	0.050
	(P	-0.391	0.492
	(O	-0.124	0.001
	(S	-0.699	-0.047
	(D	0.176	-0.150
	(H	-0.638	-0.099
MAS	(A	0.833	-0.418
	(K	-0.132	0.165
	(L	-0.366	-0.139
	MHV	0.535	0.736
	AGE	-0.061	-0.169
	FSS III	0.260	0.024

Function B provided the main distinction between the two control groups. Degree of neuroticism, Taylor's measure of anxiety and verbal intelligence all contribute to this differentiation. Specific individual scores rather than group trends must aid in the discrimination on this weaker function, accounting for only one fifth trace variance.

Since in the practical situation our 6 tests plus age, yielding 17 scores in all, provide a rather unwieldy set of calculations from which to derive a discriminant function, we decided to establish whether a subset of these scores could provide useful discriminatory power. Therefore, using the same raw data from our three experimental groups, several discriminant functions were derived depending on selected subsets of test scores.

The most successful combination of scores from just 3 tests was that using the MHQ, EPI and MAS, yielding 13 test scores. Table 4 shows that discrimination of psychiatric phobics from the control groups is little altered, but that the control groups themselves tend to be intermixed.

Table 4. Reduced variables (MHQ, EPI, MAS) discriminatory analysis 'hits and misses table'

Forecast Group	Actual Group		
	Phobic	Controls	Volunteers
Phobic	20	0	1
Controls	0	9	1
Volunteers	2	9	17

It will be noted that only one control subject, a volunteer, is misclassified as a 'patient', while 13 subjects in all are misallocated (22.0%). Since the latter discrimination is almost as efficient as the former in 'distiguishing' psychiatrically referred subjects, we provide the score weights used to yield this discrimination only.

The equation for a new subject's score is: Discriminant Function Score = (18 EPIE - 46 EPIN + 39 EPIL - 272 MHQA - 212 MHQP - 34 MHQO - 267 MHQS + 35 MHQD - 230 MHQH + 119 MASA - 43 MASK - 160 MASL) + 1000.

This score can be fitted into the scale illustrated in Fig. 1. The new subject is than tentatively designated as belonging to a phobic patient group or a population in accordance with his score on Function A. The disignation is tentative of course, until the discriminant function is cross-validated with another set of samples from the populations used.

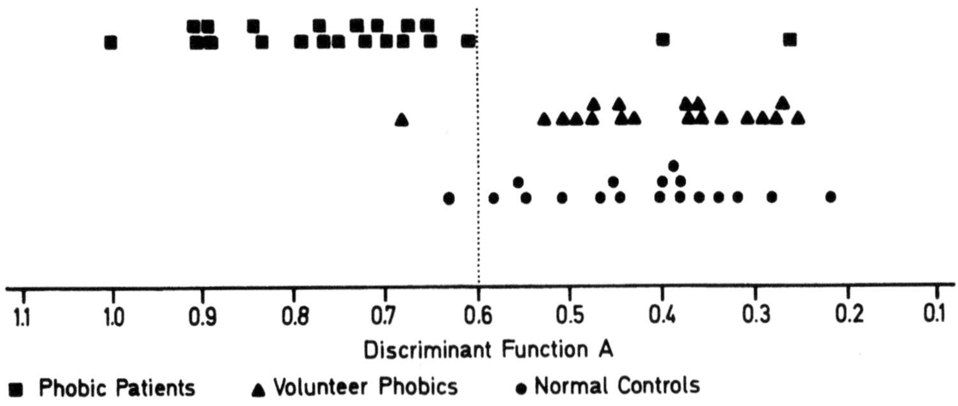

Fig. 1

IV. Discussion

It is clear that six commonly used questionnaire measures can make an impressive discrimination between a psychiatric population suffering from phobic anxiety states and two control groups, one consisting of volunteer phobic subjects, the other of normals matched to the patient group. These tests also yield reasonable discrimination between the control groups.

A selected reduction of the number of tests used to compute the discriminant function yielded almost as good discrimination between patient and control groups but not among the controls themselves.

How do we interpret these results and of what practical value are the discriminations suggested?

In each analysis of a simple set of questionnaires, commonly used in clinical settings, volunteer phobic subjects are found not to resemble psychiatric phobic patients, the latter being distinguished from them, as well as from normal controls, by high levels of neuroticism, anxiety and general symptomatology (see Fig. 1). Indeed the volunteers are much more like the control group on the measurements used, the results being a tendency to intermix these two groups in discriminant analyses.

Yet the literature indicates that firm evidence on the efficacy of systematic desensitization for the treatment of phobic anxiety comes predominantly from studies using volunteer subjects. Our findings may explain in part the disquiet expressed by a number of therapists experienced in systematic desensitization. Many patients do not appear to respond to treatment as readily as is suggested by the analogue studies.

A comparison between PAUL's summary of studies involving individual desensitization and an important report by GELDER et al. (1967) on the effectiveness of desensitization and psychotherapy with psychiatric patients illustrates this point well. In 10 of the studies using volunteer subjects, the mean number of sessions devoted to treatment was 10 spread over an average period of 4.5 weeks. After this treatment many subjects were judged completely recovered. On the other hand, GELDER et al. reported that desensitization with a phobic patient group lasted, on average, for 39 sessions, with the difference between psychotherapy and desensitization (in favour of the latter) becoming significant only after 24 treatment sessions. Only two patients, both treated by desensitization, lost their phobias completely. Self-ratings on a symptom check list correlated negatively with improvement with both types of treatment. Further the authors noted that specific or monosymptomatic phobias, such as fear of animals, respond best to desensitization. Unfortunately, in psychiatric practice it is generally agreed that, in adults, monosymptomatic phobia states are relatively uncommon.

In another study LADER (1967) compared the autonomic reactivity of a mixed group of phobics with that of anxiety states (some with depressive symptoms) and with a normal control group. Skin conductance was the physiological index of reactivity. This distinguished specific phobics from other pathological groups on both the number of spontaneous fluctuations shown on the records and on rate of habituation to 20 sound stimuli. The specific phobics resembled the normal controls by having fewer spontaneous fluctuations and demonstrating faster habituation. Further, their overt anxiety was rated as lower than that of the other patient groups.

Again LADER et al. (1967) found that few spontaneous fluctuations and rapid habituations correlated significantly with clinical improvement in desensitization and low overt anxiety; this offers prognostic indices for success with this type of treatment.

Having in mind these findings and the fact that our volunteer phobic population is distinguished from phobic patients on self-rated anxiety, neuroticism and on general neurotic symptoms, we are tempted to speculate that they resemble monosymptomatic or specific phobic patients. Discrepancies in treatment duration between volunteer specific phobics and phobic patients in general might be accounted for in this manner. Indeed, MARKS (1969) states that the more psychiatric patients with phobias resemble phobic volunteers, the closer are the results of desensitization in them to those in the volunteers.

Our evidence, and that from the literature, suggests that it is possible to distinguish two groups of phobic subjects. Descriptively, the distinction seems to contrast specific phobics with other phobic conditions on rated over anxiety, on a physiological index of reactivity and on some common self-rating questionnaires. This dichotomy would appear to have an important bearing on our expectations as regards desensitization treatment.

We would tentatively propose that the simple discriminant function provided by the EPI, MAS, and MHQ be cross-validated as a possible prognostic index. To date the evidence is purely suggestive but a cross-validation is at present under way. The investment of a short period of therapist and patient time would seem worthwhile if it allowed the prediction of whether desensitization is likely to be prolonged or successful, or if it would be better to consider some other form of treatment.

V. Conclusion

Many studies of behavioural methods for treating phobic anxiety have employed volunteer subjects in attempting to create analogues for the treatment of psychiatric patients. However, this study shows that volunteer phobic subjects differ profoundly from phobic patients on some psychometric measures on both univariate and multivariate analyses.

Volunteers show a much stronger resemblance to normal control subjects. The patients differ from both groups in their high level of neuroticism, anxiety and general psychiatric symptomatology. Although the volunteers and patients share a common disabling symptom, the differences must cast some doubt on the validity of these experiments as analogues of treatment in the clinical setting. The possibility is raised, however, that such experiments provide more useful information for the treatment of monosymptomatic phobic patients. The psychometrics used in this study provide a tentative index of severity of phobic conditions and if cross-validated may be useful in making decisions about treatment.

Acknowledgements

This work forms part of a much larger study supported by a grant from the Medical Research Council of Great Britain. It has been conducted under the general guidance and assistance of Professor J.G. Gibson, Department of Mental Health, The Queen's University of Belfast.

References

BANDURA, A., BLANCHARD, E.B., RITTER, B.: Relative efficacy of desensitization and modelling approaches for inducing behavioural, effective, and attitudinal changes. J. Person. soc. Psychol. 13, 3, 173-199 (1969).

BARLOW, D.H., AGRAS, W.S., LEITENBERG, H., WINCZE, J.P.: An experimental analysis of the effectiveness of 'shaping' in reducing maladaptive avoidance behaviour: an analogue study. Behav. Res. Ther. 8, 165-173 (1970).

CAINE, T.M., HOPE, K.: Manual of the Hysteroid and Obsessoid Questionnaire. London: University of London Press 1967.

CROWN, S., CRIPS, A.H.: A Short Clinical Diagnostic Self-Rating Scale for Psychoneurotic Patients. The Middlesex Hospital Questionnaire (MHQ). Brit. J. Psychiat. 112, 917-923 (1966).

EYSENCK, J.J., EYSENCK, S.B.C.: Manual of the Eysenck Personality Inventory. London: University of London Press 1964.

GELDER, M.G., MARKS, I.M., WOLFF, H.H.: Desensitization and psychotherapy in the treatment of phobic states: a controlled inquiry. Brit. J. Psychiat. 113, 53-73 (1967).

LACEY, J.I.: Somatic response patterning and stress: Some revisions of activation theory. In: Psychological Stress (M. APPLEY, R. TURNBULL, Eds.). New York: Appleton Century Crofts 1967.

LADER, M.H.: Palmar conductance measures in anxiety and phobic states. J. Psychosom. Res. 11, 271-281 (1967).

LADER, M.H., GELDER, M.C., MARKS, I.M.: Palmar conductance measures as predicted of response to desensitization. J. psychosom. Res. 11, 283-290 (1967).

LANG, P.J.: In: Behaviour Therapy: Appraisal and Status (C.M. FRANKS, Ed.). New York: McGraw-Hill 1969.

MARKS, I.M.: Fears and Phobias. London: Heinemann Medical Books 1969.

PAUL, G.L.: In: Behaviour Therapy: Appraisal and Status. (C.M. FRANKS, Ed.). New York: McGraw-Hill 1969.

RAVEN, J.C.: Extended Guide to Using the Mill Hill Vocabulary Scale with the Progressive Matrices Scales. London: Lewis 1958.

TAYLOR, J.: A personality scale of manifest anxiety. J. abnorm. soc. Psychol. 48, 285-290 (1953).

WOLPE, J., LANG, P.J.: A fear survey schedule for use in behaviour therapy. Behav. Res. Ther. 2, 27-30 (1964).

Response Prevention and Modelling in the Treatment of Obsessive-Compulsive Neurosis: A Study of 24 Patients

H. HEYSE

Until 1970 the literature contained only reports on single cases of obsessive-compulsive neurosis treated by behaviour therapy. V. MEYER (1970) reported on some patients who had been treated successfully in a response prevention program. Since then LEVY and MEYER (1971) published a long-term follow-up study of these cases. RACHMAN and coworkers (RACHMAN et al., 1971; HODGSON et al., 1972) reported success with 15 patients treated by flooding, modelling and a combination of these two methods. RAMSAY and SIKKEL (1971) reported improvement in 3 of 4 patients treated by a procedure similar to modelling. HEYSE (1971a) reported preliminary results of this study in 9 patients treated by response prevention.

This study was conducted between 1 November 1970 and 31 July 1972. It had two purposes. One was to repeat the successful treatment of obsessive-compulsive neurosis by either of the two behaviour therapy methods. The other was to establish whether there is a difference in the modificational effect between response prevention and modelling.

I. Patients

The 24 obsessive-compulsive neurotics (15 female, 9 male) all suffered from compulsions, and obsessive-compulsive symptomatology dominated the clinical picture. Obsessive patients with a diagnosis of depressive or schizophrenic psychosis and organic brain damage were excluded. The main compulsions were checking, washing and cleaning. The mean age was 34.4 years and the average duration of compulsions was 9 years. Using the two-sample rank test of Wilcoxon the 12 patients treated with response prevention and the 12 patients treated with modelling did not differ significantly in duration of symptoms, age or intelligence.

II. Treatment

All patients were treated as inpatients and all were hospitalized for 6 to 7 weeks with the exception of 5 who stayed longer. Eight different therapists were involved, and in addition the nurses played an extremely important role in treatment. During the first and sixth week we took a baseline; the active treatment was carried out over a period of 4 weeks. Treatment consisted of slightly modified response prevention, described by MEYER (1966; 1970; 1971) and of LEONHARD's "Individual therapy for obsessive-compulsive neurotics" (LEONHARD, 1967;

BERGMANN, 1961), which is a reassembling of the modelling procedure and which we also slightly modified.

The response prevention procedure (r.p.) was as follows:

From the beginning all rituals were prevented and there was 24-hours' supervision by a nurse. During the first 2 days everything was done so as not to aggravate the patient's condition. Starting on day 3, more and more difficulties were introduced in a hierarchic order. On days 9 and 10 the nurse faded out and the patient started the hierarchy again, this time on his own. In addition we tried to improve generalization by taking the patient out of the hospital and home step by step. In some cases most of the treatment had to be carried out at home. The therapist instructed the relatives on how to react to the patient's difficulties. In both treatment procedures the patient was occupied as much as possible in other activities such as games and social contact. Some patients got support to start work again.

In none of these cases - and this, I think, is very important - did we use any other behavioural methods systematically. Of course, principles like operant conditioning and vicarious learning were operating in an unsystematic way all the time.

The modelling procedure (m.) was as follows:

A therapist or a nurse, acting as a model, and the patient practised various situations which were arragned in a hierarchic order. The normal behaviour in a given situation was trained; then the patient was asked not to avoid or ritualize in that or a similar situation again and to repeat the situation several times on his own. Between the sessions there was no control. During the third and fourth weeks the patient got support for generalization. Alternative activities were the same as in the r.p. procedure.

III. Assessment

Patients were assessed during the first and sixth week of the stay and 4 weeks after treatment. A long-term follow-up is still going on. We chose three different ways of assessment.

1. We took a 4-day baseline before and after treatment. As far as possible, frequency and duration of compulsions were recorded in specific situations for each patient. This was repeated every day of the baseline. If possible - and in some patients this was the only way to take a baseline - the patient was asked to keep a self-record for specific compulsions.

2. There was a 5-point rating scale. This was filled in by the patient, the therapist and by two independent raters. The rating covered five aspects:
   a) Obsessions
   b) Compulsions
   c) Avoidance
   d) Anxiety
   e) General adjustment, using Marks' categories of work, leisure, sex, family relationships and social relationships.

3. Questionnaires, which have not yet been evaluated and will not be discussed here.

The practical and theoretical issues in taking a baseline on obsessive-compulsive neurotics have been discussed by HEYSE (1971b).

IV. Method of Evaluation

It was not possible to compare different symptoms directly between the patients for testing purposes. What we did was handle the data on each patient like a single case study. For the baseline data and for every aspect of the preceding ratings we tried to form an opinion about the amount of improvement. For each aspect, like baseline data, obsessions, compulsions, avoidance, anxiety and adjustment, we then used Fisher's exact test for differences between the 12 r.p. patients and the 12 m. patients.

The following is a short description of how we made the judgement about the amount of improvement. The baseline data are not independent data in a statistical sense. The washing ceremony of a patient, for example, may have some impact on the dressing rituals which follow, and mood and rituals of the first day may influence the behaviour on the second day. Therefore a test cannot be used to demonstrate statistical significance, but it is acceptable to use the test to reach a judgement on improvement. We used Wilcoxon's two-sample rank test or Fisher's exact test, depending on the type of baseline data.

In the case of the ratings, a third independent rater reduced the several ratings on every aspect to a 3-point rating: much improved, improved, and unchanged or worse. This judgement was then used for testing.

V. Results

For baseline data that are self-records and/or data on symptoms in specific situations, there is no statistically significant difference between the results for r.p. patients and m. patients. In the group in which the r.p. procedure was used, 5 patients were much improved, 3 improved and 4 unchanged; in the group treated using the m. procedure, 5 patients were much improved, 4 improved and 2 unchanged; for one patient no baseline was taken after treatment. As to the ratings for the before-therapy period and the 4-week follow-up period, there was a tendency in favour of modelling therapy for the aspects 'obsessions' and 'compulsions' (see Table 1). There was no significant difference between the procedures for the aspects 'avoidance' and 'anxiety' (see Table 1). On the general 'adjustment' rating there was significantly more improvement in the m. group (Fisher's exact test, $\alpha < 0.0124$, see Table 1).

VI. Discussion

Research in therapy presents the well-known predicament of needing to test the efficacy of one treatment method on a larger group of patients, but being able to do so only at the cost of variability in the therapeutic approaches available for individual cases. GERLINGHOFF and SCHWARZ (1972), among others, have mentioned this issue in regard to behaviour therapy with obsessive-compulsive neurotics.

Table 1. Ratings for Obsessive-Compulsive Neurotic Patients Following Treatment

	Obsessions		Compulsions	
Rating	r.p.	m.	r.p.	m.
Much improved and Improved	3	7	3	6
Not improved	6	2	8	4
No rating	3	3	1	2

	Avoidance		Anxiety	
Rating	r.p.	m.	r.p.	m.
Much improved	2	3	-	3
Improved	3	2	2	3
Not improved	6	5	9	4
No rating	1	2	1	2

	Adjustment	
Rating	r.p.	m.
Much improved	-	5
Improved	7	2
Not improved	4	3
No rating	1	2

The results of this study show both treatment procedures to be effective, though not effective enough, in the modification of obsessive-compulsive behaviour. There seems to be a slight difference in efficacy, the modelling procedure being somewhat better. Therefore the question must be raised whether response prevention should be ruled out because of the immense amount of time and personnel required. But we have to be cautious about this. We were quite astonished at the amount and speed of progress in all the r.p. patients during the period of supervision. Perhaps one could avoid a relapse in these patients by extending the duration of supervision, by a more careful transfer from supervision to self-control, and by prolonging the treatment period as a whole. As a method for getting at intense ritualistic behaviour, I think we cannot do without it. The difference between the two therapy methods was that modelling was superior in improving social adjustment, obsessions and compulsions, as shown by the ratings. It is difficult to explain this. Maybe the m. patients had more of the feeling of being responsible for their own progress.

The problems these patients have are not solved, however, by reduction of rituals and avoidance behaviour. In only a few of the cases in our sample there was a reduction in frequency and duration of obsessions. The refractoriness and persistence of the obsessions is one of the main causes of relapse. Other causes of unsatisfactory outcome are the various shortcomings of these patients in social behaviour, in work adjustment and in sexual and marital life. One could expect better and longer-lasting improvements if the specific treatment for the compulsions were combined with systematic behaviour therapy for the other shortcomings and with a method to influence obsessions more directly.

LEVY and MEYER (1971) and RACHMAN and co-workers (RACHMAN et al., 1971; HODGSON et al., 1972) did not report any such additional behavioural treatment methods. In samples of patients comparable to ours, or more incapacitated, their results were better than ours. All their patients improved. The reasons for these differences are not yet clear. According to our experience, the prognosis for behaviour therapy in obsessive-compulsive neurosis is not particularly optimistic if one focuses solely on the compulsions and avoidance behaviour and simply hopes that there is also some influence on the obsessions.

VII. Summary

24 obsessive-compulsive neurotics were treated by response prevention (12) and modelling (12). Both methods were effective in modifying obsessive-compulsive behaviour; modelling was more effective mainly in improving the general adjustment of the patients.

Acknowledgements

I thank Professor v. ZERSSEN very much for his advice, Dr. HANSERT for evaluating the data, Dr. REY, Dr. STUTTE and Dr. ULLRICH for their work as independent raters, Dr. CASTELL, Dr. HOFFMANN, Dr. KUNZE, Dr. KUNZE-TURMANN, Dr. MITTELSTEN-SCHEID, Dr. REICH, Dr. WILDNER as therapists and the nurses as co-therapists.

References

BERGMANN, B.: Individualtherapie der Zwangsneurosen. Psychiat. Neurol. med. Psychol. (Lpz.) 13, 172-177 (1961).

GERLINGHOFF, M., SCHWARZ, D.: Verhaltenstherapeutische Ansätze zur Behandlung zwangskranker Patienten in der Klinik. Nervenarzt 43, 124-129 (1972).

HEYSE, H.: Verhaltenstherapie bei Zwangsneurotikern. Paper presented at the First European Conference on Behaviour Therapy and Behaviour Modification. München 1971a.

HEYSE, H.: Issues in taking a baseline of obsessive-compulsive patients. Paper presented at the Third Annual Conference on Behavioural Modification. Wexford/Ireland 1971b.

HODGSON, R., RACHMAN, S., MARKS, I.M.: The treatment of chronic obsessive-compulsive neurosis: Follow-up and further findings. Behav. Res. Ther. 10, 181-189 (1972).

LEONHARD, K.: Individualtherapie schwerer Zwangsneurosen. Psychiat. Neurol. med. Psychol. (Lpz.) 19, 2-10 (1967).

LEVY, R., MEYER, V.: Ritual prevention in obsessional patients. Proc. roy. Soc. Med. 64, 1115-1118 (1971).

MEYER, V.: Modification of expectations in cases with obsessionsal rituals.
MEYER, V.: Paper presented at the First European Conference on Behaviour Therapy and Behaviour Modification, München 1971.
RACHMAN, S., HODGSON, R., MARKS, I.M.: The treatment of chronic obsessive-compulsive Neurosis. Behav. Res. Ther. 9, 237-247 (1971).
RAMSAY, R.W., SIKKEL, R.J.: Behaviour therapy and obsessive-compulsive neurosis. Paper presented at the First European Conference on Behaviour Therapy and Behaviour Modification, München 1971.

Three Flooding Procedures in the Treatment of Agoraphobics

R. ULLRICH, R. ULLRICH DE MUYNCK, G. CROMBACH and V. PEIKERT

I. Introduction

The experiment described was designed to test systematically the effects of in vivo flooding, combined with alprenolol, combined with a placebo, and used alone. The rationale for combining this drug with flooding is as follows:

1. Agoraphobics have been found to have markedly heightened unpleasant body sensations. This is a fact in the sense that it has not only been described repeatedly in the literature (ROBERTS, 1969; KLEIN, 1964; SNAITH, 1968; ROTH, 1959; MARKS, 1969), but has also been experimentally corroborated by means of specially developed questionnaires (ULLRICH and ULLRICH DE MUYNCK, 1972a). In comparision to patients having various other diagnoses, agoraphobics scored by far the highest on a Fear Survey Schedule (FSS) factor called 'fear of bodily symptoms'. The same study used the Emotionality Inventory (EMI), which showed that this subjectively experienced heightened somatic anxiety was more prominent in the autonomous (EMI A_2) than in the psychomotor aspect (EMI A_1) of the scale .

2. The assumption was made that such unpleasant somatic sensations can be divided into two groups: a) stimulus-dependent conditioned emotional responses and b) somatic sensations, not dependent on external phobic stimuli.

3. MARKS and co-workers have shown that with flooding procedures stimulus-dependent 'somatic' anxiety (that is, physiological as well as emotional reactions) can be reduced in a relatively short period of time (MARKS et al., 1971; WATSON et al., 1971; 1972). In our own studies this occurred mainly within a one-week period involving 10 hours of flooding (ULLRICH and ULLRICH DE MUYNCK, 1972b, c). The removal of this stimulus-related somatic anxiety may not extend to the unpleasant stimulus-unrelated sensations. Sensations of this kind (e.g. severe panic attacks) may continue to appear during or after therapy, despite successful treatment; they may also produce new avoidance behaviour and thus give the appearance of a relapse.

4. Panic attacks induced by means of sympaticomimetics such as adrenalin can be neutralized by means of antagonists on the beta-adrenergic receptors (PITTS, 1971). This group of drugs, the beta-blocking agents, was shown to reduce anxiety symptoms better than a placebo (GRANVILLE-GROSSMANN and TURNER, 1966) and to the same degree as chlordiazepoxide (WHEATLEY, 1969). The most important aspect for our study is that this effect is probably due only to the peripheral, partial blocking of the autonomous stress reaction and that there is no central tranquillizing

effect (CLEGHORN et al., 1970; BONN and TURNER, 1971; BONN et al., 1972; LADER and TYRER, 1972).

From this it would seem to follow that blocking of the autonomous reactivity (found to be heightened in agoraphobics) in combination with in vivo flooding should relieve both kinds of somatic anxiety.

Single case studies, as reported last year at the Munich conference, led us to assume that this combination of therapies would yield superior results (ULLRICH and ULLRICH DE MUYNCK, 1972c).

II. Aims of the Present Study

The present experiment was designed to test the foregoing clinical observations. We were guided by two main expectations:

1. It was predicted that the combination of beta-blocking agents with flooding procedures would be superior to flooding alone. In order to test this, three groups were used:
   A. beta-blocking agents plus flooding,
   B. placebo plus flooding, and
   C. flooding only.

It was expected that treatment A would be therapeutically superior to the other two.

2. With regard to the specifically peripheral effects of the drug, it was believed that the reduction of bodily sensations could be measured by means of the specially constructed Emotionality Inventory (EMI) and particularly by means of a factor termed 'autonomous anxiety'.

One further important question was asked. We wanted to know whether either the behaviour therapy or somatic intervention was more effective during any particular phase of therapy. It was possible that the treatments would be similar throughout the entire course of therapy, but it was also possible that the proposed specific effect of the beta-blocking agents would become especially noticeable at some particular stage of therapy. However, there was reason to assume that after habituation the specific drug effect would be seen more clearly, so we divided the analysis of the entire treatment into two phases of one week each.

III. Design

Prolonged exposure to aversive stimuli, as is typical for in vivo flooding procedures, was applied as follows to 3 groups of 8 agoraphobic patients:

A) flooding *in vivo* combined with 50 mg tablets of alprenolol 4 times a day;
B) flooding *in vivo* combined with a placebo, also 4 tablets a day;
C) flooding *in vivo* without any drugs.

The treatment period lasted for 15 days. Fourteen of these were actually therapy days. Measurements designed to test the hypotheses stated previously were taken on days 1, 8 and 15, as well as 6 weeks after completion of the experiment. On days, 1, 8 and 15 patients had been free of any drugs for 14 hs. Thus, the entire treatment period could be analysed for differential effects due to time. The significance of the difference between treatment groups was tested by means of the Mann-Whitney U-Test. For drug conditions A and B a double-blind procedure was employed.

IV. Patients

Patients were secured by writing to hospitals and specialists in the Munich area. All of the patients showed the typical phobic sequence of agoraphobic stimuli, conditioned emotional responses and avoidance behaviour. The treatment groups were matched for age, sex and the various rating scale scores used for the assessment of the agoraphobic symptomatology. The mean age was 33 years (range 21 to 50 years). There were 11 men and 13 women. Mean duration of symptoms was 6 years (range 2 to 20 years). All subjects were outpatients.

V. Treatment

1. Flooding in vivo

Under standardized conditions a training procedure (also called exposure, response prevention, differential reinforcement and paradoxical intention) was used as the basic therapy for all groups. The patients received written instructions including the following points: the connection between phobia and avoidance was explained, the patients were encouraged to conduct their exercises intensively, and were informed that the therapist was merely a 'technical counselor'. Patients had to sign a contract, undertaking to observe the conditions of the experiment in minute detail and, in particular, not to run away from any prescribed phobic situation. At the beginning of therapy two 'therapists', one of whom acted as therapist and the other as independent observer, went together to the situation judged most difficult by the patient. After one hour the patient was left to himself in the phobic situation and he had to pursue his exercises on his own. These exercises lasted for 14 days, 2 hs daily being spent on the main phobia. Altogether the patient spent about 30 hs of training on the main phobia and about 80 hs on additional phobic stimuli. The therapist spent about 20 min per day with each patient. This time was used not only to check on the daily exercises and make measurements but also to prepare the training program for the following day. The total time spent by the therapist with each patient was about 12 hs.

2. Drugs

All drugs were given with standardized instructions to the effect that they would serve only to aid training, that they would ease adaptation and that there would be no side-effects. The drug was given in a dosage of 50 mg 4 times a day, which is the dose usually given for internal diseases. Tablets were to be taken at 8 and 11 a.m. and 5 p.m.

VI. Measurements

The measurements made are given in Table 1.

Table 1. A comparison of the dependent variables at the beginning of treatment for treatment groups (Kruskal-Wasslis one-way analysis of variance) (df = 2; N = 3 x 8)

	Initial Ratings	
Observer rating	H	
A % Anxiety	1.045	NS
A + B + C Phobic behaviour	1.035	NS
D Avoidance	3.4587	NS
Heart rate	1.7337	NS
Self-rating		
SB I Task difficulty	2.5288	NS
SB II Threatening aspect	1.5608	NS
SB III Avoidance	2.1351	NS
EMI A_1 Motor anxiety	2.2785	NS
EMI A_2 Autonomous anxiety	1.9366	NS
FSS Factor agoraphobia	0.3157	NS

Two observers rated the patients independently for the following characteristics: general impression of anxiety (A%), three kinds of phobic behaviour (motor, autonomous and verbal expressions, as indicated by A, B and C) and motor and verbal avoidance behaviour (D). The heart rate was also recorded. In addition, patients completed three questionnaires. The first, termed SB (Situationsbewertung), called for an evaluation of the phobic stimulus situation in terms of task difficulty, threatening by stimuli and desire to avoid the situation (SB I, II, and III). The second questionnaire, the EMI, was designed to record the degree of psychomotor and autonomous anxiety (A_1 and A_2) experienced during the phobic situation.

Finally, the factor 'agoraphobia' taken from the FSS is also shown. All the scales shown were developed prior to this experiment and contain between 10 and 21 items. Inter-rater agreement between the two observers was well above 0.7.

As may be seen from Table 1, there were no significant differences between the three treatment groups at the outset of the experiment.

VII. Results

The general effects of treatment as assessed from the observer ratings and heart rate are shown in Fig. 1. The mean differences are given between days 1 and 15, i.e. for 14 treatment days, for the 3 behaviour rating scores in each of the treatment groups. The *p* values obtained by means of a sign test indicate that all scores decreased significantly with therapy.

The placebo condition produced the smallest changes, but none of the differences between the groups with regard to the observer rating were significant.

Fig. 2 shows the corresponding results for the self-ratings. Again it is seen that the magnitude of all scores is significantly reduced after 14 days of treatment.

The general impression gained from Fig. 2 is that, as far as the evaluative measures of the phobic situation and the FSS are concerned, beta-blocking produced the best therapeutic results, followed by flooding only. With regard to the somatic anxiety factors, group C showed the smallest improvement. Group B, receiving placebo, showed the smallest change in SB I to III and also in the FSS. As regards the total treatment period, significant improvement was already observed in the first treatment period (days 1 to 8) for all measures. During the second treatment period (days 8 to 15) only the beta-blocking group A showed further significant improvement for all rating scales. The control groups B and C remained essentially unchanged. More detailed aspects of these results are discussed below on the basis of Table 2.

Table 2 contains the results of the statistical between-group analysis for the different treatment periods of the experiment. In the left section group differences obtained for the overall therapeutic change from the beginning to the end of therapy are shown. The beta-blocking group A was significantly superior to the placebo group for several

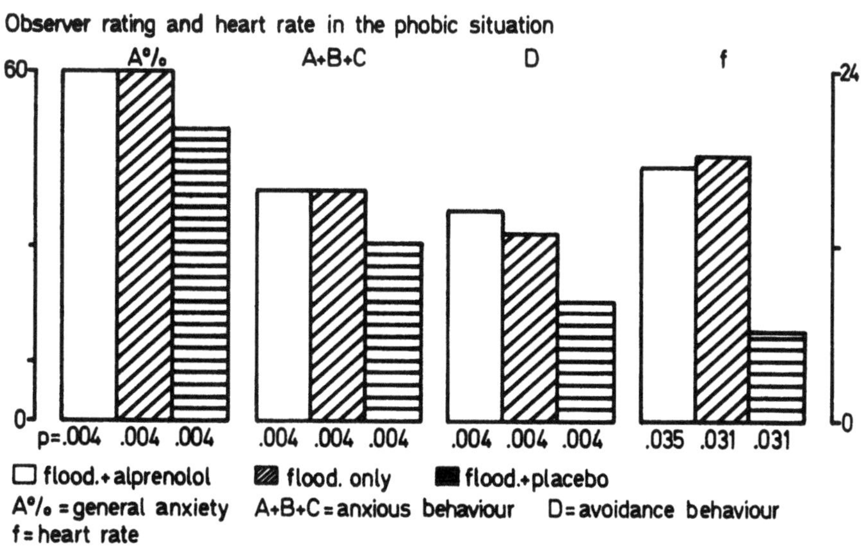

Fig. 1. Mean differences after 14 days of flooding in vivo for three treatment conditions (N = 24)

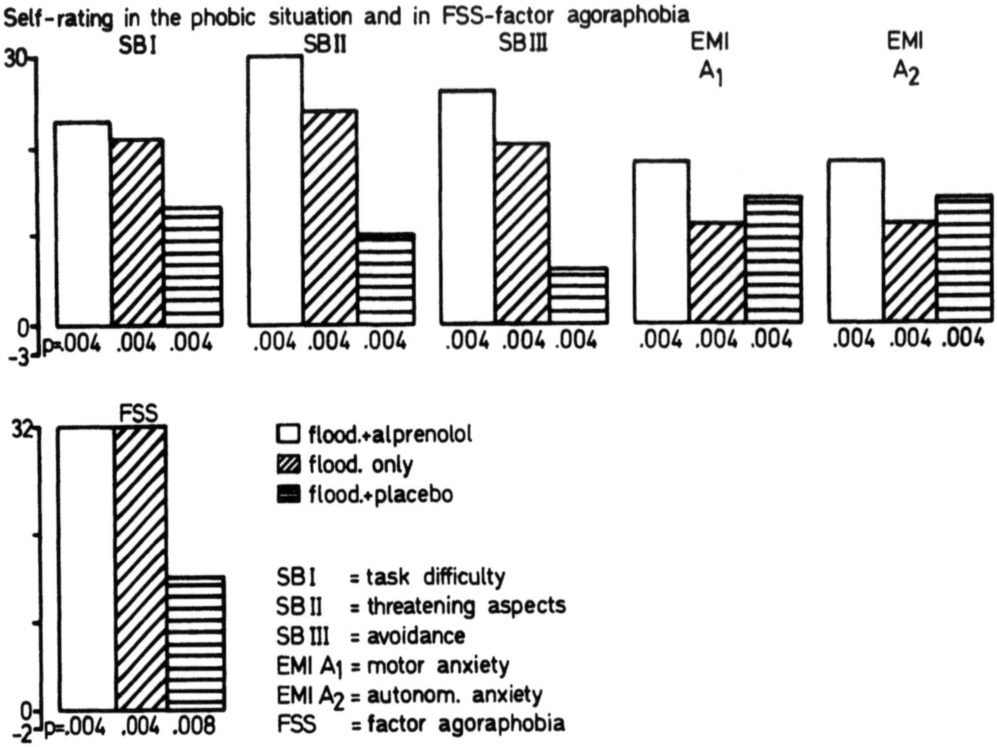

Fig. 2. Mean differences after 14 days of flooding in vivo for treatment conditions (N = 24)

variables; with regard to the flooding-only group C, this superiority was seen for autonomous anxiety. The control groups B and C did not differ significantly.

The middle section of Table 2 covers the first half of the treatment period (days 1 to 8). Drug group A was about equal to the flooding-only group C. There is a tendency for group A to be superior to the placebo group B, and this superiority is even more marked for the flooding-only group C.

In the right section the groups are compared for the second therapeutic period (days 8 to 15). Here group A is superior to both B and C in its therapeutic effect, while the two control conditions are approximately equal. There are apparent differences between the motor and autonomous aspects of somatic anxiety: the beta-blocking method was superior only for the autonomous aspect (A_2).

VIII. Discussion

Our main hypothesis was that flooding combined with a beta-blocking agent would be superior to flooding with a placebo and to flooding only. The results of the experiment showed that this was true only for the second week of therapy. Here the drug group improved further on all measures of anxiety and avoidance, and this improvement was

Table 2. Group differences for three flooding procedures (Mann-Whitney U-test)

Variables	Groups: Total Period of Treatment			1st Week			2nd Week		
	A vs.B	A vs.C	C vs.B	A vs.B	A vs.C	C vs.B	A vs.B	A vs.C	C vs.B
SB I Task difficulty	.052	NS	NS	.032[a]	NS	.041[a]	.052	.025[a]	NS
SB II Threatening aspect	NS	NS	B > C .080	NS	NS	.032[b]	.032[a]	.014[b]	NS
SB III Avoidance	.005[c]	NS	NS	.065	NS	.097	.014[b]	.014[b]	NS
EMI A_1 Motor anxiety	.014[b]	NS	NS	NS	NS	.003[c]	NS	NS	NS
EMI A_2 Autonomous anxiety	.080	.041[a]	NS	NS	NS	NS	.097	.014[b]	B > C .065
FSS Factor agoraphobia	.019[b]	NS	.052	.065	NS	NS	.019[b]	.080	NS
Heart rate	.080	NS	NS	.065	NS	NS	NS	NS	NS

a = *p* = 5 %　　A = Flooding + alprenolol　N = 8

b = *p* = 2 %　　B = Flooding + placebo　N = 8

c = *p* = 1 %　　C = Flooding only　N = 8

NS: *p* = 10 %

significant as compared to the two control groups. Results for the entire treatment period showed the same general trend: the group receiving a beta-blocking agent was significantly superior to the placebo group on several measures and superior to the flooding-only group on autonomous anxiety. This latter superiority may be specific for the drug used.

These results were shown to be time-dependent. Seen during the early stages of therapy the significant improvement on all measures of all aspects of anxiety and avoidance could be in part unspecific. Expectancy, suggestibility and the like may well have produced an initial, short-term improvement in all 3 therapy conditions. The marked improvement that occurred during the first week is probably a result of the many exercises done, which could initially have reduced stimulus-dependent unpleasant bodily sensations for all 3 groups to the same degree. If this had been the case, any additional improvement due to the drug would not have been apparent during the first week.

After the first week of treatment the chances for improvement in beta-blocking groups were no better than the chances in the other groups. The means for this group fell between those for the placebo and the flooding-only group, but the differences were not significant. By the start of the second week of treatment we could assume that the second type of unpleasant bodily sensations, i.e. the kind seen as not being stimulus-dependent, became a more important factor in the feelings of the patient and thus in relation to the maintaining or inducing of phobic behaviour, as discussed in the introduction. Beta-blocking agents can slow down such unspecific autonomous reactions and thus reduce unpleasant sensations. Therefore, the further improvement in the group receiving the beta-blocking agent - and in this group only - can be considered to be a specific effect of the drug, which was what we expected. For the reasons stated above, alprenolol is judged to make a genuine contribution to the success of flooding therapy, albeit as a supportive measure.

Finally, we would like to mention the difficulties experienced in assessing studies in which similar treatment methods are compared. These difficulties were due not only to the time-dependent effect but also to the sensitivity of the measurement methods used. The general effect of therapy was registered by all the methods used, including observer ratings and physiological parameters; however, a finer differentiation was possible only with the self-ratings, which were superior to the observer ratings.

IX. Summary

Three groups of eight agoraphobics, matched for age, sex and various measures of anxiety and avoidance, were treated for two weeks with flooding *in vivo*. In one group, flooding was combined with alprenolol, a beta-blocking agent, and in one with a placebo. A third group was treated with flooding *in vivo* only. In this double-blind study overall significant improvement was already seen during the first week in all three groups on verbal, motor, autonomous, physiological and behavioural measures of anxiety and avoidance. In the second week the group receiving alprenolol was the only one that showed further overall improvement and was superior to both control groups. The conclusion is drawn that alprenolol is a real adjuvant in flooding therapy.

References

BONN, J.A., TURNER, P.: D-Propranolol and anxiety. Lancet 1971 I,1355-1356.
BONN, J.A., TURNER, P., HICKS, D.C.: Beta-adrenergic-receptor blockade with practolol in treatment of anxiety. Lancet 1972 I, 814-815.
CLEGHORN, J.M., PETERFY, G., PINTER, E.J., PATEE, C.J.: Verbal anxiety and the Beta-adrenergic-receptors: A facilitating mechanism? J. nerv. ment. Dis. 151, 266-272 (1970).
GRAINVILLE-GROSSMANN, K.L., TURNER, P.: The effect of propranolol on anxiety. Lancet 1966 I, 788-790.
KLEIN, D.F.: The delineation of two drug-responsive anxiety syndromes. Psychopharmacologia 5, 397-408 (1964).
LADER, M.H., TYRER, P.J.: Central and peripheral effects of propranolol and sotalol in normal human subjects. Brit. J. Pharmacol. 45, 557-560 (1972).
MARKS, I.M.: Fears and Phobias. London: Heinemann 1969.
MARKS, I.M., BOULOUGOURIS, J.C., MARSET, P.: Flooding versus desensitization in the treatment of phobic patients: A crossover study. Brit. J. Psychiat. 119, 353-375 (1971).
PITTS, F.N., jr.: Biochemical factors in anxiety neurosis. Behav. Sci. 16, 82 (1971).
ROBERTS, A.H.: Housebound housewives - A follow-up study of a phobic anxiety state. Brit. J. Psychiat. 110, 191-197 (1969).
ROTH, M.: The phobic anxiety depersonalization syndrome. Proc. roy. Soc. Med. 52, 587 (1959).
SNAITH, R.P.: A clinical investigation of phobias. Brit. J. Psychiat. 114, 673-697 (1968).
ULLRICH, R., ULLRICH DE MUYNCK, RITA: Behandlungsmethoden bei Agoraphobikern. Paper presented at the 4th Conference of the GVT, Münster 1972a. To be published.
ULLRICH, R., ULLRICH DE MUYNCK, RITA: Modelos terapeuticos complejos en análisis y modoficación de conducta. In: PELECHANO, V. (Dir.): Adaptacion y conducta. Bases biologicas y procesus complejos, S. 59-100. Madrid: Marova 1972b.
ULLRICH, R., ULLRICH DE MUYNCK, RITA: Klinische Probleme bei der Anwendung der Reizüberflutungsmethode. Paper presented at the 1st European Conference on Behaviour Modification. Munich 1971. To be published: München: Urban & Schwarzenberg 1972c.
WATSON, J.P., GAIND, R., MARKS, J.M.: Prolonged exposure: A rapid treatment for phobias. Brit. med. J. 1971 I, 13-15.
WATSON, J.P., GAIND, R., MARKS, J.M.: Physiological habituation to continuous phobic stimulation. Behav. Res. Ther. 10, 269-278 (1972).
WHEATLEY, D.: Comparative effects of propranolol and chlordiazepoxide in anxiety states. Brit. J. Psychiat. 115, 1411-1412 (1969).

The Efficiency of a Standardized Assertive Training Program (ATP)

R. ULLRICH DE MUYNCK and R. ULLRICH

I. Introduction

The methods and goals of assertive training vary according to the definition of 'assertion' used. WOLPE (1958; 1969) introduced the concept of 'assertive responses', basing himself on SALTER's theory (1949) and adapting the term to his theoretical network. WOLPE and LAZARUS (1966) believe that 'failure to assert... is manifest wherever anxiety has been conditioned'. In insecure persons this anxiety is associated primarily with personal failures. It expresses itself as a fear of failing in the eyes of others and of subsequently being held in less esteem (ROTTER, 1954; SPIELBERGER, 1966). A stepwise hierarchic procedure in the sense of systematic desensitization (WOLPE, 1958) would, according to this concept, offer itself as an assertive training method.

Nonassertion or insecurity is not, however, always related to anxiety or inhibition but may also represent a deficit in the behavioural repertoire. Because of a faulty learning history the individual has never learned to cope with particular 'critical' problem situations. He does not behave assertively and thus suffers the resulting negative consequences. ROSE BRANDZEL (1963) trained social skills in a group of mentally and physically handicapped youth who were seeking employment. She reported that within the first 3 months of role-playing training the number of jobs accepted rose from 50 to 91 %. Apart from the treatment of social skills, the attitude a person has toward himself seems to be a significant factor in assertive training. 'Assertion' is, as a rule, directly related to observable behaviour. However, this seems to be an oversimplification because self-assertiveness frequently depends on self-evaluation. Overemphasis on achievement, extreme caution and inappropriate self-devaluation or criticism are frequently the roots of insecure behaviour. Accordingly, ELLIS (1962) with his 'rational-emotional therapy', KELLY (1955) with his 'fixed-role therapy' and DOROTHY SUSSKIND (1970) believe that cognitive restructuring of the self-image may lead to permanently self-assured behaviour. REHM and MARSTON (1968) found evidence for this. They conditioned self-reinforcement in men having social contact problems. Self-ratings and observer ratings showed that the results were better in this group than in a similar group treated by means of non-directive therapy and another control group. These considerations suggest that the nomological network of the concept of insecurity and, consequently, the most salient aspects of assertive training may be adequately represented by 3 main categories:

a) attitude toward self or self-evaluation;
b) social anxiety and inhibition;
c) social skills.

II. The Assertive Training Program (ATP)

A standardized assertive training program was developed for use with groups. This program consists of 110 social situations which were classified according to their level of difficulty and their content. These situations were systematically arranged in hierarchies. They were obtained empirically in sessions conducted with patients. All situations were standardized on 4 variables: actual social behaviour, partner, reaction of partner and place of action. In each of these variables there were up to 9 levels of difficulty. With this procedure a great many situations with widely varying levels of difficulty can be described precisely. The situations in the program consist of four hierarchies:

a) inability to press for demands;
b) inability to refuse and to criticize others;
c) inability to establish contact;
d) fear of failure and of public exposure.

The basic item structure is complemented by standardized instructions designed to establish a system of self-control over behaviour, to improve effective social strategies, to improve social communication, and to yield rules for the application of differential reinforcement. The training exercises are conducted both by role-playing in the hospital, including role reversal, and "on location" in the group. Homework is also assigned. There are non-verbal as well as verbal training exercises. Training occurs in groups of 5 to 7 patients with 2 instructors. The instructors serve as models during role-playing. At the beginning of a training session each situation is rated by the patients for difficulty. Those patients who consider this situation to be particularly easy begin the role-playing; they are succeeded by the other patients later on. Diverse procedures of operant conditioning are used throughout in order to foster the learning of new behaviour and the extinction of undesirable behaviour.

III. Aims of this Experiment

The two chief aims of the experiment described here were (1) to find out whether ATP is an effective method for reducing insecurity as defined earlier and (2) to see whether the therapeutic results achieved are maintained over an acceptable period of time.

IV. Methodology

Twenty patients hospitalized at the Max Planck Institute for Psychiatry in Munich were treated for a peroid of 6 weeks with the ATP described. The program consisted of 30 hours of training and some additional exercises 'on location'. The experimental group consisted of a mixed group of neurotics with the following diagnoses: agoraphobia, neurotic depression, social anxiety, writer's cramp, torticollis spasticus, stuttering, alcohol and/or drug dependence, sexual problems and deviations, and anorexia nervosa.

This experimental group was divided into 4 separate groups. The groups underwent the same assertive training program but each group was directed by a different therapist.

The control group consisted of 20 hospitalized neurotics with diagnostic labels comparable to those in the experimental group. In case of rare conditions such as writer's cramp or torticollis spasticus, patients were assigned at random to the experimental or control group, the more frequently occurring diagnostic categories being distributed equally to the two groups. Treatment costs for all patients in both groups were covered by compulsory health insurance. Both groups showed comparable socio-economic characteristics. All patients in the control group had individual therapy daily, involving various therapeutic procedures such as desensitization, operant conditioning and/or therapeutic discussions. However, none of these control patients received any treatment with regard to social problems during the experimental period of 6 weeks.

Several tests were given to both groups. Initially all patients were tested with a questionnaire on Personal Insecurity (U), an Inventory on Emotionality (EMI), the Fear Survey Schedule (FSS) (WOLPE and LANG, 1964) and an additional battery of personality tests which were given for an unrelated purpose. The insecurity questionnaire had been developed by the authors specifically to record therapeutic effects. The questionnaire includes items on self-evaluation about social matters, on feelings connected with problematic social interaction and on social skills. A factor analysis yielded 7 factors; 3 of these have to do with general attitudes (general insecurity, guilt feelings and over-politeness), while the other 4 record behaviour as observed in training sessions (fear of failure, inability to refuse, contact anxiety and inability to press for demands). The emotionality inventory was also developed by the authors. In this case, factor analysis again yielded 7 factors; 4 of these are related directly to the events occurring during training (inhibition, psychomotor anxiety, autonomous anxiety and psychological anxiety). The three remaining factors, which are less specific with regard to the training sessions, are aggression, exhaustion and depression.

During the experimental period the patients completed the questionnaires four times, the items of the scales being rearranged at random each time. At the end of the 6 weeks the whole test battery was given again. Six months after discharge, a follow-up study of the experimental group was conducted. Unfortunately, the control group could not be investigated in this way because in the interim some of the patients in this group had to be treated by means of assertive training.

V. Results

1. Insecurity Questionnaire (U)

Fig. 1 shows the 4 specific insecurity factors for the control group. Note that none of the 4 factors changed appreciably during the course of therapy. Again for the control group, Fig. 2 shows the scores for the less specific insecurity factors. Again, no significant differences were found. Fig. 3 and 4 show the results for the experimental group. Fig. 3 shows those factors which were trained specifically in therapy sessions. Between A and D 'fear of failure' changed appreciably and this change is significant at the 0.2 % level. This improvement was maintained for additional 6 months. With regard to 'inability to refuse' the difference between A and D is also significant at the 0.2 % level. This effect was also maintained over an additional period of 6 months, with the score dropping further, although not significantly. With regard to 'contact anxiety', the improvement from A to D is

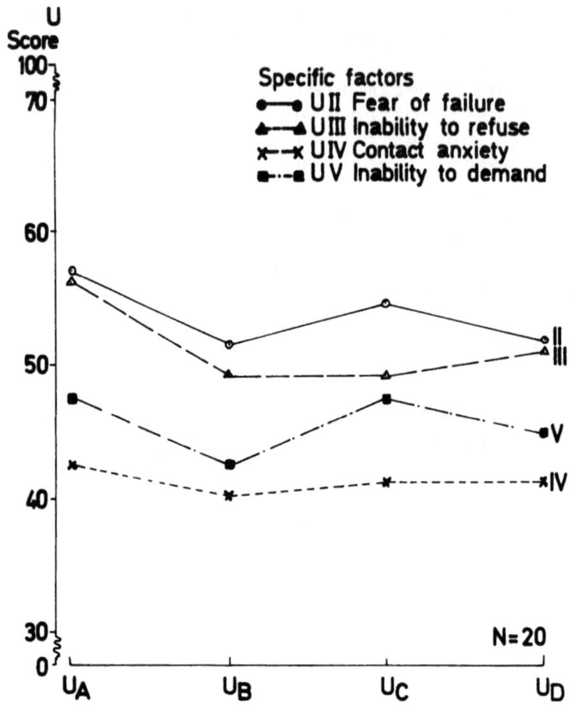

Fig. 1. Control group without social training

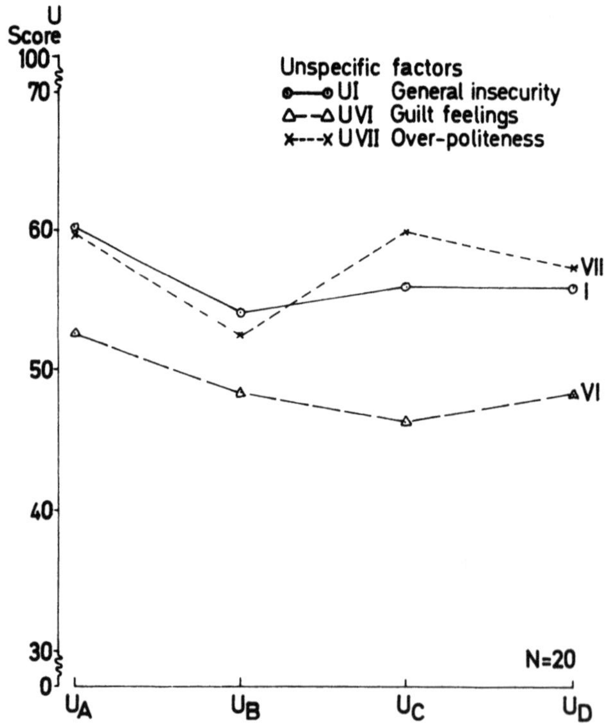

Fig. 2. Control group without social training

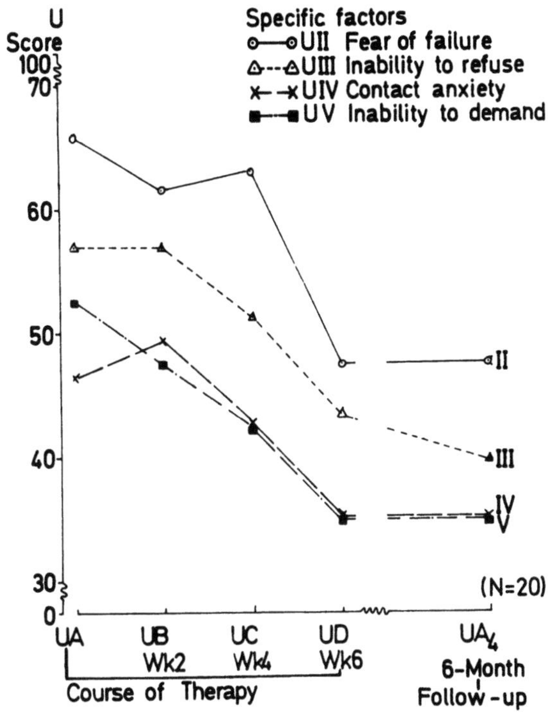

Fig. 3. Assertive Training Program (ATP). Therapy control and follow-up

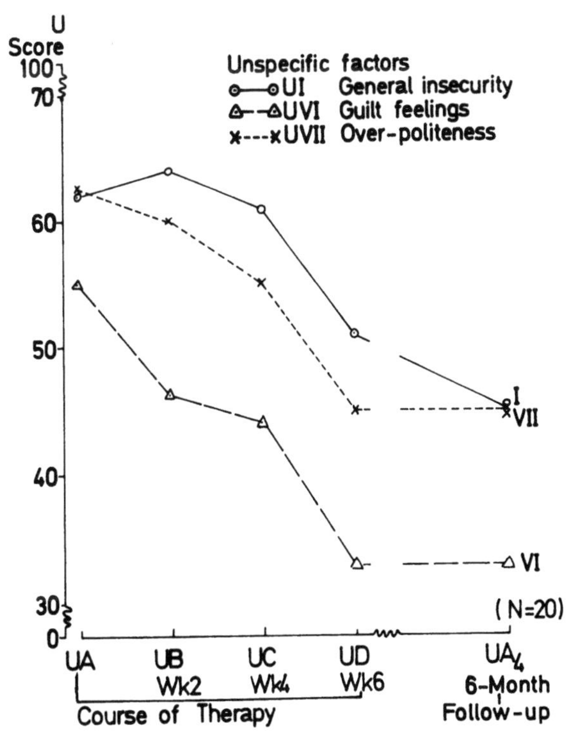

Fig. 4. Assertive Training Program (ATP). Therapy control and follow-up

significant at the 0.1 % level, and this effect was still seen after 6 months. For 'inability to press for demands' results are even more significant; in this case the difference was significant at the 0.1 % level, and the improvement was maintained during the following 6 months.

Fig. 4 shows the general factors, i.e. those which with regard to training were unspecific. 'General insecurity' improved from A to D at a rate significant at the 0.1 % level. After another 6 months this course dropped further, and the additional improvement is almost significant at the 5 % level. With regard to the factor 'guilt feelings', the difference from A to D is significant at the 0.1 % level; the improvement here was also maintained during the subsequent 6-months period. Finally, for the factor 'overpoliteness' the improvement from A to D is significant at the 2.5 % level and remains stable. The trend here of course signifies that the patients became less dependent on social norms and more independent for themselves.

2. Emotionality Inventory (EMI)

In the control group all emotionality factors remained unchanged. The results for the experimental group are shown in Fig. 5. In the upper section are the results for the specific emotionality factors that play a role in training exercises. These results are very clear in the sense that inhibition, psychomotor and autonomous anxiety show differences between A and D which are significant at the 1 % level. In the case of the fourth factor, psychological anxiety, the difference is highly significant (0.1 % level), follow-up after 6 months did not show any further change. The middle portion of Fig. 5 shows the unspecific emotionality factors. For none of these factors the difference between the scores obtained at the beginning and end of therapy was significant. Likewise, there was no significant change during the follow-up period.

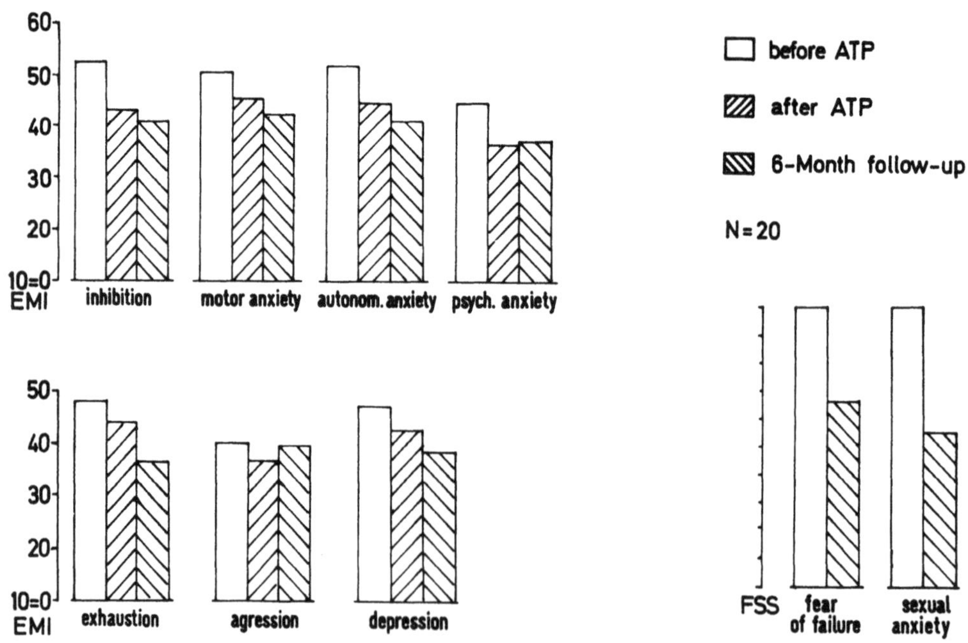

Fig. 5. Assertive Training Program (ATP). Therapy control and follow-up

3. Fear Survey Schedule (FSS)

The bottom part of Fig. 5 shows two factors from the FSS for the experimental group. These factors are 'fear of failure' and 'sexual anxiety', which means anxiety when faced with heterosexual contant. By mistake in the execution of the experiment a number of patients were not given the FSS at the end of the 6 weeks of therapy. Therefore, no statistical test was applied to the A-to-D period. However, the difference between the A and follow-up 6 months after the end of therapy could be tested for significance. This difference is significant at the 0.1 % level in the case of 'fear of failure' and at the 1 % level for 'sexual anxiety'.

VI. Discussion

The results of the study show clearly that the two main aims of the study were accomplished: ATP was effective in reducing insecurity in the three areas described earlier, and the improvement achieved was maintained over a period of at least 6 months. Particular significance is attached to the observation that not only those factors that were trained showed improvement but also that attitudes and feelings about social interaction became more positive. In the course of training marked progress was made in the development of social skills such as the capacity to press for demands. Moreover, the decrease in insecurity was steady and rapid throughout the training program.

The results obtained on the emotionality inventory are also noteworthy. Training appears to have alleviated somatically experienced anxiety as well as psychological anxiety and inhibition. This indicates that the general well-being of the disturbed patients also improved. This result is also considered to be a direct consequence af the training program, for none of the patients received drugs or any other additional therapy. The mere effect of hospitalization cannot be held responsible for the improvement since the control group, which was also hospitalized, did not improve significantly.

That the control group remained unchanged with regard to the insecurity questionnaire as well as to the emotionality inventory, seems to be due to the experimental conditions. During the experimental period of 6 weeks no therapy concerning social problems was allowed. This experimental restriction meant that the therapy of the control patients was not representative of single-case therapy as usually done in a clinical setting. Thus the comparison between the experimental group and the control group may only be made with regard to the unspecific therapeutic milieu, such as time spent with the therapist, hospitalization and other activities shared by all ward patients.

The maintenance of training effects achieved also deserves mention. Elsewhere we reported on a pilot study in the first group of patients treated using the ATP (ULLRICH DE MUYNCK and ULLRICH, 1971). The social behaviour and social adaption of these patients were rated by independent observers and data are available for a one-year follow-up period. The improvement achieved was maintained, and the patients themselves also rated their situation after discharge regarding occupation, leisure time, family and friends as much improved.

In this study 4 therapists were involved in the training. In view of the consistency of the results, it is assumed that improvement was achieved independent of the therapists and can therefore be considered as an outcome of the program itself. Similar results were obtained in another study with 10 different therapists, nearly all of them still in training, who treated 58 neurotics (ULLRICH de MUYNCK, 1972).

Finally, the fact that these good therapeutic results were obtained in a group of neurotics with extremely diverse symptomatology probably indicates that various kinds of patients received specific attention in a program that is essentially very complex and provides for treatment of various kinds of symptoms. This observation encourages the treatment not only of various types of neurotics with programs such as ATP but also of people with other types of psychiatric disorders such as psychosis (ULLRICH, 1972).

In conclusion, the assertive training program is an effective method for modifying social disturbances for the benefit of the patients.

References

BRANDZEL, ROSE: Role playing as a training device in preparing multiple-handicapped youth for employment. Group Psychotherapy 16, 16-21 (1963).
ELLIS, A.: Reason and Emotion in Psychotherapy. New York: Lyle Stuart 1962.
KELLY, G.A.: The Psychology of Personal Constructs. New York: Norton 1955.
REHM, L.S., MARSTON, A.R.: Reduction of social anxiety through modification of self-reinforcement: An instigation therapy technique. J. consult. clin. Psychol. 32, 565-574 (1958).
ROTTER, J.B.: Social Learning and Clinical Psychology. Englewood Cliffs/ N.J.: Prentice Hall 1954.
SALTER, A.: Conditioned Reflex Therapy. New York: Capricorn 1949.
SPIELGERGER, C.D.: Anxiety and Behaviour. New York, London: Academic Press 1966.
SUSSKIND, DOROTHY: The idealized self-image (ISI): a new technique in confidence training. Behav. Ther. 1, 538-541 (1970).
ULLRICH, R.: Indikationsstellung und klinische Relevanz des Assertive Training Program (ATP). Paper presented at the 4. Conference on Behaviour Therapy and Modification, Münster 1972.
ULLRICH DE MUYNCK, RITA: Selbstsicherheitstraining: Modelle und Effizienz. Paper presented at the 4. Conference on Behaviour Therapy and Modification., Münster 1972.
ULLRICH DE MUYNCK, RITA, ULLRICH, R.: Standardisierung des Selbstsicherheitstrainings für Gruppen. Paper presented at the 1. Conference of the European Assoc. of Behaviour Therapy and Modification, Munich 1971. München: Urban & Schwarzenberg (in press).
WOLPE, J.: Psychotherapy by Reciprocal Inhibition. Stanford Univ. Press 1958.
WOLPE, J., LANG, P.J.: A fear survey schedule for use in behaviour therapy 2, 27-30 (1964).
WOLPE, J., LAZARUS, A.A.: Behaviour Therapy Techniques.Oxford: Pergamon Press 1966.

Behaviour Therapy and Bereavement

R.W. RAMSAY

I. Introduction

In clinical practice one often sees clients with various social problems which a psychoanalytically trained therapist would immediately diagnose as an unresolved, pathological mourning process. Behaviour therapists do not seem to notice this, as there is little literature on the subject of grief and mourning from this corner of psychotherapy. The article by McAULEY and QUINN (1971) is the only one in the field which could be found to deal with mourning. LAZARUS (1968), LIBERMAN and RASKIN (1971) and WOLPE (1971) deal with the theoretical aspects of clinical depression, and BURGESS (1968) and LEWINSOHN et al. (1968) deal with behaviour therapy and depression. But depression and mourning are not the same, even if depression plays a major role in mourning. This dearth of behaviour therapy literature, in contrast to the extensive psychoanalytic literature, may be due to the fact that, like unresolved oedipal conflicts, unresolved pathological mourning processes may exist only in the eye of the beholder. Our contention, after treating a number of clients in the manner described below, is that the problem does exist, but we are in possession of a treatment and are looking for a theoretical basis for this type of treatment.

II. Characteristics of Mourning and Grief

There is little or no agreement in the literature as to how to define the various terms, and also no agreement as to how to explain what happens. The only agreement is that mourning and grief are widespread human experiences, which are extremely painful.

The characteristics of mourning according to FREUD (1917) are a profoundly painful dejection, loss of the capacity to love, inhibition of all activity, and a loss of interest in the outside world in so far as it does not recall the dead one.

BOWLBY (1961; 1963) uses the word mourning to denote the psychological processes that are set in motion by the loss of a loved object and which commonly lead to the relinquishing of the object. The word grief BOWLBY uses to denote the subjective states that follow loss and accompany mourning. AVERILL (1968) described bereavement behaviour from cultural, biological and psychological aspects. He sees in bereavement behaviour two components: mourning and grief. The former, according to him, is of cultural origin, while grief is the product of biological evolution. He summarizes the major features of grief as follows:

a) grief is a complex but stereotyped response pattern which includes such psychological and physiological symptoms as withdrawal, fatigue, sleep disturbances, and loss of appetite;

b) it is elicited by a rather well-defined stimulus situation, namely, the real or imagined loss of a significant object (or role), and it is resolved when new object relations are established;

c) it is a ubiquitous phenomenon among human beings and appears in other social species as well, especially in higher primates;

d) it is an extremely stressful emotion, both psychologically and physiologically, and yet behaviour during grief is often antithetical to the establishment of new relations, and hence the alleviation of the stress (p. 744).

No attempt will be made to differentiate between normal and pathological mourning; it is assumed to be normal unless it is so severe or prolonged as to need clinical intervention, then it is pathological. SIGGINS (1967) in her review states: 'I myself regard mourning as pathological if any of the reactions are excessively intense or if the process of mourning is unduly prolonged. Such a prolongation of mourning may be due to a delay in beginning the process, or to a retarding of the process once it has begun, or both'.

In our coverage of mourning we will make no distinction between bereavement due to death of a loved one, or other forms of forced loss of objects. Bereavement can also be severe when the object is lost due to divorce, or when the object is more abstract, e.g. job, homeland, way of life, etc.

III. Phases

There seem to be certain phases in the mourning process which can be distinguished from each other and which are necessary for proceeding further in the resolution of the problem.

a) Denial: the person denies that there has been any loss and lives as if the loved object still exists. This often necessitates dissociation from the real world in order to preserve the fantasy.

b) Depression: as denial starts breaking down the person begins to experience the full force of the loss and the painfulness and emptiness of life without the loved one.

c) Guilt: the person begins to blame himself for the loss, or for not making it easier for the loved one before parting.

d) Aggression: the person is aggressive toward others for not being able to ease the pain, for not having done enough to prevent the loss. There is also sometimes aggression against the loved object itself for having caused the pain.

e) Anxiety: the guilt and aggression always contain elements of anxiety, and there may also be anxiety for the uncertainties of a different life in the future.

f) Re-integration: the person organizes a way of life in which the lost object has no place.

There is no agreement on this classification in the literature. However, it does seem to be of value to try and identify what takes place and to know what to expect. It might be better to view this sequence as components of reactions that will occur, rather than as phases which follow each other in a systematic order.

IV. Where is the Behaviour Therapist?

It may be that behaviour therapists, due to their training in dealing with the here-and-now, are not concerned with antecedents. Thus something like a mourning process does not exist: the client is depressed, the client is anxious, etc., and these problems are treated by existing behaviour therapy techniques. However, where a number of problems seem to form a clinical syndrome with a rather well-defined antecedent stimulus situation that has relevance for the here-and-now behaviour of the client, it might be worthwhile to try to view the syndrome in its entirety and to treat it accordingly.

V. Treatment

Our approach is a combination of what the Gestalt therapists may call confrontation, what Albert Ellis would see as strongly rational and what the behaviour therapist would see as implosive emotional-expressive therapy. The aim of the therapist is to elicit high levels of emotion and to continue for long periods of time to allow the emotions to exhaust themselves.

Some prerequisites to a therapy for bereavement are that the therapist and client should have a good working relationship with each other, the client should know in advance that the treatment will be painful, and both therapist and client should be prepared once they start to put in long sessions with a minimum of time between sessions. Our experience has been that sessions last about 1 1/2 to 2 hours and should be daily.

Typically, after some history taking, after deciding on a bereavement therapy (a point to be discussed later), and after the other prerequisites have been met, the therapist in the first session will ask the client to get comfortable in a chair, to close his eyes and to describe in words the loved one: appearance, mannerisms, what they did together, etc. The purpose of this is for the client to bring the loved one as vividly as possible to mind and for the therapist to assemble details which may be used later. The therapist after some minutes starts trying to break through the denial by saying things like: 'but now she is dead, that's all finished now, you'll never see her again, etc.'. Usually the client will burst out crying, and the therapist encourages the client to cry, waits till the crying subsides and then continues to ask about the loved one and to confront the client with the fact that she is dead. Such a sitting should continue until the client does not cry any more, then the therapist feeds back the various details of the loved one coupled with such phrases as 'but now she is dead'. The therapist must continue going over the same ground, again and again, but must work up in an hierarchic manner to more and more details of an intimate nature: holidays together, quiet evenings at home, evenings out together, mutual interests, sexual contacts, etc. If the client has trouble crying or feeling sadness, he is asked to describe what happened at the funeral, to remember all the people there, to see them crying, and to try and allow himself to feel like them. Some useful suggestions on emotional-expressive training can be found in SERBER et al. (1968).

When the crying starts to diminish, the client will probably for some time become deeply depressed, the depth and duration of the depression varying with the severity of the problem. The therapist should at this stage be alert for possible suicide, and sometimes hospitalization is essential. The therapist should go on with the therapy as rapidly as possible at this point, to bring the duration of the depressive phase to a minimum.

The next stage is to elicit and explore the aggression against the self (guilt?) and against others. The therapist suggests and encourages anger against others such as the doctors who didn't do enough, the friends who were not helpful, the parents who thought only of themselves, the client himself who could have made things easier, could have given the deceased more love, etc. The range of possibilities depends on the therapist's knowledge of details of the relationship, plus his inventiveness. Obviously not all the things suggested will be applicable, but some will 'click', and then the therapist goes over this ground again and again until the anger is extinguished. Once again, suggestions from SERBER et al. (1968) are useful in cases where the client has difficulty in feeling anger, and the therapist will probably have to model extensively.

The last part of the aggression, which does not always appear and does not seem to be a necessary part of this phase, is aggression directed against the deceased, for leaving, for being dead and at rest, for causing the pain and anguish of the bereavement. The therapist should always explore this avenue, but our experience has been that it is only in some cases that this anger appears.

The anxiety mentioned in the previous section will also be present during the guilt and aggression phases, in fact most clients swing back and forth between depression, guilt, anxiety and aggression. The anxiety can be due to a number of factors, and it will not be possible, or necessary, to isolate them and desensitize in the normal manner. The approach is more implosive than desensitizing, and any one session should go on until anxiety or any strong negative emotion is extinguished.

The therapist has to go on attempting to elicit emotions until the client is no longer depressed and does not react in an emotional way when talking about the loved one. This decreased arousal state must be reflected in behaviour outside of the therapy situation. Various possessions which belonged to the loved one should no longer occupy a revered position in the house, and the client should be able to discuss plans for the future which show that other people can take the place of the loved one. The implementing of these plans is the last, re-integration phase, and is usually a slow process, no longer intensive therapy. The client may be able to do it alone, or with support on an infrequent basis from the therapist.

VI. Case Study

As illustration, a particularly difficult therapy will be described. This is not typical of what we have done so far, in that the therapy took a relatively long time, but it shows the possibilities of the technique.

Mrs. S. (34) married in 1961, became pregnant in 1963; both husband and wife did not want children, and at 3 months a spontaneous (?) abortion occurred. At the end of 1969 she again became pregnant, this time the wife wanted a child but the husband was strongly against having children as he was asthmatic and was afraid that any child would be the same. There were fights between husband and wife which included physical damage to the wife. At 7 months pregnancy she had to go to the hospital, there were fights between the husband and the hospital staff after which the husband was barred from the hospital. The child was born dead in the hospital. Ten days after leaving the hospital, the client heard that her mother had cancer, and a month later the mother died. At about the same time two horses that the husband and client owned had to be destroyed. At the beginning of 1971 the client again became pregnant, and there ensued more violent scenes between husband and wife. In August 1971 the husband died in the hospital during a severe asthma attack. Ten days later the client gave birth to a daughter. Mrs. S. reported that she had not cried at the husband's death or at the funeral.

In April 1972 the client visited her G.P., who referred her to a psychiatrist, but on the day of the appointment the psychiatrist was killed in a traffic accident. She was referred further to a psychiatric outpatient department. The presenting problems were depression, inability to deal with the child, a fear that she would hurt the child, and the fact that the events of the past year kept going through her head like a film which she could not turn off.

VII. Therapy

Arrangements were made to have friends look after the child, and Mrs. S. was admitted as an inpatient to the psychiatric ward of a general hospital. The therapy strategy was explained to her by the psychiatrist who had taken the case history, and she agreed to take part in an intensive programme to be carried out daily by the author and the admitting psychiatrist, and a nurse was assigned to be with her when necessary. At the beginning of therapy the client was asked to close her eyes, to imagine her husband, to describe him and then to say to herself such phrases as 'but now he's dead, I'll never see him again'. The saying of these phrases did not work, as she reported that he was constantly present, they conversed with each other and even went to bed together. She was then instructed that if he did not go away she was to try and send him away, to tell him that he was dead and must go. This did not work either, as he refused to leave. She was then instructed to forcibly send him away, to fight with him if necessary. This also failed to work, even though the emotional reactions were intense. She lost every fight with him. She was then instructed to fight with him, and the therapist would help her to win. All this took about 2 weeks, in session of 1 1/2 h daily, and she became extremely agitated in every session. During the 3rd week of treatment she finally succeeded in sending the husband away temporarily, but then became severely depressed, aggressive towards the therapists, wanted to stop the therapy, to leave the hospital and to do away with the child and herself. The hospital staff were prepared to detain her against her will but this proved not to be necessary. Within a few days she was again prepared to continue the therapy, although she was still very depressed. At this stage she stated that she had come to realize that it was not that he refused to leave, but that she did not want to let him go.

This phase of breaking down the denial took weeks, with constant shifting into aggression, guilt and anxiety. The aggression was directed against the doctors who had treated the husband, against the therapists, the child, and against the husband himself. During this time, the 'film' that had been playing through her mind gradually became fragmented and fainter, but one scene remained strong: a fight that she and the husband had had just before his death. She was asked to remember this, to go through it in her mind, and it took 5 long and violent sessions to extinguish the anxiety that was coupled with these memories. Each session produced more and more details of the fight, with the last detail being that the husband had almost murdered her by holding a pillow over her face.

After 6 weeks of treatment she wanted to see the child again, but was still afraid, and could not hold the child close to her. At the same time she started going home again for short periods, but suffered severe anxiety attacks in the home. This was treated by forced prolonged exposure during which she had to clean up the house and put away all the husband's belongings. They owned 2 cats which the husband had liked very much, and it took 2 sessions for her to bring herself to tell the cats that the husband was dead. It took another 3 sessions to be able to tell the child that the father was dead, and still 3 more sessions to tell herself that he was dead. Each session was a highly emotional experience. Most of the sittings were recorded on videotape, with her consent.

After 2 months of intensive work the client was discharged from the hospital, and therapy was no longer intensive. The 'film' had ceased to exist, the anxiety attached to the child had not completely disappeared but had been considerably reduced, and the panic attacks at home had ceased. She reported that for the first time in a year she occasionally felt lonely and sought out contact with other people. Therapy will continue into the re-integration phase. Intensive therapy time in the 2 months totalled 60 sittings of 1 1/2 h average duration, plus a full-time nurse for 4 weeks.

VIII. Other Cases

Not all cases are as severe as the one described above. Some bereavement problems can be dealt with in one session, others in 3 or 4 sittings. One client, a woman of 29 who after a divorce had had severe social problems with men, was able to remarry after 4 implosive sessions. In total, some 10 patients have been treated by the author and colleagues, and the results have been impressive and gratifying.

IX. Comments

In carrying out therapy such as this, we have been impressed by the violence of the emotional outbursts, and in some cases the therapist has needed support in going on with the presenting of the stimuli until the response extinguishes. The therapist must expect strong reactions: crying fits, angry outbursts, panic reactions and threats of suicide, and the therapist <u>must</u> in any one sitting continue to present the stimuli which elicit an outburst until the reaction subsides. This may take a number of hours, but it is considered essential that the reactions subside before a sitting is ended. This can be exhausting for both client and therapist.

A further problem which has arisen is that the therapist is often frightened or reluctant to deal with the concepts of death. The therapist finds sometimes that his own bereavement experiences hinder him in the therapy, and that he has to face his own fears of breaking the taboo of dealing openly with death.

X. Discussion

Until now, no experimental work has been done in this area. The theoretical background is vague and confused, the technique of treatment is not clearly formulated, the indications for when to use this technique are no more than clinical hunches, and the assessment of results is completely subjective. However, in spite of these criticisms, it is felt that it is worthwhile going further into these problems.

The theoretical behaviour therapy articles on depression barely touch on the effects of bereavement, and much serious work will have to be done in order to understand depression and mourning, and the differences and similarities between them.

Diagnosis and indications for treatment is another field sorely in need of careful work. A behaviour analysis of a client will indicate many problem areas, but to relate these problems to each other and to show that they form a syndrome which we may call pathological mourning is not easy. Even assuming that we can show that such a syndrome exists, we are still faced with the choice of treatment focused on the precipitating event or an anhistorical treatment of the here-and-now lack of positive reinforcement, anxiety, aggression and conditioned helplessness that WOLPE (1971) advocates. BELLAK and BERNEMAN (1971) in their criticism of WOLPE state: "With regard to behavioural therapy, our impression is that it is not only simplistic and reductionistic, but also based on an overvaluation of the psychologic concept of transfer of training: a concept which experimental psychologists treat with reservations, particularly with regard to the range of its applicability".

The technique described in this article apparently works with some patients, but it needs to be more carefully worked out into a treatment package which others can use. The question of whether this is one man's technique which only he can use had already been answered: until now to our knowledge 7 therapists have used this approach with success. It will still have to be worked out in detail though so that therapists without contact with the author can use it.

It will be necessary to show experimentally whether this method has more to offer in terms of efficiency than other, more conventional forms of therapy and to find out in more detail what these other therapies consist of so that comparisons can be made. A forthcoming book, edited by PARKES (1972), may help here. Controlled studies will have to be carried out using different approaches in order to evaluate the behaviour therapy attack.

Despite all these criticisms and problems it is felt that the form of therapy described here is worthwhile; it can fit into the framework of behaviour therapy and can be offered as a valuable form of treatment for certain problems.

XI. Summary

In this paper an attempt is made to come to grips with the process of mourning within a behaviour-therapeutic context. The psychodynamic literature on the subject of mourning and psychotherapy is loose and unstructured, and the behaviouristic literature is almost non-existent. With the use of concepts from implosive therapy and emotional expressive training, a possible behaviour therapy approach to the treatment of unresolved grief reactions is suggested, and some case studies are described. It is felt that this form of treatment can broaden the range of therapeutic tools available to the behaviour therapist, but the theoretical background needs elaboration.

References

AVERILL, J.R.: Grief: its nature and significance. Psychol. Bull. 70, 721-748 (1968).

BELLAK, L., BERNEMAN, N.: A systematic view of depression. Amer. J. Psychother. 25, 385-393 (1971).

BOWLBY, J.: Processes of mourning. Int. J. Psycho-Anal. 42, 317-340 (1961).

BOWLBY, J.: Pathological mourning and childhood mourning. J. Amer. psychoanal. Ass. 11, 500-541 (1963).

BURGESS, E.P.: The modification of depressive behaviour. In: RUBIN, R., FRANKS, C. (Eds.): Advances in Behavior Therapy. New York: Academic Press 1968.

FREUD, S.: Mourning and Melancholia. S.E., Vol. 14 (1917).

LAZARUS, A.A.: Learning theory and the treatment of depression. Behav. Res. Ther. 6, 83-89 (1968).

LEWINSOHN, P.M., WEINSTEIN, M.S., SHAW, D.A.: Depression: a clinical research approach. In: RUBIN, R., FRANKS, C. (Eds.): Advances in Behavior Therapy. New York: Academic Press 1968.

LIBERMAN, R.P., RASKIN, D.E.: Depression: a behavioral formulation. Arch. gen. Psychiat. 24, 515-523 (1971).

McAULEY, R., QUINN, J.T.: Behavioural analysis treatment and theoretical implications of a case of depression. Paper presented at the Dublin Conference on Behavioural Modification 1971.

PARKES, C.M.: Bereavement: Studies of Grief in Adult Life. London: Tavistock Publications 1972.

SERBER, M., GOLDSTEIN, A., PIAGET, G.W., KORT, F.: The use of implosive-expressive therapy in anxiety reactions. In: RUBIN, R., FRANKS, C. (Eds.): Advances in Behavior Therapy. New York: Academic Press 1968.

SIGGINS, L.D.: Mourning: a critical survey. Int. J. Psychiat. 3, 418-432 (1967).

WOLPE, J.: Neurotic depression: experimental analog, clinical syndromes, and treatment. Amer. J. Psychother. 25, 362-368 (1971).

Models of Depression

R. McAULEY and J.T. QUINN

I. Behavioural Models of Depression

This paper attempts to critically summarize current behavioural ideas on depression. Three chronic grief reaction case studies are presented at the end of the paper. Consequently some reference is made to the literature on grief reactions in the theoretical section of the paper.

One of the most adequate behavioural definitions of depression is that offered by BECK (1962): "It is a constellation of behaviours among whose most characteristic elements are motor and verbal retardation, crying, sadness, loss of mirth, loss of interest, self-devaluation, sleeplessness, and anorexia". This extensive definition covers both operant and respondent changes. Adequate assessment of the relative importance of each of these changes in each case should have some bearing on the type of treatment strategy adopted. Such considerations will be reflected in the eventual outcome. However, it seems that most workers have failed to reach this ideal. For instance, FERSTER (1965), LAZARUS (1968), LIBERMAN and RASKIN (1971), PATTERSON and ROSENBERRY (1969), and LEWINSOHN et al. (1969) have all tended to concentrate more on social or operant theory than on respondent theory. It is hoped that the models outlined below will demonstrate some of the forgoing shortcomings.

II. Social-Reinforcement Model

In 1966 FERSTER suggested three possible mechanisms that might explain the reduced social behaviour observed in depression :

1. loss of social-reinforcement
2. shifts in reinforcement contingencies
3. punishment and aversive control.

The first two statements form the basic premises of the social-reinforcement theory of depression. Loss of social reinforcement or in other terms loss of discriminative stimuli for positive reinforcement may follow such situations as loss of spouse, loss of job, loss of privileges etc.. Often, as LIBERMAN (LIBERMAN and RASKIN, 1971) emphasizes, loss may be quite subtle. For instance, promotion at work may be associated with loss of reinforcers, such as praise for good work and the security of a well-supervised job. A further example: MADDISON and WALKER (1967) noted that young widows tend to exhibit the most severe grief reactions. KREITMAN et al. (1970) noted that normal couples tend as they grow older to spend more time in the company of others. Thus the repertoires of younger couples may be more closely dependent than that of older couples, hence death in younger marriages may be associated with a relatively greater loss than in older marriages. Shifts in reinforcement contingencies may produce similar effects. The most obvious difference between this situation and loss of social reinforcement is that, whereas the latter results in time-out effects, shifts in reinforcement contingencies may involve extinction situations.

Generally, it may be suggested that in persons with wide social repertoires relatively large losses would be required to precipitate depression, while in those with poor or socially inadequate repertoires small losses may result in marked depression.

Both PATTERSON and ROSENBERRY (1969) and LEWINSOHN et al. (1969) emphasise the importance of the environment in the genesis and maintenance of depressive behaviour. Some forms may be maintained by positive reinforcement from persons in the immediate environment; in other cases the depressive behaviour may be maintained by situations which result in negative reinforcement. In other words, the individual who finds himself socially rejected may in future attempt to avoid pontenially rejecting situations.

These brief remarks emphasise the complexity of some forms of depressive behaviour. When exploring the histories of such behaviour one must always account for the following:

1) present loss (amount)
2) previous social repertoires
3) the significance of environmental factors.

However, in spite of the complexity of the preceding model, one must not fail to remember that it only accounts for the operant changes of depression.

Only a few behavioural workers have considered the emotional components of depression. We are sure that there is no doubt about their importance, since techniques such as desensitisation have been successfully employed. DENGROVE (1966) and RAMSEY (1972) have used these techniques in the treatment of grief reactions. WOLPE (1971) also reported the successful use of desensitisation in relation to some cases of neurotic depression. We referred earlier to three situations listed by FERSTER (1965), which could result in reduced social behaviour. Such situations are usually aversive and may thus result in or elicit emotional behaviour. Such behaviour may in several ways promote a further reduction in social behaviour (i.e. anxiety may be related to social avoidance, and freezing may be observed as paucity of action). Such effects further add to the complexity of the total model, in that we now have operant and respondent changes which will effectively result in reduced social behaviour. Two emotional models are now considered.

III. The Avoidance Model

As already noted, desensitisation has been used in the successful treatment of some forms of grief and depression. It is noticeable that grief is often typified by such avoidance behaviour as denial of the reality of loss and, at times actual illness. Thus it is possible to classify some depressions and grief reactions as phobias and treat them accordingly. However, it must be noted that avoidance of this order may make assessment and hence classification difficult. For instance, if the patient denies the events associated with the illness, we may be unable to make a reliable formulation of the underlying processes involved in the illness. Such events may only come to light during desensitisation if we decide on that course of action.

IV. Conditioned-Emotional-Suppression Model

This model centres around the well-substantiated Estes-Skinner Effect (ESTES and SKINNER, 1941) and can be summarised as follows. When non-contingent shock is applied to ongoing behaviour, we often observe excessive suppression of emotion and response. When a signal is paired with the shock, the signal will eventually itself acquire some of the properties of the non-contingent shock. This is why it is called "Conditioned Emotional Suppression". The effect is dependent on the parameters of the aversive stimuli, past experience, and probably heredity. In regard to past experience, CHURCH (1969) demonstrated that the past aversive history will to some degree determine whether sensitisation or adaptation occurs in the new aversive situation.

This model can be utilised to explain some of the behaviour observed in both normal and abnormal grief reactions. Death of a spouse is often unexpected and therefore can be viewed as non-contingent. Cues associated with the dead person now become conditioned stimuli for eliciting conditioned emotional suppression. In the large majority of grief reactions adaption appears to occur quickly. It is possible that sensitisation plays an important part in those illnesses which are prolonged. There are no studies in the literature on grief that would support such a claim, but MADDISON and WALKER (1968) do suggest the possibility that persons with prolonged grief reactions have had previously ambivalent and therefore aversive relationships with the dead person. Such an aversive history may pave the way for sensitisation effects.

V. Learned Helplessness

The last model to be considered is 'Learned Helplessness'. During investigations of conditioned emotional responses, MAIER et al. (1969) demonstrated that approximately 80 % of experimentally naive dogs failed to escape or avoid shock in a shuttlebox following a series of inescapable shocks given in a harness. This failure to escape in the shuttlebox was demonstrated in the first instance up to a maximum of 24 h after the unavoidable shocks. Following the failure to escape in the shuttlebox, it was possible to demonstrate the effect for several months and in some cases longer. The effect was demonstrated over a wide range of shock parameters. The workers suggested that this effect was most like a learned one, i.e. the animal had learned that, no matter what it did, shock was unavoidable, and therefore it failed to escape when introduced into the shuttlebox. The behaviour was considered to result from an extinction of motor responses, and it was shown that to experimentally reverse the effect, it was necessary to drag the animals physically from side to side of the shuttlebox, until eventually, after many trials, they learned to escape the shock. WOLPE (1971) offers this as a possible model for neurotic depression and suggests the use of shaping techniques and desensitisation to overcome learned helplessness.

The explanations offered for these experimental observations fail to take account of several factors:

1. They do not consider that the behaviour may be freezing and thus respondent in nature.
2. They do not adequately account for environmental cues, which might be important in such behaviour. They suggest, on the basis of presentation of a single signalling stimulus for shock, that the environmental cues present do not affect the experimental animal's responses. We suggest that present experimental knowledge does not adequately separate learned helplessness from conditioned emotional suppression.

We think conditioned emotional suppression and learned helplessness are probably related in that they lie at opposite ends of a continuum. Further, it would seem important for therapeutic reasons to be able to differentiate these models, since learned helplessness suggests shaping prodecure, whereas conditioned emotional suppression suggests primarily extinction of emotional responses. WOLPE (1971) regularly uses both shaping and desensitisation techniques when treating cases of neurotic depression. The above argument would tend to suggest that using both procedures may be unnecessary in some cases; thus, adequate assessment and selection of the most effective treatment procedure (whether shaping or desensitisation) might reduce both treatment and therapist time.

We have now built a fairly extensive model of depression, which gives coverage of both the emotional and operant aspects of depression. It can clearly be seen that some depressive histories may be quite complicated, and this again clearly stresses the need for detailed assessment procedures.

The most elaborate diagnostic methods are employed by PATTERSON and ROSENBERRY (1969) and LEWINSOHN et al. (1969). Following their initial assessment they carry out detailed objective observations on the patient in his natural environment. More recently, LEWINSOHN et al. (1971) have employed group interaction as a diagnostic (and therapeutic) tool. The behaviour of both patients and other persons in the environment is identified, coded and recorded in terms of frequency, duration and intensity. As well as establishing a diagnosis, these procedures establish baselines that are of value in assessing therapeutic progess. Obviously, in the routine clinical setting, such procedures are unrealistic. However, attempts to approach them will, as LAZARUS (1968) points out, prevent misclassification; this is especially important in cases of endogenous depression, which in the first instance requires physical methods of treatment. In a section on assessment KANFER and SASLOW (1965) suggest defining the target behaviour in terms of deficits and excesses, e.g. in depression, reduced motor behaviour is a deficit whereas high anxiety is an excess. This approach, which may be applied not only to the patient but also to his environment, implies basic treatment strategies. While behavioural excesses may be removed by extinction, behavioural deficits may be corrected by shaping techniques. Summaries of the models outlined and treatment strategies are provided in Figs. 1 and 2.

VI. Case Examples

Case 1: A 50-year-old woman presented 2 1/2 years after the death of her husband with a persistent grief reaction. She has 4 daughters and appears to be extremely dependent on them, as she was on her husband.

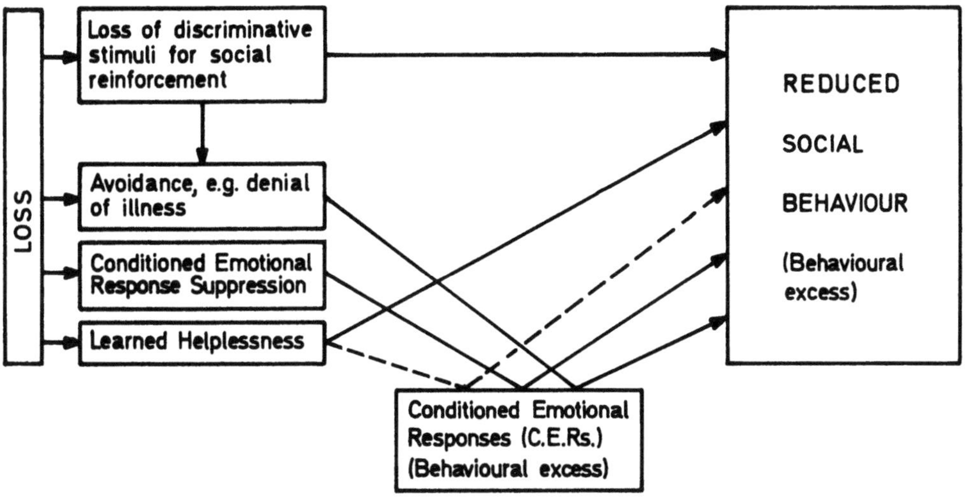

Fig. 1. Summary of the effects of loss. The arrows indicate the possible mechanisms of reduced social behaviour as seen in depression. The broken arrow from Learned Helplessness indicates doubt about the importance of emotional behaviour in relation to this particular model

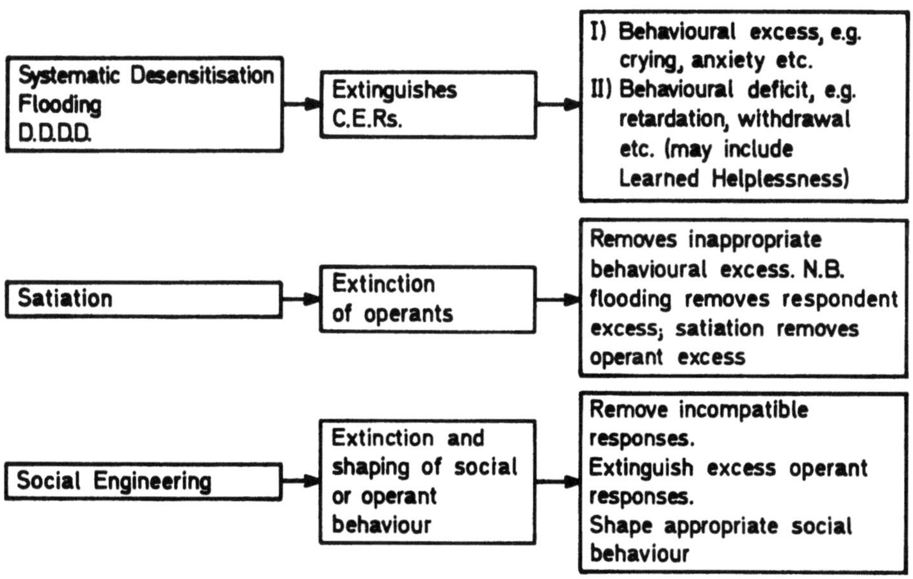

Fig. 2. Summary of treatments. C.E.Rs. = Conditioned Emotional Responses. D.D.D.D. = Declining Drug Dose Desensitisation. For further explanation, see text

Her children were tired of her persistent complaining and were often angry and hostile toward the patient. Afterwards they usually felt remorseful and consequently allowed the patient to talk at length about her depressive behaviour thus indirectly reinforcing such behaviour. (A potentially aversive situation has become a discriminative stimulus for positive reinforcement). The patient exhibited high levels of hostility and neuroticism on psychological testing. She is of low average intelligence. Following observation in the hospital setting, it was felt that much of her excessive grieving behaviour was attention-seeking, and thus was emitted (or operant) rather than elicited (or respondent). Consequently, a treatment strategy of satiation of grieving behaviour was planned. This was to be followed by appropriate reinforcement of adaptive behaviour by her daughters in the home setting. The satiation programme lasted 6 h per day for 3 weeks. During these sessions the patient talked to nurses about her grief, wrote essays and listened to herself on a tape recorder talking about her grief. A dramatic and sustained improvement followed after two weeks of treatment. The dramatic improvement occurred on an anniversary date. At present, 3 months after treatment, it has been found unnecessary to carry out the second half of the treatment procedure. The patient remains extremely well.

Comment: Some might argue that we used a flooding rather than a satiation technique. However, we suggest that this does not seem to be the case, since during the treatment the observable emotional components were minimal, even when the patient was talking about the potentially most painful topics. The patient was not having drugs at this time.

Case 2: A 26-year-old woman presented following an overdose 10 months after the sudden death of her husband. His death was preceded by the loss of some close in-laws three months previously. She had known her husband for 6 years prior to marriage and was apparently extremely dependent on him. Since her husband's death she had been depressed, tense and anxious. She was convinced that nothing could be done to help her and that further traumatic events were inevitable. In the hospital she was uncooperative and refused to let us interview her relatives. She also refused to complete her psychological assessment. A Declining Dose Drug Desensitisation treatment (McCORMICK and O'GORMAN, 1971)

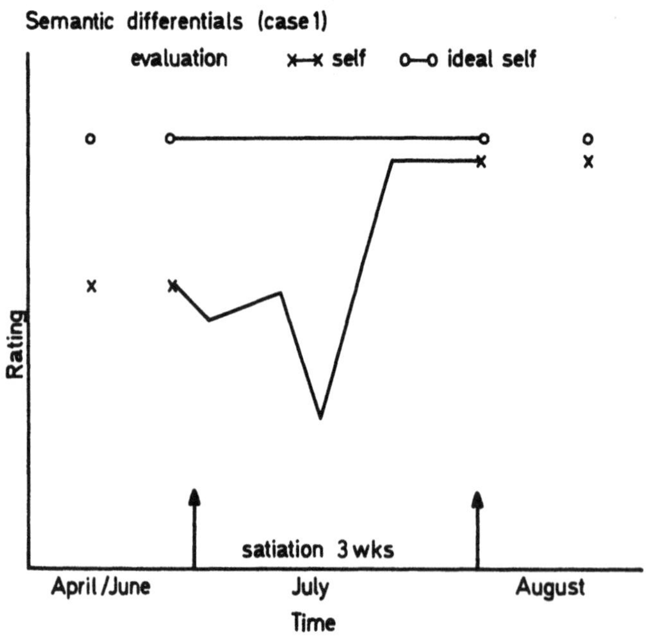

Fig. 3. This graph shows the marked changes which occurred in self-evaluation during the period of treatment

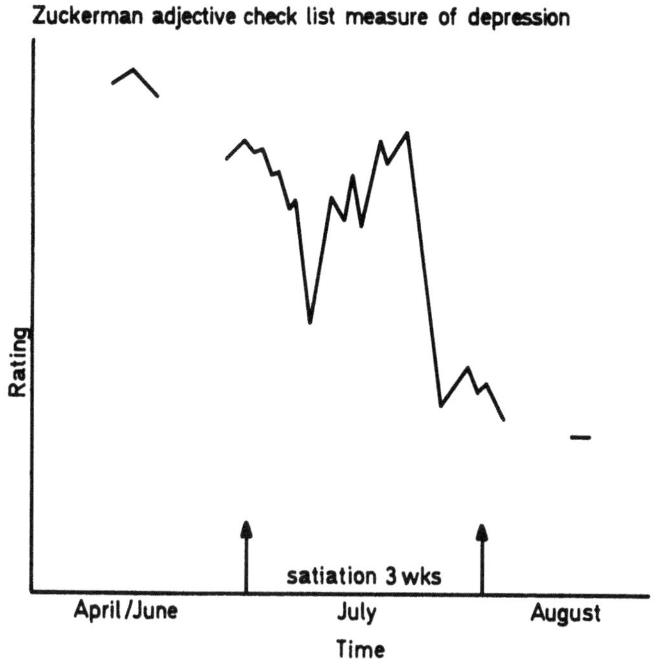

Fig. 4. This graph represents changes in depressive behaviour as recorded by means of Zuckerman adjective lists. This measure, which also rates general anxiety, yielded results for anxiety which were very similar to the ratings for depression

followed by shaping of new behaviour was planned. She refused to cooperate and several weeks later discharged herself. Since that time she has apparently improved spontaneously and is now working again.

Comment: The nature of the patient's behaviour fits the model 'learned helplessness', as illustrated by such remarks as: 'It's useless; there is nothing I can do to help myself'. Apart from the fact that the order of treatment strategies may have been wrong in their emphasis, it would appear that any attempt at treatment would have failed simply because the patient was completely non-cooperative.

Case 3: A 60-year-old man presented 4 months after the sudden death of his brother. He is single and of low intelligence. Psychological testing revealed high general hostility and high defensiveness. The history did not suggest that the relationship with his brother was in any way very close or conflictual. On admission he was reluctant to discuss the death, and he persistently denied feeling anxious or depressed. Objectively he frequently wept, and always appeared tense and anxious. He was regarded as a considerable suicide risk. A Declining Dose Drug Desensitisation was attempted. Fourteen 2-h sessions, in which he was prompted to discuss the death, were carried out over 2 weeks. He showed no clinical improvement. At this stage he was assessed indepentently and E.C.T. was recommended. Nine E.C.Ts. were applied without any success. Memory disturbance was marked following E.C.T.. Assessment for brain damage was carried out 3 months later and the results suggested possible organic impairment. At the time of reporting he has made little improvement.

Comment: This case illustrates the difficulty of making a full behavioural formulation in cases which are marked by avoidance behaviour such as denial of illness. Further, it would appear in this case that avoidance behaviour was a fairly standard way of responding, even outside illness. It may be important in such cases to strengthen the avoidance behaviour rather than remove it, since it is such a well-established coping mechanism.

References

BECK, A.T.: Depression: Clinical Experimental and Theoretical Aspects, p. 275-276. New York: Harper and Row 1962.

CHURCH, R.M.: Response suppression. In: CAMPBELL, B.A., CHURCH, R.M. (Eds.): Punishment and Aversive Control. New York: Appleton Century Crofts 1969.

DENGROVE, E.: Treatment of non-phobic disorders by the behaviour therapies. Lecture to the Association for Advancement of the Behaviour Therapies. New York 1966.

ESTES, W.K., SKINNER, B.F.: Some quantitative properties of anxiety (Estes-Skinner Effect). J. e. Psychol. 29, 390-400 (1941).

FERSTER, C.B.: Classification of behavioural pathologies. In: Research in Behaviour Modification (KRASNER, L., ULLMAN, L.P., Eds.). New York: Holt, Rinehart, and Winston 1965.

KRIETMAN, N., COLLINS, J., NELSON, B., TROOP, J.: Time sharing and social activity. Brit. J. Psychiat. 117, 47 (1970).

KANFER, F., SASLOW, G.: Behavioural analysis. Arch. gen. Psychiat. 12, 529-538 (1965).

LAZARUS, A.A.: Learning theory and the treatment of depression. Behav. Res. Ther. 6, 83-89 (1968).

LEWINSOHN, P.M., WEINSTEIN, M.S., SHAW, D.A.: Depression: A clinical research approach. In: RUBIN, R., FRANKS, C. (Eds.): Advances in Behavior Therapy. New York: Academic Press 1969.

LEWINSOHN, P.M., WEINSTEIN, M.S., ALPER, T.: A behavioural approach to the group treatment of depressed persons: A methodological contribution. J. clin. Psychol. 26, 525-532 (1970).

LIBERMAN, R.P., RASKIN, D.E.: Depression: A behavioural formulation. Arch. gen. Psychiat. 24, 515-523 (1971).

MADDISON, D., WALKER, W.L.: Factors affecting the outcome of conjugal bereavement. Brit. J. Psychiat. 113, 1057-67 (1967).

MAIER, S.F., SELIGMAN, M.E.P., SOLOMON, R.L.: Pavlovian fear, conditioning and learned helplessness. In: CAMPBELL, B.A., CHURCH, R.M. (Eds.): Punishment and Aversive Behaviour. New York: Appleton Century Crofts 1969.

McCORMICK, W.O., O'GORMAN, E.O.: Declining Dose Drug Desensitisation. Proceedings of the Behavioural Engineering Conference 1971.

PATTERSON, G.R., ROSENBERRY, C.: A social learning formulation of depression. Paper presented at the International Conference on Behaviour Modification, Banff/Alberta 1969.

RAMSEY, R.: Behaviour Therapy and Grief. Proceedings of the Second European Conference on Behaviour Therapy, Wexford/Ireland 1972.

WOLPE, J.: Neurotic depression: experimental analog, clinical syndromes, and treatment. Amer. J. Psychother. 25, 362-8 (1971).

III. Behaviour Treatment of Sexual Dysfunction

The Masters and Johnson Approach to Marital Sexual Problems in a National Health Service Setting

J. BANCROFT

Masters and Johnson's results in the treatment of marital sexual problems are generally superior to those of other workers. The contribution they have made in this area is enormous; however, there are a number of questions that arise from their work.

(1) Can their technique be shown to be superior to others in a properly controlled comparative study? (2) What are the essential components of their complex multifaceted method, and (3) Can it be modified to make it feasible in a National Health Service setting?

In this paper I will describe a modification of their technique which is practicable in a National Health Service setting, briefly reporting the results observed with the first 10 married couples treated. This represents the preparatory stage of a controlled study which is due to begin shortly. I will first indicate the basic Masters and Johnson principles that have been incorporated in this method, give clinical details of the 10 couples and their response to treatment, and finally describe the treatment procedure in more detail, illustrating with examples from the 10 cases.

The basic Masters and Johnson principles which have been used are:

a) Treat the couple, not the individual;
b) Identify and aim to modify relevant sexual attitudes;
c) Give authoritative direction for sexual behaviour
   1. in a non-specific way, establishing so-called "sensate focus";
   2. in specific ways, according to the type of sexual difficulty encountered.

There is a further basic Masters and Johnson principle which is not listed here. This is the use of a male and female therapist team. A female co-therapist was involved, in part only, in 4 of the 10 cases, but her involvement came to an end when she left the area. It is, of course, more difficult to provide two therapists than one, and it is of some importance to know to what extent the success of this approach depends on having two therapists. The technique evolved has for the most part been used by one therapist only.

Clinical details of the 10 couples are given in Table 1. The follow-up varied from 1 year to 2 months. Of the 4 unsuccessful cases, one (Rat.) should have responded according to most criteria, but the husband withdrew from treatment when things seemed to be going well. Another couple (C) presented a long-standing marital problem of which the sexual relationship was only part. Their first 8 sessions were associated with a considerable improvement in their general relationship as well as the virtual disappearance of the wife's long-standing agoraphobic problem. However, they were reluctant to come to grips with the sexual relationship for fear that it would spoil their new-found happiness. They withdrew from treatment when I started to put pressure on them.

The other two failures were problems of long standing. In both cases considerable progress was made but non-sexual factors operating in the relationship served to prevent the outcome from being successful. It is because the early stages were so encouraging that treatment in each case was so prolonged. In the 'improved' couple (S) - the first couple treated - the Masters and Johnson principles were not properly applied until 7 sessions had gone by. In these early stages a hierarchic approach to ejaculating in the presence of the female partner was used. The man was asked to masturbate in gradually closer proximity to his wife. This was successful in his case but produced a negative reaction in his wife. From that point the approach was changed and thereafter they both made satisfactory progress. Treatment was cut short, however, when the husband changed his job and left the country. This case underlines the importance of treating the couple rather than the individual.

The procedure I have used is as follows:

1st and 2nd Sessions

a) Each partner seen separately for history-taking
b) Couple seen jointly (5-10 minutes); instructions for:
   1. "Sensate focus"
   2. Ban on intercourse

3rd Session onwards - couple seen jointly.

In each session:

a) Discuss attainment of behavioural goals set previous session
b) Explore relevant attitudes
c) Attempt modification of relevant attitudes
d) Facilitate communication between couple during session
e) Set new behavioural goals.

Taking the history individually from each partner emphasises the dyadic nature of the problem; it also provides the therapist with the basis of an understanding of the aetiology and relevant attitudes involved. However, the initial history is only of limited value in this respect, which is why there is so much emphasis on identifying attitudes in the subsequent treatment sessions. Occasionally the initial history can be misleading. This was illustrated in Couple J. Here they colluded in their initial accounts in order to place the blame clearly on the husband. It became clear later in treatment that the initial failure to consumate the marriage on the honeymoon was due as much to vaginismus in the wife as to erectile impotence in the husband.

The various types of behavioural goals can be categorised as follows:

Hierarchic approach used throughout

a) "Sensate Focus" plus good communication (verbal and non-verbal)
b) Specific Techniques
   1. "Diversionary" approach (continuation of sensate focus) for erectile impotence and orgasmic dysfunction
   2. "Conditioning" approach (Squeeze technique) for premature ejaculation
   3. "Deconditioning" approach (graded delators) for vaginismus
   4. "Unblocking" approach (superstimulation) for ejaculatory incompetence.

The initial ban on sexual intercourse, which is given at the first session with the couple together, frequently induces a striking sense of relief in the couple, who report that their relationship with one another has been more relaxed than for some considerable time and that the early attempts at sensate focus have been rewarding in a way which is either novel for them or reminds them of their experiences before they were married. In this sensate focus stage, emphasis is placed on giving pleasure to one's partner rather than receiving it. This approach underlines the essence of this part of the treatment, which is commmunication. One must communicate either verbally or non-verbally to find out what is enjoyable for one's partner. Frequently the quality of communication in the marriage becomes very clear at this early stage. Resentment linked to the sexual relationship will also become obvious and will need to be resolved before significant progress with this stage is made; as often as not, resolution depends on being able to communicate feelings of hostility.

Initially the couple is instructed to avoid contact with genitalia in this 'giving of pleasure' to each other. When they are able to relax and enjoy this degree of contact they are permitted to involve the genitalia also, although they are encouraged to continue with the more general body contact. Also at this stage, agreement is reached with the couple as to a reasonable frequency for physical contact to occur.

In dealing with this 'specific' stage, I use the term 'diversionary' to emphasise the key principle of treatment when tackling problems of erection in the male or orgasm in the female. This approach is in fact a continuation of the sensate focus stage in which it is emphasized that erections and orgasms are spontaneous responses which do not require special attention and which will occur of their own accord provided the situation is right. Treatment therefore aims at diverting the couple's attention away from those specific physiological responses, and towards the giving and receiving of sensual pleasure, thus freeing them from the previously inhibiting goals of orgasm or erection. In the case of erectile impotence, the therapist asks no questions about erection. When the couple reports that erections are occurring, however, the therapist responds calmly as though this were an inevitable occurrence, given time. At this stage some attention to erection is encouraged in order that the couple can experience the waxing and waning of erection. This is to counter the fear that as soon as erection occurs it will be lost if it is not used promptly.

I have used the term 'conditioning' to describe Masters and Johnson's squeeze technique for premature ejaculation because it does appear to be the closest thing to a straightforward learning procedure in their approach. However, I do not intend to say much about this because the only case in this series of 10 in which premature ejaculation was a problem, was the couple (Rat.) who dropped out after 8 sessions before we reached this part of the treatment.

I have used the term 'deconditioning' to describe the use of graded dilators in treating vaginismus. The severe case of vaginismus of 11 years' duration that I have reported here (I) gives a history which is very suggestive of a conditioned response. Whatever the factors which caused vaginismus in the first place, and there were several fairly obvious ones in this girl, the pain caused as a result of the spasm and the repeated attempts for the next 11 years to overcome the spasm would be sufficient to account for this self-perpetuating problem, although her response to treatment indicated that there were important personality factors contributing also. In addition, this technique clearly involves a hierarchic approach, firstly with the change from dilating finger to increasing sizes of glass dilators, and secondly in the changing from dilation by the doctor, who will be considered either safe or proper, to the husband who will have been considered either potentially dangerous or wrong.

The 'unblocking' approach for ejaculatory incompetence is something which is quite different again from any of the three previous approaches. The intense stimulation of the penis which is encouraged with the aid of lubricating jelly is appropriate physiologically for these males who appear to need far more intense stimulation than the average man. In addition, when ejaculation finally occurs, this has the quality of a key experience leading to a dramatic reduction in inhibition. Thereafter the level of stimulation required appears to be very much less. Hence the analogy of relieving an obstruction.

The setting of these appropriate behavioural goals in relatively small hierarchic stages serves an additional important function. In each session difficulties in achieving the set goals are discussed and this frequently highlights crucial attitudes which will themselves require modification if treatment is to be fully effective. For this purpose the couple's attempts to reach the behavioural goals must be questioned in uncompromising detail.

The following are examples of attitudes revealed in this way:

a) Episodes involving physical contact may be infrequent and fall short of the agreed frequency. Close questioning reveals that one or both partners not only regard sex as something that only happens immediately before going to sleep but also that they have, probably as a result of the sexual problem, made a permanent habit of staying up late watching television or working irregular hours. It is emphasised that time must be allocated for this particular purpose. Infrequent sexual contact between sessions may also reveal a passive attitude to therapy which assumes that all that has to be done is to attend the treatment session, the therapist being responsible for the rest. It is emphasised that the bulk of the work for success must be done at home; the visits to the therapist are primarily briefing sessions.
Paucity of such contact may also reveal a tendency of one partner (particularly the male) to cope with interpersonal difficulties by opting out or withdrawing. In 3 of the couples the attitude was very much in evidence.

b) Questioning may reveal that the early stages in the hierarchy of sexual contact produce a negative response in one or other partner in spite of the ban on sexual intercourse. In one case in which the wife reacted this way, this was because the husband was too timid and not assertive enough in his approach. Further questioning revealed that there was a considerable descrepancy between the wife's fantasy of the ideal lover, who would dominate and take her sexually, and her real-life husband. Such descrepancies between ideals and reality are often important.

c) Reluctance to initiate activity by the wife may reveal the attitude that the woman should be passive and not demonstrate too much in the way of sexual feelings.

d) Lack of progress in the sensate focus stage may reveal communication problems of either a straightforward kind or stemming from an inability to express resentment satisfactorily. One wife was against speaking during loveplay because it seemed "too cold-blooded". In another couple no progress was made until they were helped to have rows.

Stages in the hierarchy close to vaginal entry may reveal the fear that once the sequence goes beyond a certain point the woman will have no control over the situation. In such a case further progress is organised to ensure that she does have control.

The use of a lubricating jelly may reveal a fastidiousness in either the man or the woman which results in either vaginal secretion or ejaculation considered as unpleasant. Masters and Johnson in fact found the couple's response to lubricating jelly a very useful prognostic indicator of outcome.

Such key attitudes will become clear if the therapist steadfastly pursues those goals and asks for accounts in sufficient detail. There is no place for the embarrassed evasion of tricky topics.

Recognition of key attitudes such as these may, however, be easier than their modification. The following are some examples of ways in which one may attempt to modify them. The 'confessional' function of helping an individual to reveal feelings or behaviour which for many years had been guiltily hidden and to which the therapist reacts with calm reassurance, can be effective. In one case (Rai.) the wife was eventually able to reveal that she had been masturbating since the age of 6 whenever anything bad or frightening had occurred. She had come to associate sexual arousal with bad things. This habit was placed into a reasonable perspective by some rational and uncritical discussion.

Simply encouraging the couple to talk about previously taboo topics will tend to counteract inhibited attitudes.

Inertia in one or both partners can be countered by the threat to terminate treatment or the statement that if no further progress is made the couple will have to seriously consider the alternatives open to them, one of which would be separation. It is important in such cases for the therapist to avoid accepting responsibility for the apparent or impending failure of treatment.

On the other hand, too unrealistic expectations may also be a problem, progress being limited by the feeling that things were not happening quickly enough. In such cases a timetable of progress which has anxiety-reducing effects can be agreed upon with the couple. In one pair with ejaculatory incompetence (M) it was agreed that no ejaculation would be expected for at least 6 months. In fact it occurred two weeks later.

By patient debate the intelligent spouse may be persuaded of the relevance of an attitude to the sexual problem which previously had been denied. In the same couple with ejaculatory incompetence the husband valued his attitude that it was 'wrong to wear one's heart on one's sleeve'. This same reluctance to show too much emotion to others seemed relevant to the sexual situation. His eventual acceptance of this relevance preceded the 'breakthrough' in treatment.

In all of these approaches the therapist must guard against appearing to side with one partner against the other.

Treatment sessions last from 40 to 60 minutes during which on average one third to one half is spent on behavioural goals, the rest on relevant attitudes. Initially, I started on a weekly basis, and in most cases it is probably advisable to continue with at least this frequency. In some cases, however, it becomes clear that the rate of change is going to be relatively slow, and then 2 or even 3 weekly appointments may be appropriate; 15 sessions seem a reasonable course of treatment for the majority, - comparing well with the 14 successive days of the Masters and Johnson course.

My initial impression, therefore, is that not only can this treatment be modified to fit into a National Health Service and be given by one therapist but it is likely to be effective in a reasonable proportion of cases.

Research is now needed (1) to establish that such an approach is superior to other behavioural techniques such as systematic desensitization, and (2) to clarify the crucial components of this method as well as useful prognostic criteria.

How important is it to involve both partners, how necessary is it to have two therapists? Is the 'sensate focus' stage unnecessary? Can one simply concentrate on behavioural goals and let attitudes take care of themselves?

Hopefully we will be able to answer some of these questions at a later conference.

Table 1. Clinical details of the ten couples under treatment

Couple	Age M F	Presenting Problem	Problems in Spouse	Duration	1° or 2°	Previous Treatment	No. of Sessions	Outcome
Ry.	28 27	M Erect. Imp.	F Vaginismus	5 yrs	1°	++	12	Successful
J.	35 29	M Erect. Imp.	F + Vaginismus	9 yrs	1°	++	32	Failed
Rat.	34 32	M Erect. Imp. Prem. Ejac.	-	3 yrs	2°	-	8	Failed
E.	46 45	M Erect. Imp. Ejac. Inad.	F + Attitude	3 yrs	2°	-	15	Successful
Rai.	41 34	M Erect. Imp.	F + Attitude	6 yrs	1°	-	13	Successful
C.	40 39	M Erect. Imp.	F + Attitude	5 yrs	2°	-	9	Uncertain
S.	28 30	M Ejac. Inad.	F + Attitude	3 yrs	1°	-	14	Improved
M.	39 30	M Ejac. Inad.	F $\pm$	1 1/2 yrs	1°	-	12	Successful
N.	25 25	F "Frigidity"	-	1 1/2 yrs	2°	-	12	Successful
I.	28 27	F Vaginismus	-	11 yrs (5)	1°	++	22	Failed

The Relevance of the Masters and Johnson Methodology to the Treatment of Sexual Disorders in an Outpatient Clinic

P.T. BROWN and A. KOLASZYNSKA-CARR

During the past 9 months, first by accident and more recently by design, we have been accumulating couples whose presenting problems appear to be amenable to a therapeutic attack within the Masters and Johnsons framework for dealing with human sexual dysfunction (MASTERS and JOHNSON, 1970). We wish to report briefly upon 10 of these couples. During the course of our work with them we have had to alter some of Masters and Johnson's treatment proposals to fit the circumstances of outpatient services in the N.H.S. Without wishing to overgeneralise at this stage, we can begin to draw some tentative conclusions about the management of this type of disorder, which we hope to verify or reject as time goes on. At this early stage we would like to state our experience and views to provide a basis for discussion among people who are feeling their way in the same clinical area.

The group consists of 10 couples in the age range of 21 to 35 years (mean age 25.9 for the women, 27.5 for the men). The duration of disorder varies from 6 months to 15 years, with an average of 4.3 years. The dysfunction has been present throughout the marriage in all but two of the pairs. Eight of the 10 pairs have been seen within the last 6 months. The sources of referral have been: general practitioners - 4, Marriage Guidance Council - 3, psychiatrists - 3.

Five of the pairs presented with primary male dysfunction and five with female dysfunction. Among the men, there were 2 cases of premature ejaculation, one of secondary impotence, and 2 of low sexual tension; among the women, there was one case of vaginismus and 4 showing various forms of orgasmic inadequacy (one coital, one situational, and two random). Three of the men were from professional backgrounds, five were semi-skilled operatives and clerks, one was a farmer and one was a bus driver. Occupationally, the group was therefore fairly mixed, unlike the Masters and Johnson group which was overweighted from the professions.

In the treatment of the 10 couples the senior author was involved with 5 different co-therapists, of whom 3 were clinical psychologists in the process of qualifying, one a marriage guidance counsellor, and one a student social worker. Three of the couples have had a change of female co-therapist during the period of treatment involvement. We return to a discussion of this.

The essential difference between an N.H.S. outpatient setting and the highly specialised situation which Masters and Johnson describe appears to us to be in a) the amount of time available and b) the relatively clinical and impersonal nature of outpatient facilities. The British National Health outpatient system is characterized by good clinical care despite overstretched staff resources and often crowded physical conditions. In contrast, Masters and Johnson describe a honeymoon hotel where for two intensive weeks nothing is more important than the sexual development of the presenting couple, which the whole atmosphere is designed to facilitate. With regard to the nature of N.H.S. outpatient facilities, we think that the personal quality of the encounter with the co-therapists can overcome all but the most depersonalising conditions. Some sessions we have conducted have been in competition with the vocal distress of cows during a market afternoon, and we think to no detriment!

The problem of time, however, carries more implications and is more serious than the physical amenities of the treatment setting; it involves consideration of both therapist and patient time commitments. We have incorporated couples presenting with sexual dysfunction into the routine work of busy clinical lives, in marked contrast to Masters and Johnson who concentrate upon sexual dysfunction to the exclusion of any other clinical interest. Our typical procedure on the first occasion is to meet the presenting couple together. We quickly adopt Christian name terms between therapists and couples, and between therapists, though we have not yet had a couple breaking the professional barriers spontaneously. The first meeting lasts about 30 minutes and is designed to be reassuring and encouraging. We deliberately express a great deal of optimistic interest in the presenting disorder. More importantly, the aim is to disabuse the presenting couple of any idea that they are patients. The negative returns from continued attempts at intercourse are discussed, and the session ends with an injunction to refrain from intercourse. The couple leaves the first session understanding that they will attend for 3 further sessions before a firm commitment to any achievement is undertaken on either side. The 3 sessions comprise two of co-therapy enquiry and a concluding round-table discussion.

The question of disabusing the presenting couples of the idea that they are patients deserves further exploration. The whole paraphenalia of the primacy of G.P. referral and the general atmosphere of an outpatient clinic combine to encourage the presenting couple into a belief that they have an illness, for which the cure may be difficult but is in principle likely to be similar to the other cures a dispensing N.H.S. encourages passive recipients to take. We have found it very helpful to use Bannister's idea of persuading a couple in a treatment setting where their development as individuals is involved to conceive of themselves as in a research-student relationship, where the supervisor (the therapist) has a certain amount of knowledge and experience of similar problems which he conveys over time to the research students (couple) who gradually become more expert in the area of research (personal development) than the supervisor. We find that couples respond very readily to such a concept, and the use of Christian names encourages the breakdown of illness-orientated expectations.

At the next two appointments, the couple are seen individually, first by the therapist of the same sex and then by the therapist of the opposite sex. The couple may or may not be seen by the therapist pair during the same session on their further attendances, but are enjoined not to discuss the content of co-therapy interviews with each other during this period, which typically lasts 3 weeks. In the allocation of time to these co-therapy interviews we wonder whether the extremely detailed type of personal history enquiry which Masters and Johnson advocate is entirely necessary. We normally find that an hour's interviewing time for each occasion of meeting is adequate, and this in itself is so much more than people with previous outpatient experience expect that it serves to emphasize the non-patient aspect of the couple's involvement.

The time commitment of the couple themselves is perhaps the most important aspect of management in the outpatient context. Attending a hospital has the advantage that individuals can be released from work fairly easily without too many questions being asked. We try to capitalise on this to keep co-therapy appointments within the confines of the normal clinical day. However, the fact that the couple continue to go to work and (in marked contrast to the procedure adopted by Masters and Johnson) live at home has extensive ramifications for what we call the commitment of personal time, and we shall return to a consideration of this shortly.

The two individual interviews, round-table discussion and the keeping of appointments created considerable problems in managing avoidance of intercourse and development of the sensate focus stage. It is in this stage that the problem of the couple's commitment of personal time becomes most apparent.

We have observed that, even where there is no relationship disturbance, couples presenting with sexual dysfunction have typically organised their lives in such a manner that the opportunity for sexual encounter arises very little. This may be exacerbated by the exigencies of shift working. Taking the intermittencies of menstruation into account and a 3-week day/night shift system, one couple had opportunity for sexual encounters for one week in a 6-week cycle. The period of the sensate focus involves for us above all a readjustment of the individual's time commitment to the partner. We feel that couples who simply do not set time aside will not respond, and it is probable that in the early stages of treatment any observed unwillingness to set aside adequate time portends an unsuccessful outcome.

The sensate focus period may be extended over several weeks. In ideal circumstances we see it as lasting for not more than a month. But accident, family illness, and the hazards of keeping regular outpatient appointments while maintaining home and job may combine to extend this period up to 10 weeks in our experience. Perhaps such an extension might only be tolerated in a couple with low sexual tension, while for other couples it would carry more serious implications. We do, however, think it important to recognise real-life difficulties which may prevent adequate concentration upon the sensate focus development, and to design the flow of treatment with these difficulties in mind rather than to insist upon the finer details of early physical involvement when emotional energies are necessarily in use elsewhere.

It is possible that the extension of the sensate focus period, and indeed the initial enquiry period, may allow one to form gradual judgements about the strength of the relationship of the presenting couple that will be more accurate than a rapid approach permits. It is also possible that a time-extended procedure will permit a couple with relationship difficulties to involve themselves in co-therapy procedures, whereas in a more intensive setting they might be unable to do so.

We have not yet observed the effect of time extension sufficiently to comment on this in detail. We have, however, deliberately untertaken to see 2 couples who presented primarily with a disturbance of their relationship rather than sexual dysfunction, though the disturbance of the relationship had destructive implications for their sexual relationship. We wished to see whether it would be possible to improve the qualitiy of the personal relationship by attacking it from the point of view of the development of the couple's physical trust for each other within a sensate focus framework. Of the 2 couples we have seen in this framework, one has been manifestly unsuccessful, the other obviously successful. Hence, a vulnerable relationship might be strengthened if approached gradually within a co-therapy format.

We noted early that in seeing the 10 couples we chose to make up this group, 5 female co-therapists participated, and 3 couples experienced a change of female co-therapist during their treatment involvement. We doubt whether Masters and Johnson would approve of changing one of the therapists during the course of the treatment procedure, and we ourselves would not approve of changing both. However, insofar as the interaction between the co-therapists acts as a model for the marital pair, we see no reason why their observation of one co-therapist in relationship with more than one other co-therapist should not also be beneficial.

What of the extent of involvement of the co-therapists with each other? Masters and Johnson imply that co-therapy is a way of life and that an intimate understanding of each co-therapist's sexual value system by the consenting co-therapist partner is a desideratum of successful marital co-therapy. If this is the case, then marital co-therapists will have to develop a unique range of professional commitments. Our experience is that a reasonable degree of mutual professional and social respect is sufficient to enable co-therapists to work effectively in this area without adverse effects upon the co-therapy experience. Insofar as the outpatient procedure we outlined is less intense than that which Masters and Johnson have developed, so the relationship between the co-therapists and the marital pair is similarly less charged. It would nevertheless be extremely difficult to engage in co-therapy encounters with a co-therapist from whom one felt socially or personally estranged.

We have said nothing so far about the outcome of treatment. Of this group of 10, 3 couples have been unsuccessful in overcoming their difficulties while 5 of the remaining 7 have been successful and the other two look set fair. The 3 unsuccessful cases all have in common a wife who had experienced a successful extra-marital relationship, and also an impoverished or strongly negative personal relationship with the husband. While we have seen one or the other of these characteristics in successful couples, we have not seen a combination.

BANCROFT (1972) observed that Masters and Johnson's co-therapy treatment programme is essentially a pragmatic procedure, and is none the worse for that. We would entirely agree. It is, however, worth considering the possibility that some of the more formal aspects of behaviour modification might usefully be incorporated. The principles of the reduction of anxiety and desensitization have clear implications for, say, the modification of secondary impotence or the improvement of vaginismus. We would not wish, however, to see a learning-theory "takeover" of Masters and Johnson. Its pragmatism is appealing.

The small sample that we have presented here is of a middle to lower-middle working class cultural background. It is a group, which without N.H.S. outpatient facilities, could probably not avail itself of treatment procedures in this area, and we ourselves feel that, given a sensitive awareness of the value and limitations of the co-therapy format approach to the treatment of sexual dysfunction, it is transferable in style, if not entirety, to an N.H.S. outpatient setting.

References

BANCROFT, J.: Paper presented to a meeting of the Behaviour Therapy Association, London 17th April 1972.

MASTERS, W.H., JOHNSON, VIRGINIA E.: Human Sexual Inadequacy. London: Churchill 1970.

Treatment of Frigidity by Group Desensitization[+]

E. O'GORMAN, H. McALLISTER, J.T. QUINN, P.J. GRAHAM and J.J.M. HARBISON

Systematic desensitization is a widely used treatment for sexual frigidity (LAZARUS, 1963; FAULK, 1970). LAZARUS (1961) reported the successful use of group desensitization in the treatment of phobic patients, and in 1968 he described a small group of frigid patients treated by group desensitization, 3 out of 4 patients being much improved by the treatment. STONE and LEVINE (1950) advocated group discussion of sexual problems as a psychotherapeutic technique in cases of sexual difficulties. The present study reports the use of group desensitization combined with limited group discussion of sexual problems in the treatment of frigid patients.

The 15 female patients were aged between 18 and 40 years, had been married for at least one year, and complained of sexual difficulty not related to any physical cause or associated with a sexual deviation. Symptoms included loss or absence of a desire for sex, dyspareunia and non-consummation. Their spouses were also seen.

I. Treatment Method

The 15 patients included in the study were divided into 3 groups; spouses were also allocated to 3 corresponding groups. The patient groups met twice a week for one hour for 20 sessions. In the early sessions patients were taught and then practised deep muscular relaxation; in the first part of later sessions they were treated by systematic desensitization to a standard hierarchy of sexual behaviour. The hierarchy was constructed on the basis of individual interviews with patients and their spouses and then agreed to by the group. The second part of all sessions was used for group discussion of sexual information and in the early stage for agreeing upon the joint hierarchy.

At the beginning and end of treatment the patients completed the Sexual Interest Questionnaire, SIN (HARBISON et al., 1973).

The spouses met for one hour a week while their wives were in treatment. The purpose of these meetings was mainly educative. They were conducted in a directive manner and the topics discussed were related to the sexual problems in the marriages and how these problems affected the husbands. As treatment progressed, the husbands were encouraged

[+] This research was supported by the Northern Ireland Hospitals Authority and the Medical Research Council. Four of us (J.J.M. H., P.J. G., J.T. Q. and H. McA.) constitute a research team; no seniority of authorship is implied by the order of names on this paper.

to discuss the progress of the wife's treatment and the planning of graded real-life sexual behaviour. Simple advice was given to encourage the husband to reinforce the wife's progress in real-life sexual behaviour.

II. Results

Fifteen patients started the treatment. 4 did not finish it. Of these, one did not really start and 3 failed to complete the course: one patient lapsed because she was involved in a car accident, another because of the distance she had to travel to the treatment centre, and the third because she was pregnant. The other patient terminated treatment at the end of the first session without giving any reason. Of the 14 patients who finished or spent a reasonable time in the programme, 7 rated the outcome as excellent or very good, 2 as good and 5 as fair or poor.

Twelve of these patients completed the Sexual Interest Questionnaire (the questionnaire had not been developed at the beginning of this study). Seven of these 12 rated the results of treatment as very good or excellent and 5 as fair or poor. Table 1 shows the results of the sexual interest scores before and after therapy from patients who rated improved outcome as excellent, very good, or good, and from those claiming little benefit from treatment, who rated outcome as fair or poor.

Table 1. Total SIN scores for improved and unimproved frigid patients

	Before Treatment	After Treatment
Control Females	150	150
Improved (n = 7)	69	127
Unimproved (n = 5)	64	60

Table 1 also shows the scores obtained on this test by normal females. Prior to treatment all patients had scores within the frigid range; those who rated themselves as improved scored a substantial rise in sexual interest, while those who rated the treatment as only fair or poor showed no increase (the difference between the pre- and post-treatment scores in the successful group is significant at the $p = 0.05$ level). It is interesting that while there was a substantial rise in sexual interest in the successful group, it is still well below that found in normal females. The results of the preliminary study reported here suggest that group desensitization is a promising treatment in frigidity.

III. Discussion

A number of points about the programme appear worthy of comment. The inclusion of desensitization in a group setting, group discussion of sexual problems, and the participation of husbands in a group makes treatment rather complex. The inclusion of the spouse in a group desensitization programme is not reported elsewhere. However, the incorporation of the spouse in the treatment of sexual disorders has been discussed by other workers, e.g. MADSEN and ULLMAN (1967) and MASTERS and JOHNSON (1970) involve husbands in treatment procedures.

An interesting part of the present study is the use of the new sexual interest questionnaire; the scores agreed well with the rated outcome of the treatment. The advantage of a quantified measure of sexual interest is illustrated by the fact that, while sexual interest scores increased in those patients who improved they can still be differentiated from those of a normal group of women.

It is clearly more efficient to treat patients in groups rather than individually. The results obtained do not suggest that there has been any important loss of efficiency with the group desensitization method. The results of the study appear to compare favourably with those of BRADY (1967) and COOPER (1970), who both use individual desensitization.

In the procedure reported above relatively small groups were treated. There appears to be no reason why the group should not be increased to 8 or 10, thereby increasing the efficiency of the treatment programme still further.

References

BRADY, J.P.: Brevital-relaxation treatment of frigidity. Behav. Res. Ther. 4, 71-77 (1966).

COOPER, A.J.: Frigidity, treatment and short-term prognosis. J. Psychosom. Res. 14, 133-147 (1970).

FAULK, M.: Factors in the treatment of frigidity. Brit. J. Psychiat. 119, 53-56 (1971).

HARBISON, J.J.M. et al.: A questionnaire measure of sexual interest. Arch. Sex. Behav. in press (1973).

LAZARUS, A.A.: Treatment of frigidity by systematic desensitization. J. Nerv. Ment. Dis. 136, 272-278 (1961).

LAZARUS, A.A.: Group therapy of phobic disorders by systematic desensitization. J. abnorm. soc. Psychol. 63, 505-510 (1963).

LAZARUS, A.A.: Behavior therapy and marriage counseling. J. Amer. Soc. Psychosom. Dent. Med. 15, 49-56 (1968).

MADSEN, G.H., ULLMANN, L.P.: Innovations in the desensitization of frigidity. Behav. Res. Ther. 5, 67-68 (1967).

MASTERS, W.H., JOHNSON, V.E.: Human Sexual Inadequacy. London: Churchill 1970.

STONE, A., LEVINE, L.: Group therapy in sexual maladjustment. In. J. Psychiat. 104, 195-202 (1950).

Aversion Therapy with Sexual Deviants

J.B. ASHCROFT and D. EAVES

I. Introduction

From 1965 onwards, FELDMAN and MacCULLOCH et al. produced a series of papers based on the use of anticipatory avoidance in the treatment of homosexuality. These authors reviewed the experimental evidence on anticipatory avoidance learning with the aim of defining a treatment procedure that would take full account of the variables that have been found effective in increasing resistance to the extinction of a conditioned response. Their original procedure may be briefly described as follows. The sexually deviant patient (for this purpose, a homosexual) is instructed to look at a male picture that is presented to him, for as long as he finds it attractive. If, after 8 sec, he has not rejected this picture by pressing the switch provided, he receives an electric shock. He can avoid this shock if he rejects the slide within the 8-sec. period. However, a schedule of reinforcement is used, i.e. not all his attempts at avoidance are successful. One third of the trials allow the subject to avoid immediately (IA), one third allow avoidance after a variable amount of delay (DA), and the remaining one third are unsuccessful, i.e. the patient receives a shock. On a number of random occasions a female slide is presented for 10 sec., unaccompanied by shock, and the patient can press a switch to have the slide returned. In 1967 they reported that 58 % of patients who had completed treatment and had been followed up for a minimum of a year were sufficiently improved for treatment to be considered successful. Moreover, they presented evidence to show that particular patterns of avoidance responding have a high value as predictors of outcome. They showed that very variable response latencies, together with a high proportion of trials on which subjects failed to avoid at all, usually predicted failure.

It has been argued that the FELDMAN-MacCULLOCH procedure may owe its success partly to the use of a treatment paradigm that includes avoidance rather than punishment, or a classic paradigm. Elsewhere, it has been argued that avoidance responses, i.e. key presses in the FELDMAN-MacCULLOCH treatment programme, have only a tenuous relationship to sexual approach or avoidance responses and that the changes that occur have little to do with this. It has also been pointed out that, since the patient is asked to press the key only when he no longer finds the slide sexually attractive, there is a direct link between sexual response and key press. However, even though FELDMAN and MacCULLOCH show that key-press responses are prognostic indicators, it does not necessarily follow that key presses are de facto avoidance responses. They are merely signals by the patient that some change is taking place in his sexual attitude to the slide.

One recognized method of studying avoidance behaviour with animals has been the use of the yoked pair. In an attempt to evaluate the importance of the avoidance response, we carried out a yoked-pair study in which stimulus conditions were identical for each patient but key presses did not affect stimulus conditions for the yoked subject.

II. Apparatus

A solid-state device was used for the presentation of two slides (male CS1 and female CS2) and shock. The design of this device was reported in 1970; it was programmed to operate according to the original FELDMAN-MacCULLOCH schedule, i.e. one third of trials were non-reinforced, one third DA, and one third IA. In addition, half the trials were followed by a female slide and half of these had opportunity for recall. Since it was not possible to carry out the experiment with more than one subject at once, it was necessary for effecting the yoked control to record the sequence and timing of stimulus presentations. This was done by the use of a two-channel stereo tape recorder with remote control and an electronic oscillator (Fig. 1). The upper channel of the tape carried a sine-wave tone of 400 Hz and the lower channel a sine-wave

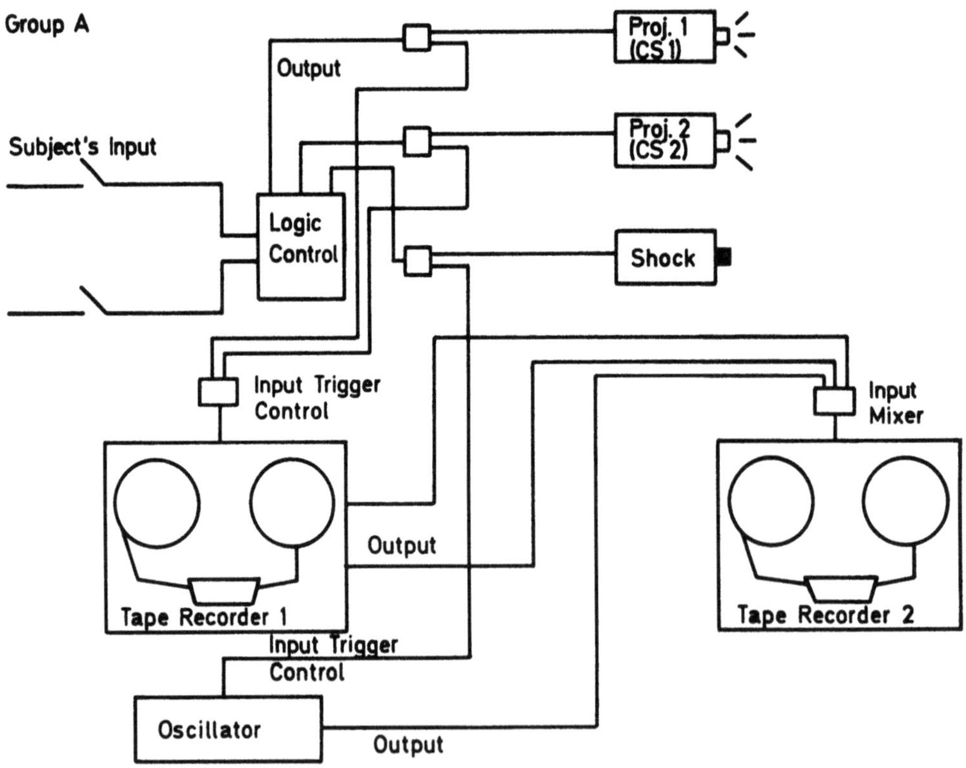

Fig. 1. Apparatus design - Group A. Operation of CS1 triggers tape recorder 1 and selects channel 1 on which is recorded a 400 Hz tone. This is recorded onto tape recorder 2, which is running continuously, for as long as CS1 is presented. Similarly, presentation of CS2 triggers and records a 600 Hz tone. Operation of shock stimulus triggers the oscillator set at 625 Hz and is similarly recorded

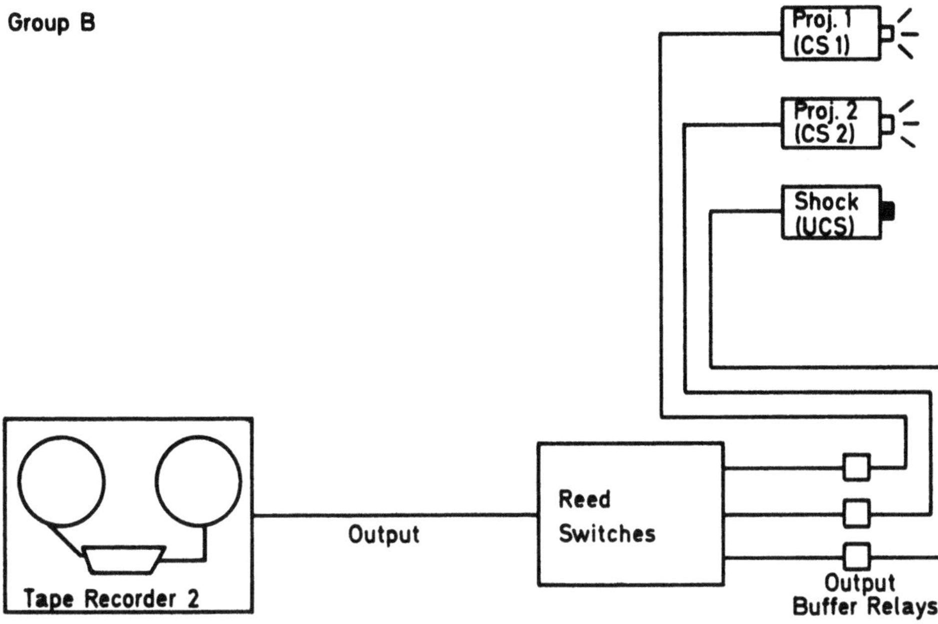

Fig. 2. Apparatus design - Group B. Tape recorder 2 feeds the appropriate signals into the bank of reed switches which are set to trigger CS1 if a 400 Hz signal is presented, CS2 if a 600 Hz signal is presented, a shock if a 625 Hz signal is presented

tone of 600 Hz; the oscillator was set at 625 Hz. The layout was so arranged that the tape recorder was automatically triggered and played back the 400 Hz tone when the CS1 (male slide) was presented, and the 600 Hz tone when the CS2 was presented; the oscillator was triggered to play the 625 Hz tone when the UCS was presented. The output was fed into another continuously running tape recorder so that the whole session could be recorded as a series of differently pitched tones (Fig. 2). To facilitate duplication of any particular session, this recording was fed into a series of reed-box switches that operated 3 relays. The reed boxes operated differentially to close the relay contacts according to the pitch of the tone presented. The slide projectors and shock box were coupled to the relays so that the operation of a particular relay would switch on the appropriate stimulus.

III. Method and Subjects

The experiment consisted of two groups with two patients in each group. Group I patients underwent the original FELDMAN-MacCULLOCH anticipatory avoidance schedule, i.e. each patient selected a series of 15 slides of attractive males and 15 slides of females. These were ranked according to their attractiveness to the subject. He was then given the following instructions, which are a variation of the original version: "On several occasions you will see a picture that you have selected. At some state in the session you may receive an electric shock. You will receive a shock when the screen is blank. To attempt to remove the shock and picture, press the button on the right side and say "NO".

You may at any time press the button and say "NO" to request that the picture be turned off, but you are asked not to do this if the picture is at all sexually attractive".

When the subject had made 3 consecutive button-press responses the initial training session was terminated. Any response immediately switched off the slide. He was given the same instructions before the next session with the addition of: "Occasionally the first picture will be followed by a second picture. This will stay on for a short time. You can request to see the picture again by pressing the button on the left side and saying "YES PLEASE". You may do this whenever you wish."

The subsequent sessions consisted of the schedule proper, progressively working up the hierarchy of male slides and down the hierarchy of female slides. Male slides were changed after a session when the mean latency times were less than 2 sec. and female slides, when the subject consistently pressed the return key.

Latency times, frequency of key presses, S.O.M. scores and S.D. scores were recorded.

Group II subjects similarly selected a hierarchy of 15 male and 15 female pictures. They were given precisely the same instructions, but the sequencing and timing of stimulus presentations were identical to those of the yoked partner in Group I, and the subject's key presses did not affect this. Again, latency times, frequency of key presses and S.O.M. scores were recorded.

The subjects were 4 homosexual males, all of whom had voluntarily requested treatment of their homosexuality. The first two to arrive were assigned to Group I, the second two to Group II. The mean age of Group I was 32.5 and that of Group II 38.5 (not significantly different). We have the relevant clinical data.

IV. Results

1. "Avoidance" Responses

a) Latencies

Subjects AI and AII. As can be seen from Fig. 3a and b, the latency times for these two subjects were very similar, and statistical analysis shows no significant differences between the two. Both had low variability and showed a pattern similar to FELDMAN and MacCULLOCH's successes.

b) Response Rates

Subjects AI and AII. AI gradually reduced his rate of responding to about one key press per trial. Since the stimulus conditions are in no way changed by the number of key presses above one, the most economical response frequency is one response per trial. However, AII's rate of responding increased markedly throughout the therapy period, despite the fact that the stimulus conditions in his case were not response-contingent.

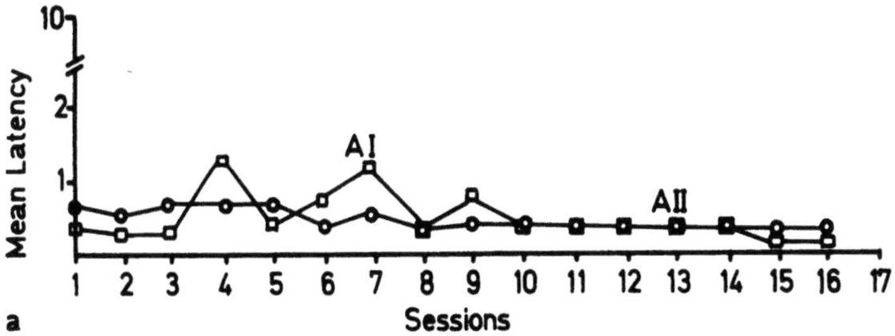

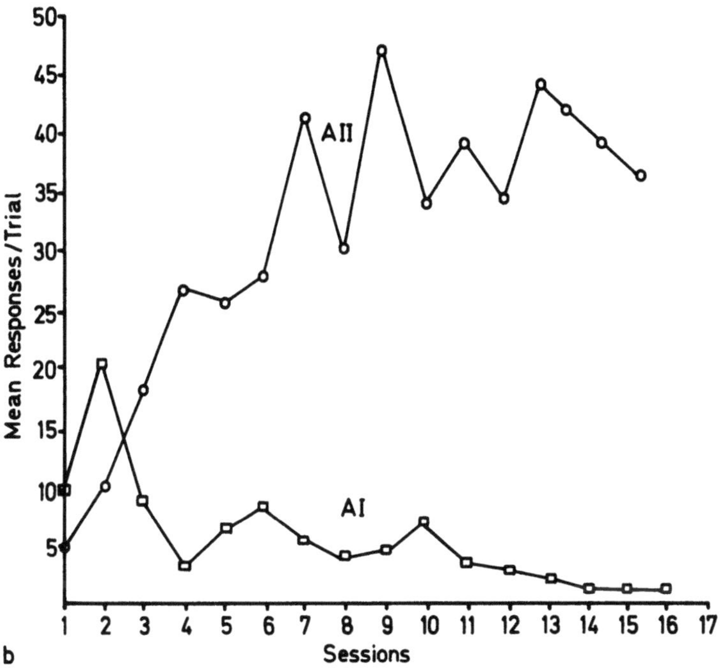

Fig. 3a and b. (a) Avoidance response latencies. Mean avoidance latency for subjects AI and AII showed no difference. Both subjects responded fairly quickly on most trials. (b) Avoidance response rates. Subject AI gradually reduced his rate of avoidance responding to about one key press per trial. Despite stimulus conditions being non-response contingent for subject AII, his avoidance response rate increased markedly throughout the therapy period

c) Latencies

Subjects BI and BII. As Fig. 4a and b show, BII showed a very variable pattern of responding, with high latency times, a pattern very similar to FELDMAN and MacCULLOCH's successes.

d) Response Rates

Subjects BI and BII. BI very quickly settled down to the most economical response rate and maintained this throughout therapy, whereas BII's rate of responding was much more variable, finally collapsing altoghether. This is a pattern described by FELDMAN and MacCULLOCH as being typical of failure.

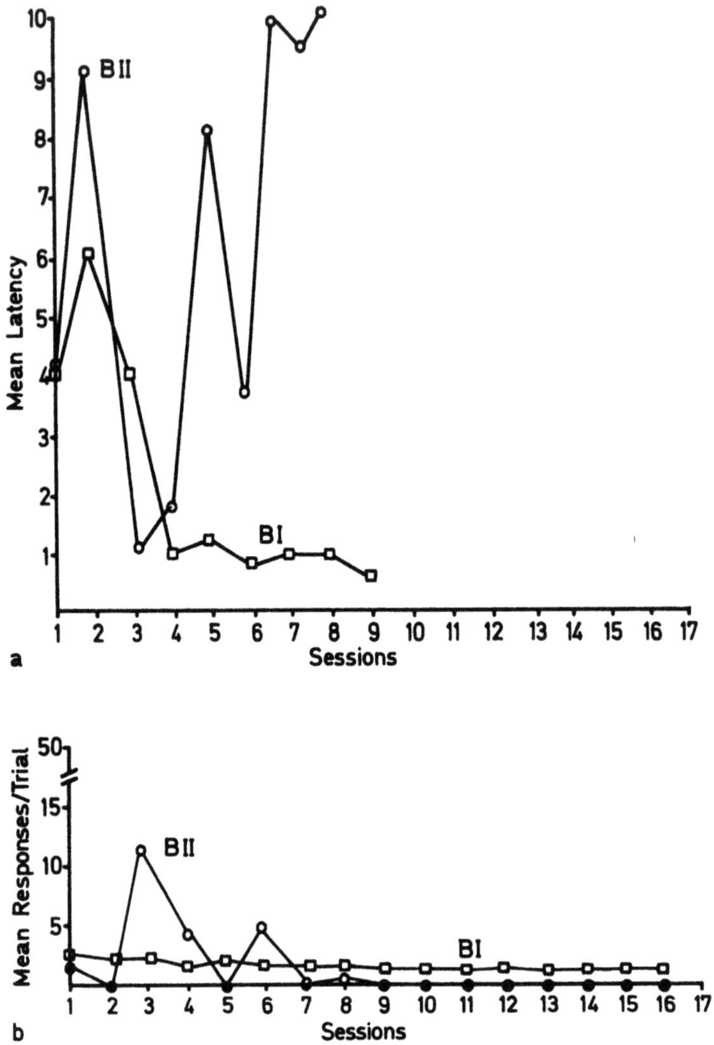

Fig. 4a and b. (a) Avoidance response latencies. Subject BI quickly settled down to a low response latency. A pattern similar to FELDMAN and MacCULLOCH's successes, whereas BII maintained a variable pattern of avoidance response latencies. (b) Avoidance response rates. Subject BI quickly settled down to an economic rate of response whereas BII's response rate was much more variable, finally collapsing altogether

2. "Approach" Responses

Subjects AI and AII. As can be seen from Fig. 5, subject AII's response rate was significantly higher than AI's but both subjects responded at a comparatively high mean rate.

Subjects BI and BII. These subjects responded at a low rate throughout, with BI responding at the most economical level virtually throughout. Again BII's response rate collapsed completely (Fig. 6).

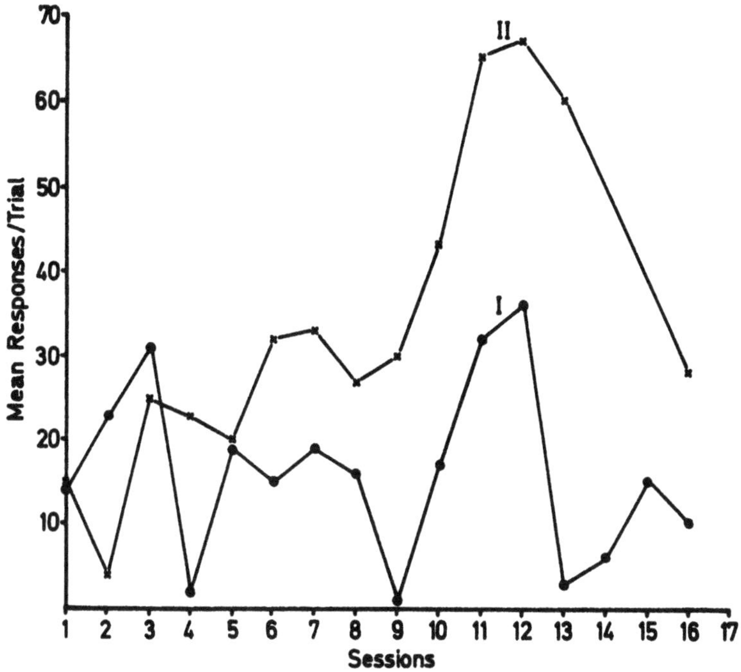

Fig. 5. Approach response rates. Both subjects' approach responses were at a fairly high mean rate, with AII's being significantly higher than AI's

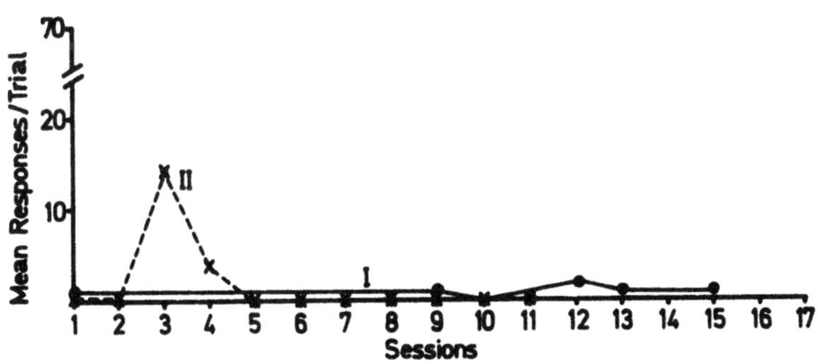

Fig. 6. Approach response rates. Both subjects' approach responses were at a low rate, BI responding at optimum economy and BII's responses collapsing completely

3. S.O.M. (Sexual Orientation Method) Scores

Final, absolute S.O.M. scores reflect accurately the outcome of treatment. Subjects AI and AII both show large reductions in the attractiveness of males with corresponding increased attraction to females. Subject BI showed low attraction to males before treatment and maintained this throughout, whereas BII started high and stayed high (Fig. 7).

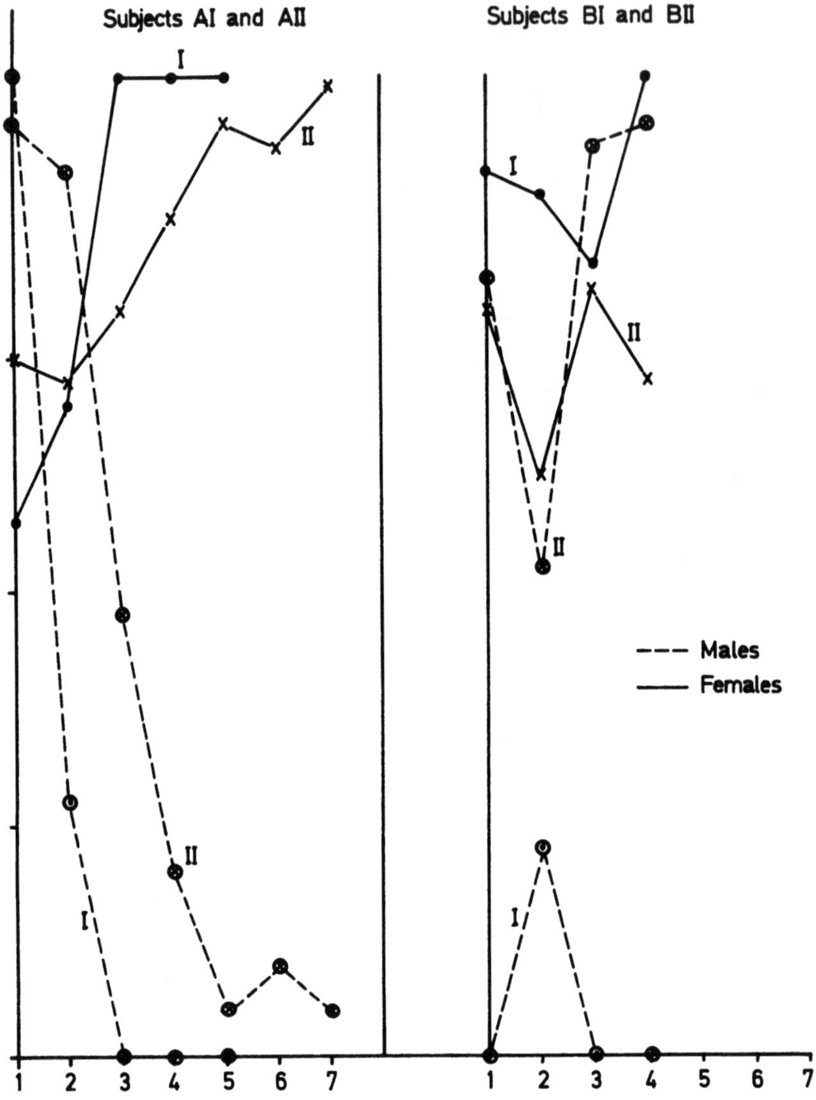

Fig. 7. Sexual Orientation Method. Subjects AI and AII showed large reductions in measured attraction to males and corresponding increases in attraction to females. Subject BI showed low attraction to males before treatment and throughout therapy. Subject BII's attraction to males started high and stayed high throughout therapy

V. Conclusions

The two subjects in Group I (original schedule) show response latency patterns very similar to those of FELDMAN and MacCULLOCH's successful subjects. Patients in Group II, however, showed responses which were different from each other but had a distinct similarity to those of FELDMAN and MacCULLOCH's patients, one being successful, the other not. This experiment was a pilot study and used only 4 subjects, but the results suggest that the schedule, as such, does not appear to affect the key-pressing response significantly. It would appear that the instructions given to the subject before treatment are of more importance and that his expectations consequent upon these instructions determine the responses. That changes do occur with successful cases is undoubted, and reductions on response latency would appear to be useful prognostic indicators. However, the way those responses affect stimulus conditions would appear to be irrelevant to outcome.

Recent work by FELDMAN and MacCULLOCH has, of course, shown that, with patients who have had precious pleasurable heterosexual experience, classic conditioning is just as effective in changing sexual preference as anticipatory avoidance. This may well be reflected in the results obtained in this pilot study, in that the classic component of anticipatory avoidance may be the important one.

References

AZRIN, N.H., HOLTZ, W.C.: Punishment. In: W.K. HONIG (Ed.): Operant Behaviour. New York: Appleton-Century-Crofts.

BIRK, L., HUDDLESTON, W., MILLER, E., COHLER, B.: Avoidance conditioning for homosexuality. Arch. gen. Psychiat. 25, 314-323 (1971).

CAMPBELL, B.A., CHURCH, R.K.: Punishment and Aversion Behaviour. Century Psychology Series - Appleton-Century-Crofts 1969.

CHURCH, R.: The varied effects of punishment. Psychol. Bull. 70, 269-402 (1963).

EAVES, D., ASHCROFT, J.B.: Behavioural treatment of sex offenders. Sexual Medizin. Accepted for publication (1972).

FELDMAN, M.P: Aversion therapy for sexual deviations: A critical review. Psychol. Bull. 65, 65-79 (1966).

FELDMAN, M.P., MacCULLOCH, M.J.: The application of anticipatory avoidance learning to the treatment of homosexuality. I. Theory, technique and preliminary results. Behav. Res. Ther. 2, 165-183 (1965).

FELDMAN, M.P., MacCULLOCH, M.J.: Homosexual Behaviour, Therapy and Assessment. Oxford: Pergamon Press (1971).

HERRNSTEIN, R.J.: Method and theory in the study of avoidance. Psychol. Rev. 76, 1, 49-69 (1969).

MacCULLOCH, M.J., FELDMAN, M.P.: Aversion therapy in management of 43 homosexuals. Brit. med. J. 1967II, 594-597.

RACHMAN, S., TEASDALE, J.: Aversion Therapy and Behaviour Disorders: An Analysis. London: Routledge and Kegan Paul 1969.

RACHMAN, S., TEASDALE, J.: Aversion therapy: an appraisal. In: C.M. FRANKS (Ed.): Behaviour Therapy: Appraisal and Status. London: McGraw Hill 1969.

A Controlled Investigation of the Efficacy of Conjoint Marital Therapy: Interpretative Versus Directive

M.J. CROWE

The field of interpretative family therapy and its cognate discipline of marital psychotherapy have been well reviewed by BEELS and FERBER (1969). This form of marital therapy is practised according to two main theoretical models: psychoanalysis and systems theory. In both, the therapist's time is mostly occupied in listening and in interpreting inconscious processes of here-and-now observed interaction; little direct advice is given. Within both theoretical frameworks, there are big variations in technique, some therapists prefering a more dominant central role, while others sit back and make infrequent comments or interpretations. BEELS and FERBER have actually observed family therapists at work and give good, clear descriptions of their activities, which in some cases are similar to published descriptions, and in others seem to be much wider-ranging. No clear answer is given to the question: "Is the therapeutic intervention effective?" According to WELLS et al. (1972) only one of the many trials of family therapy was adequately controlled. This trial, by LANGSLEY et al. (1969), showed that, with random assignment of patients thought suitable for emergency admission to a psychiatric hospital, those who were assigned to outpatient family therapy did just as well as those who were admitted on all general criteria, and better on the criteria of time lost from work and further time spent in hospital. Other, less well-controlled studies showed that between 70 and 80 % of presenting problems can be expected to improve, though in the marital sphere this figure is a little lower.

A newer departure, directive of 'operant-interpersonal' marital therapy, has been introduced by STUART (1969). His approach is to attempt to find some behaviour in each partner that would be rewarding to the other: he then persuades the partners to 'exchange' such rewarding behaviour on an equal basis. The simple theory on which this treatment is based states that, while normal, functioning marriages embody a considerable amount of such exchange of rewards, disturbed marriages do not, but instead rely on coercion (e.g. threats, nagging and violence) as the means of obtaining desired behaviour from each other. Working on similar principles, was used video tape feedback to point out to couples where they have, or have not, been rewarding each other for desired behaviour. No controlled studies of this approach are available, but STUART seems to have obtained reasonable improvement in 4 couples without any psychiatric problems, who were on the brink of divorce.

Obviously the two approaches, interpretative and directive, have certain similarities. In both, the couple are seen together and, in both, the aim is to improve the interaction between them and as a by-product to get rid of any psychiatric symptoms. Psychoanalytically orientated workers would emphasize insight as an important goal, systems theorists would emphasize understanding of the power structure and communication in the relationship, and directive therapists would emphasize appropriate reward for behaviour. Differences between the interpretative and directive approaches are also important. In the directive approach, the therapist sets himself up as the expert and takes responsibility for telling the couple what to do; he also sets tasks for them to complete before the next appointment. In the interpretative approach, he helps them to find their own answers, but puts the responsibility on them to make appropriate use of his insights. In the directive approach, the emphasis is always on harmony and mutual reward: in the interpretative approach there may be much discussion of anger and hostility, and the therapist may become angry intentionally, to motive an emotional interchange between the partners.

The aim of the present study is to evaluate these two approaches, interpretative and directive, in the treatment of couples with marital problems and to compare them with a control procedure of common-sense counselling. Subjects for the study are patients referred with their spouses from the various units at the Bethlem-Maudsley Hospital, in whom marital difficulties are thought to be important factors, but excluding psychotic, organic or very long-standing personality problems.

The therapy is largely carried out by one therapist (M.J.C.), although other therapists are also treating cases in the study, so that it is not just a test of one person's skill, or lack of it, in a particular approach. Couples are assigned at random to (1) an interpretative approach, based on that of SKYNNER (1969) and some of the systems theory techniques; (2) a directive approach, based on that of STUART, plus some MASTERS and JOHNSON sexual techniques; and (3) a control procedure in which the therapist acts as a non-involved peacemaker, trying to get the couple to understand each other's point of view. The sessions are tape-recorded, and random sessions will be assessed by an independent judge to see if he can allocate them according to the treatment approach being used.

Therapy sessions are held for an hour once a week or once every two weeks, depending on patients' wishes and availability. The aim in all cases is to have 10 therapy sessions, but it may be possible in some cases to stop before the 10 sessions and in others it may be necessary to continue up to 15, if progress is being made and there are still problems to clear up.

Regular and frequent assessment is carried out by means of questionnaires and interviews at intervals of about 4 weeks during therapy. The questionnaires are filled in separately by each partner and cover the following areas: presenting or 'target' problems, general psychiatric symptoms, attitudes toward significant figures, adjustment in the marital, work, leisure, social and sexual spheres, and a careful enquiry into the behaviour of both partners since the last assessment. In addition, the independent assessor, who is blind to treatment contingencies, carries out structured interviews separately with each partner based on the adjustment questionnaires mentioned above, and holds joint interviews with both partners to assess their target symptoms and to make a rough assessment of the interaction between the partners. The assessor's interviews take place at the beginning and the end of therapy.

Examples of Cases Treated by the Two Major Approaches

1. Directive approach: Mr. and Mrs. O. 13 sessions. Married 3 yrs. In 20's.

Problems: Wife's depression
Husband's inability to ejaculate
Minor problems: Wife's lack of interest in newspapers etc.
Husband's ignoring of wife and her conversation

In the first session, the principles of mutual reinforcement were explained. They then kept a diary of joint activities, as a result of which the following plan was made: the husband had to help with the washing up, take his wife out for a meal on some evenings, help her to understand the news items and kiss her nicely (she was the judge). The wife had to take an interest in the news, help him with his photographic work, help him with the Masters and Johnson technique for failure to ejaculate, and be more active in sexual intercourse. The couple cooperated well with this regime and three of the problems rapidly dropped out of the picture - wife became less depressed, and their interests began to coincide. Concentration on the sexual problem, however, while increasing their admitted attractiveness for each other, did not enable him to ejaculate, and they are currently working on a method of artificial insemination, using his nocturnal emissions.

2. Interpretative approach: Mr. and Mrs. M. 5 sessions. Married 9 yrs. In 30's. Two children.

Problems: Husband's irresponsibility
Wife's over-indulgence in drugs and alcohol
Minor problems: Husband's transvestism (one episode)
Wife's dyspareunia, abdominal pain, insomnia

In the first session, we explored the relationship. I pointed out that the husband was behaving like a guilty little boy, promising to turn over a new leaf, while the wife was the stern taskmistress and was the final judge of his behaviour. She pointed out how her husband had been a mother's boy, whereas she had carried her own family after the death of her mother. She was still doing the same. I pointed out that everyone has an adult and a childish side, and she was denying the child in her, while he was not recognising his adult responsibilities. She then said that, on the contrary, she enjoyed herself greatly, was the life and soul of the party, but got severe headaches the day after. I pointed out that she was very tense in the session and wondered if at parties she took the responsibility for seeing that everyone had a good time. She agreed that she was tense and pointed out that, when her husband dressed in her panties, she felt that she was the only man in the house. I pointed out that she was taking the lead in the session, too. She said that her husband seemed incapable of telling her what to do. At this point, the husband sat up and stated that he would be completely independent if necessary - he could look after himself. I approved his tone and manner, and when she asked at the end if I could help her, I said I could help her husband to do so.

In subsequent sessions, much the same sort of interchange took place, and the husband partially asserted himself and took over some monetary responsibilities, while the wife, with my commendation, began to take a back seat and allow him to do the talking. She remained in some pain, especially after intercourse, but gave up using sedatives, obtained a voluntary post at a local old people's home, and encouraged the husband in his new-found responsibilities.

A pilot study, in which 9 couples have been treated by each of the two major methods and two by the control procedure, has been assessed on purely clinical grounds. Four of the interpretative group couples lapsed before the end of treatment, while only one of the directive group couples did so. Two couples in the interpretative, one in the directive and one in the supportive group were rated much improved, in that their adjustment was good and the main problem was lost. One 'interpretative' couple and three 'directive' couples were rated improved, in that adjustment was improved but the main problem remained. Four interpretative couples, 4 directive and one supportive couple were rated slightly improved (including two interpretative couples who defaulted). The other 3 defaulting couples were rated unchanged. The only couples who showed reluctance to terminate therapy were 3 of those in the directive group.

In summary, it may be said at this stage that interpretative marital therapy seems to have more dramatic results in some cases, but is less reliable in that more of the couples seem to default before the end of treatment. On the other hand, the directive approach produces less dramatic, but more consistent, gains, while in some cases causing an excessive dependency on the therapist, as shown by reluctance to terminate therapy.

References

BEELS, C., FERBER, A.: Family therapy: A view. Family Process 8, 280 (1961).

LANGSLEY, D.G. et al.: Follow-up evaluation of family crisis therapy. Amer. J. Orthopsychiat. 31, 753 (1969).

SKYNNER, A.C.: A group-analytic approach to conjoint family therapy. J. Child Psychol. 10, 81 (1969).

STUART, R.B.: Operant-interpersonal treatment for marital discord. J. consult. clin. Psychol. 33, 675 (1969).

WELLS, R.A., DILKES, T.C., TRIVELLI, N.: The results of family therapy: A critical review of the literature. Family Process 11, 189 (1972).

Marital Interaction in Sexual Dysfunction+

J.J.M. HARBISON, H. McALLISTER, J.T. QUINN and P.J. GRAHAM

In previous communications (GRAHAM et al., 1973; QUINN et al., 1973) we discussed the use of the Interpersonal Perception Technique (DREWERY, 1969) in the study of marriages in which a sexual problem exists. This technique attempts to measure how accurately a spouse perceives his partner and how accurately he can predict the partner's perception of him. Each partner fills out the Edwards Personal Preference Schedule three times (see Table 1): once as he would fill it in for 'himself', once as his spouse would fill it in, and once as he expects his spouse to fill it in for him. Using the 6 questionnaires obtained in this way, it is possible to derive 7 correlations between the scores for husband and wife. DREWERY and RAE (1969) have used this technique to descriminate between good and bad prognosis marriages in alcoholic subjects. In the pilot study referred to above, GRAHAM et al. (1973) suggested that the technique had promise in the assessment of marriages in which a sexual problem existed. The preliminary results from 10 marriages showed significant differences between the marriages of impotent patients and DREWERY and RAE's control subjects. The present paper reports an extension of this work.

I. Subjects

The Interpersonal Perception Technique was used with 4 groups of marriages. There were 21 marriages in each of the four groups, consisting of a control group, a group of frigid patients, a group of impotent patients, and a group of psychiatric patients in whom sexual problems were not the major presenting problem. The spouses of all the subjects were also assessed.

II. Results

The results are shown in Table 2. This table presents product moment correlation coefficients for the 7 ways in which the scores from the 3 sets of questionnaires can be compared. For example, (BXA1) is a comparison between the wife's perception of herself and how her husband

---

+ This research was carried out as part of an M.R.C.-supported project (M.R.C.) G970/340/C) under the general direction of Professor J.G. Gibson. Four of us (P.J.G., J.T.Q., H.McA., J.J.M.H.) constitute a research team. No seniority of authorship is implied by the order of names on this paper.

Table 1. Interpersonal Perception Technique: Ways wife/husband have to complete questionnaire

Husbands' protocols coded	Respondent asked to describe	Wives' protocols coded
A	Myself as I am	B
A 1	My spouse as I see him/her	B 1
A 2	Myself as I think my spouse sees me	B 2

Table 2. Mean intercorrelations from I.P.T. on groups of normal, psychiatric impotent and frigid marriages (N = 21 in each sample)

Comparisons	Normal	Psychiatric	Impotent	Frigid
A X B	.40	.39	.37	.43
B X A1	.50	.43	.51	.50
B1 X A2	.61	.50	.60	.65
A X A2	.49	.38	.40	.45
A X B1	.49	.42	.44	.46
A1 X B2	.63	.68	.59	.65
B X B2	.25	.14	.19	.15

perceives her. Simple inspection of this table shows that the results do not bear out the findings of the pilot study.

Table 3 presents a discriminant function analysis of the product moment correlation coefficients for all of these four groups. Discriminant function analysis is a technique that maximises differences in data between groups that are already self-defined and is appropriate for application to the 4 groups in our study. The discriminant function itself is a weighted combination of the original data. The analysis uses this function to allocate groups to the opposite end of a statistically derived continuum. The 'hits-and misses' comparison in Table 3 illustrates how unsuccessful the analysis has been in this case in allocating marriages to their self-defined groups. These results bear out the impressions gained from Table 2, that the technique is not discriminating between the 4 groups.

Table 3. Discriminant analysis based on I.P.T. intercorrelations for groups of normal (n = 20), frigid (n = 21), impotent (n = 21) and psychiatric (n = 21) marriages

		Actual Group			
		Normal	Frigid	Impotent	Psychiatric
Forecast Group	Normal	6	4	6	4
	Frigid	9	12	9	6
	Impotent	3	1	4	4
	Psychiatric	2	4	2	7

III. Discussion

It would appear that our initial optimism about the Interpersonal Perception Technique is not borne out, at least at the level in discriminating between criterion groups. It is, of course, possible that this technique will discriminate between good and bad prognosis marriages; however, we feel the technique requires further refinement. For example, DREWERY and RAE have not, to our knowledge, carried out an analysis designed to detect whether the instructions to fill out the questionnaires in these different ways are effective. An analysis of variance of our data would suggest that the instructional effect is weak and complex. While the details of this analysis will be reported in later publications, it appears that the most likely explanation for the failure to discriminate between the 4 groups may be that the test itself is not effective as a measure of interpersonal perception. If this suggestion is true, its usefulness as a prognostic index should be seriously questioned.

It is salutory to remember that the test is cumbersome and expensive in terms of patient time. The patients and their spouses spend approximately 6 hours completing this test. This in itself might call into question the utility of the technique, and when the time expenditure is put against the apparent weakness of the test, we would suggest that more useful measures of marital interaction can be provided by other techniques.

Other psychometric instruments exist, for example, semantic differentials, repertory grids and in particular dyad grids. We will also report elsewhere the value or otherwise of comparisons between simple psychometric measures on husbands and wives separately. Further, it appears plausible that interactional measures can usefully be developed by using such techniques as interactional games and observation of intermarital reinforcement patterns.

References

DREWERY, J.: An inter-personal perception technique. Brit. J. Med. Psychol. 42, 171-181 (1969).

DREWERY, J.B.: A group comparison of alcoholic and non-alcoholic marriages using the inter-personal perception technique. Brit. J. Psychiat. 115, 287-300 (1969).

GRAHAM, P. JOAN, HARBISON, J.J.M., McALLISTER, H., QUINN, J.T.: The use of measurement in the assessment of the patient's social environment. In: BRENGELMANN, J.C., TUNNER, W. (Eds.). Behavior Therapy. Munich: 1973.

QUINN, J.T., GRAHAM, P. JOAN, HARBISON, J.J.M., McALLISTER, H.: The Assessment of Sexual Function. New York: Appleton Century Crofts (in press) 1973.

IV. Approaches to Specific Behaviour Problems

Systematic Desensitization and Self-Control Training in the Treatment of Speech Anxiety

W. TUNNER, C. OELKERS, R. FERSTL and N. BIRBAUMER

I. Summary

This experiment deals with the modification of physiological, subjective and motoric aspects of anxiety, evaluated by 4 different measures during the course of 2 different but parallel therapy programs.

Speech anxiety in student clients was chosen as the target problem: 20 subjects were matched in 2 therapy and two control groups. One therapy group was given systematic desensitization (SD), the second obtained self-control training (SC), during which the client was primarily trained to control the physiological symptoms of anxiety.

The therapeutic results were measured by in vivo tests given before therapy, at half-time (6 sessions), at three-quarter time (9 sessions), at the end of the program, and 7 months after the end of the therapy. The tests consisted of public speaking situations before an audience of 20 to 25 students. During the subject's performance in this situation we recorded the following anxiety indices

1) physiological measurement (GSR)
2) behaviour observation during public speaking
3) analysis of subjective anxiety with the help of 2 questionnaires.

The following results were obtained:

During the course of therapy there was a significant reduction in all 3 aspects of anxiety for both therapy groups. Summarizing, we can state that a general effectiveness of both methods (SD and SC) was demonstrated by our evaluations of the 3 aspects of anxiety, and that it was maintained until the follow-up.

II. Introduction

Analysis of external anxiety-evoking stimuli is one condition for SD. The stimuli are characterized by their specific contents and classified in an anxiety hierarchy according to their capacity for provoking anxiety. Whereas investigators have submitted item contents to painstaking analysis, they have settled for a fairly subjective classification of degrees of intensity in characterizing the anxiety response.

The emphasis on a thorough analysis of external anxiety-evoking stimuli evolved from the initial interpretation of SD as a classic deconditioning procedure (WOLPE, 1958). It is consistent with Pavlov's experiments, suggesting that human subjects condition more or less passively to stimuli.

The preceding interpretation of desensitization is supported by a number of experiments. Nevertheless, clinical experience and research results have repeatedly shown positive therapeutic desensitization effects, which could not be completely explained by the initial interpretation. For example, it is not clear why successful desensitization of rat, snake, and speech anxiety has positive effects on various other social situations in the sense of stimulus generalization.

Of the proposed interpretations of these effects, we prefer the one that regards SD as a method by which the client learns to discriminate anticipation of anxiety stimuli and to respond with self-instruction and relaxation (GOLDFRIED, 1971; SUINN and RICHARDSON, 1971). We believe that, above all, the proprioceptive feedback of anxiety response should be the discriminating factor and induce relaxation. Thus, both the approach to the previously feared object and cognitive coping mechanisms are facilitated, and the learned escape or avoidance responses are inhibited and eliminated.

Hence, our therapy programme is aimed at achieving discrimination and control of the various components of the physiological aspect of anxiety response. The specific response criteria are considered to be relatively independent of the variable forms of external stimuli.

Our interpretation requires 3 steps in therapy:

1. definition of proprioceptive anxiety-evoking stimuli,
2. practice of relaxation response that is incompatible with anxiety,
3. inhibition of proprioceptive anticipation stimuli through relaxation.

Whereas classic SD defines external stimuli and incorporates them into the anxiety hierarchy, the first phase of our program deals only with the definition of proprioceptive anxiety-evoking stimuli. During the second phase, as in classic desensitization, muscle relaxation exercises are performed according to JACOBSON (1964). In the third phase, proprioceptive excitation is provoked in the therapeutic situation and then eliminated by self-instruction in relaxation. These therapeutic procedures correspond essentially to the concept of self-control, as suggested for the modification of various forms of maladaptive behaviour (GOLDFRIED, 1971; GOLDFRIED and MERBAUM, 1972; KANFER, 1970; KANFER and KAROLY, 1971).

The following study was designed to examine the effects of the foregoing therapy phases on modification of speech anxiety and to compare it with the classic SD. Speech anxiety is defined as a distrubance of the motoric, autonomic and subjective aspects when speaking in public. Therefore, in our study we considered anxiety to be multidimensional, just like any other stress response and, according to the relevant social and objective situation, to consist of various components of physiological tenseness, subjective phenomena and motoric reactions.

In order to register the changes in motoric, subjective and autonomic anxiety responses in correlation with therapeutic sessions, various evalutations were made during the course of therapy as well as before and after the program. On the basis of clinical experience, it was very obvious that the rate of reduction of the motoric, subjective and autonomic aspects of anxiety response differed. These discrepancies could, in effect, shed light on the processes underlying the therapeutic procedure.

In our study the following broad questions were examined:

1. What effect does therapy based on self-control of anxiety response have, and in what way does it differ from classic SD?
2. How do motoric, subjective and autonomic anxiety responses alter during these different therapy programs?

III. Method

1. Sample Selection

On the basis of a test battery, 20 out of 35 applicants who responded to a bulletin-board notice in the Psychological Institute of the University of Munich and were between the ages of 20 and 30, were eligible for therapy of speech anxiety. They were matched in 4 groups of 6 persons. In order to gain a qualitative understanding of each person's individual problems, a standard interview was also held with each client. Besides various personal problems, a general fear of autority was found; 19 showed maximum anxiety shortly before speaking in public. Over half consequently avoided the critical situation of public speaking. Almost all (17) feared being laughed and jeered at. Autonomic anxiety responses such as trembling of the hands (17), increased perspiration (15) and blushing (12) were reported.

2. Instruments

a) Questionnaires

1. A German translation of the questionnaire for analysis of speech anxiety (PRCS): PAUL's (1966) shortened form of the "Personal report of confidence as a speaker".
2. The questionnaire for analysis of habitual anxiety (TRAIT); this questionnaire was developed by SPIELGERGER (1969) and examines the relatively stable dispostion for anxiety response (German version).
3. The questionnaire for the analysis of vegetative lability (VELA). Fahrenberg's questionnaire, analyzed according to Rasch (FERSTL, 1968), was used to determine physical dysfunctions.
4. The social anxiety scale by DIXON et al. (1967). This scale enables a general survey of average social anxiety (PICHOT, 1967).
5. The Fear Survey Schedule (FSS) in a shortened form by LANG (1963) (German version).
6. The actual feeling scale (B-S) by ZERSSEN et al. (1970). This schedule is composed of two parallel forms.
7. The questionnaire for analysis of actual anxiety (STAIT) "State Anxiety Inventory" by SPIELBERGER (1969). This inventory determines the degree of actual anxiety against habitual anxiety (German version).

b) Behaviour Observation

Timed Behavioural Checklist for Performance Anxiety (TBCL) by CLEVENGER and KING (1961) in the shortened form by PAUL (1966). Behaviour patterns defined in an observation list were checked and recorded by various trained observers at 30-sec intervals during the first 5 minutes of the speech (German version).

c) Analysis of Autonomic Reactions

Spontaneous fluctuations and basal resistance of psychogalvanic skin response (PGSR) were chosen for evaluation of autonomic activity and

<table>
<tr><th>groups \ tests</th><th>before therapy</th><th>1 in vivo test</th><th>2 in vivo test</th><th>3 in vivo test</th><th>4 in vivo test</th><th>after therapy</th><th>5 in vivo test follow-up</th></tr>
<tr><th></th><th></th><th></th><th colspan="2">therapy: SD,SC</th><th></th><th></th><th></th></tr>
<tr><td>SD-group (N=5)</td><td rowspan="4">PRCS
TRAIT
VELA
Soc.Anxiety
FSS</td><td rowspan="4">STATE
B-S
GSR
TBCL</td><td rowspan="3">STATE
B-S
GSR
TBCL</td><td rowspan="3">STATE
B-S
GSR
TBCL</td><td rowspan="4">STATE
B-S
GSR
TBCL</td><td rowspan="4">PRCS
TRAIT
VELA
Soc.Anxiety
FSS</td><td rowspan="2">STATE
B-S
GSR
TBCL</td></tr>
<tr><td>SC-group (N=5)</td></tr>
<tr><td>CG_1 (N=5)</td><td rowspan="2"></td></tr>
<tr><td>CG_2 (N=5)</td><td></td><td></td></tr>
</table>

SD = Desensitization

SC = Self-Control

1. in vivo test: before therapy
2. " " : after 6 sessions
3. " " : " 9 "
4. " " : " 12 " = after therapy
5. " " : 6 months after therapy

Fig. 1. General experimental design and procedure (for explanation of abbreviations see p. 129)

interpreted as anxiety. The experimental design of the assessment is shown in Fig. 1.

3. Experimental Procedure

The 4 groups were divided into 2 therapy groups (SD and SC training) and 2 control groups (placebo and waiting list).

a) Desensitization (SD)

Desensitization was performed according to the suggestion of WOLPE (1958) and comprised 4 phases:

a) brief explanation of reciprocal inhibition and desensitization,
b) relaxation training of JACOBSON (1938),
c) construction of anxiety hierarchy,
d) presentation of anxiety hierarchy during relaxation.

Each person was shown 6 to 12 scenes involving public speaking. The criteria for the scenes were exactly defined as to size and type of audience, difficulty of text, etc. Each person was given a total of 12 sessions of approx. 30 min each. In 3 sessions before therapy began, muscular relaxation exercises were practised and anxiety hierarchies were constructed.

The sessions were distributed among 2 therapists.

b) Self-Control Training Group (SC)

This program consisted mainly of 4 phases:

a) a brief introduction to the principle of self-control of nervous reactions

b) relaxation exercises according to JACOBSON
c) exercises for discrimination and control of nervous reactions
d) encouraging the client to try out discrimination and self-control of real-life situations and to discuss these exercises in each therapy session.

In order to practise discrimination and control of nervous reactions, anxiety-provoking situations had to be produced; this was achieved by electric shocks to the forearm. The following instructions were given: "In these sessions you should learn to distinguish your nervous reactions in their varying degrees and to eliminate them by use of self-relaxation. First, we'll try to identify your nervous reactions when confronted with an unpleasant situation. In order to learn to perceive and cope with these reactions, you will be threatened with an electric shock. After the tape count-down of 10 to 0 you will actually receive a shock on your forearm from the electrodes placed there. During the count-down you are to watch for the first sign of tenseness. As soon as you notice any, you are to raise your right index finger, the count-down will then be interrupted and you will be granted enough time to eliminate tenseness by self-relaxation. When you have succeeded in relaxing, you can make a sign and we will discuss your experiences. Then we will begin the exercise again".

Each session consisted of approx. 8 exercises. Every person showed some nervous reactions during the count-down, mainly expressed in physical disorders, such as augmentation of heart beat, increased sweating, respiratory difficulties, tension build-up in certain muscles, etc. As in desensitization, 12 therapeutic sessions were given plus 3 sessions for explanation of self-control training and relaxation exercises. Each of the 15 sessions lasted approx. 20 min. These sessions were also distributed among 2 therapists.

c) Placebo (Control Group I)

Placebo therapy consisted of regular meetings with the therapist, in which the client talked about his general psychological problems. The therapist did not intervene with interpretation or instructions. These sessions served mainly to motivate the clients to take part in the assessment procedure.

d) Waiting List (Control Group II)

After having filled out the pre-tests, this group of persons were put on the waiting list. Therapy began after the "post-therapy" tests, i.e. after an interval of 3 months.

4. Assessment

Measures were taken in both therapy groups and in the placebo group after sessions 6, 9, and 12. Like the pre- and post-therapy tests, they consisted of (1) behaviour observation, (2) analysis of autonomic reactions (GSR), and (3) the questionnaires (see Fig. 1).

IV. Procedure

Each client received a newspaper clipping of 4 sheets plus a brief index of the contents. We instructed them as follows: "You are given a text on which you are to report to a larger audience. You can keep the index list, but we must ask you not to take any further notes. Your report should last approx. 5 min; you have 15 min to prepare your speech". After 15 min the client was taken to a room where the GSR of his middle and index finger tips was measured. He was already accustomed to this situation since we had tried it out once before the pre-test. Changes in resistance were registered by the pen in the usual way, simultaneously showing activity and changes in basal resistance (constant current).

The following instructions were given before measurement: "Please make yourself as comfortable as possible. I will measure your skin resistance during 5 min. In front of you you see a stop watch, which will ring when the 5 min are up. After filling out 2 brief questionnaires you will then make your speech to the audience".

After these measurements the 2 questionnaires concerning actual anxiety (STAIT) and actual feeling (B-S) were filled out and the client was taken to a room where the audience and observer were waiting. The test was over after 5 min of extemporary speaking.

Post-therapy test and follow-up:

Immediately after the 12 therapeutic sessions we undertook the post-therapy test with all 4 groups (SD, SG, CG I, CG II) and 7 months later, the follow-up with the 2 therapy groups (see Fig. 1).

V. Results

In comparing the 4 groups we examined mainly the following questions:

1. Can statistical differences be found in the various evaluations during the course of therapy?
2. Can a definite trend be distinguished in the therapy process? Linear and curvilinear components in the data were considered for this purpose.
3. The data obtained in the course of therapy should be examined in respect to the various evaluation criteria at different points in the program.
4. The data derived from the pre- and post-therapy tests as well as from the 7 months later follow-up should be checked for a possible generalization effect.

a) Analysis of Significant Changes in the 3 Different Anxiety Aspects (Wilcoxon Test for Matched Samples)

Data on the 3 aspects were checked by non-parametric tests in the first to fourth *in-vivo* tests for all 4 groups, as well as in the first to fifth tests (see Fig. 1) for the two therapy groups. We were able to show a significant change in the first to fourth, as well as in the first to fifth tests for the two therapy groups by the Wilcoxon test for matched samples (SIEGEL, 1956) (see Tables 1 and 2). The two control groups showed no significant changes for the first to forth *in-vivo* tests (see Table 1). Fig. 2a to d shows graphs of the average changes in the various anxiety measures for the first to fourth *in-vivo* tests for all 4 groups. Fig. 3 clearly demonstrates the changes in the first to fourth tests for the SD and SC groups, as well as for the two control groups (CG I, CG II).

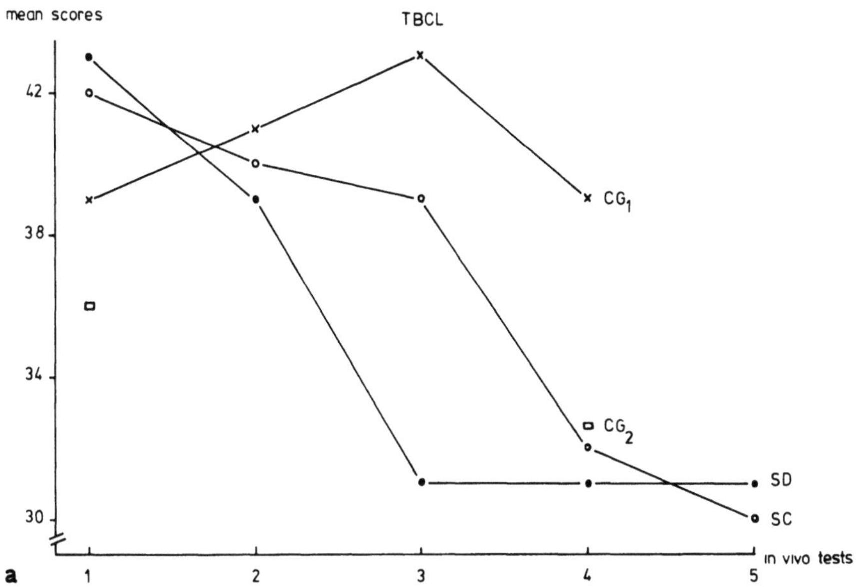

Fig. 2a-d. (a) Mean Timed Behavioural Check List for performance anxiety (TBCL) - changes from pre-treatment to 5th in-vivo test for the 2 therapy groups, and from 1st to 4th tests for Control Group I (CG I), and from 1st and 4th tests for Control Group II (CG II). (b) Mean changes on Questionnaire for Analysis of Actual Anxiety (STATE) from pre-treatment to 5th in-vivo test for the 2 therapy groups, and from 1st to 4th tests for CG I, and from 1st and 4th tests for CG II. (c) Mean changes on Actual Feeling Scale (B-S) from pre-treatment to 5th in-vivo test for the 2 therapy groups, and from 1st to 4th tests for CG I, and from 1st and 4th tests for CG II. (d) Mean GSR changes from pre-treatment to 5th in-vivo test for the 2 therapy groups, and from 1st to 4th tests for CG I, and from 1st and 4th tests for CG II

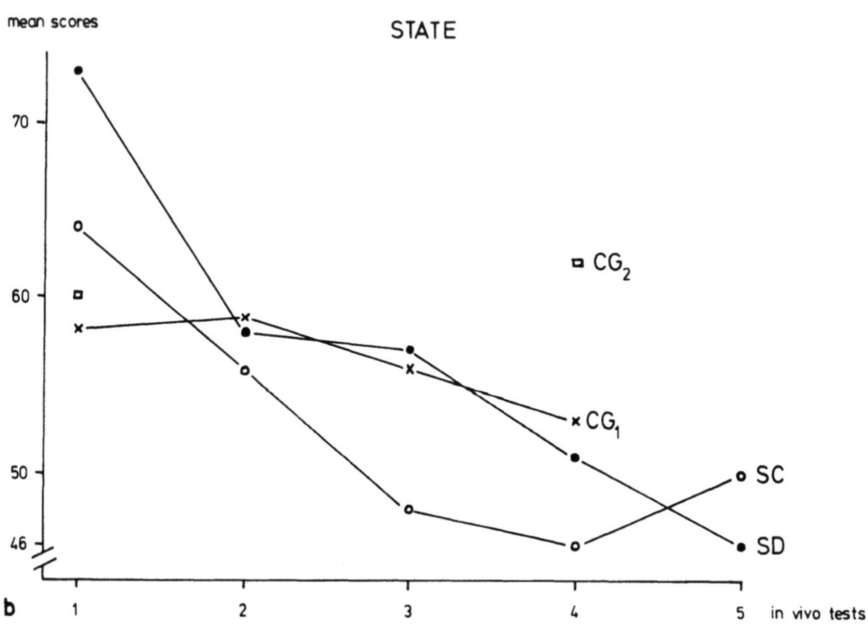

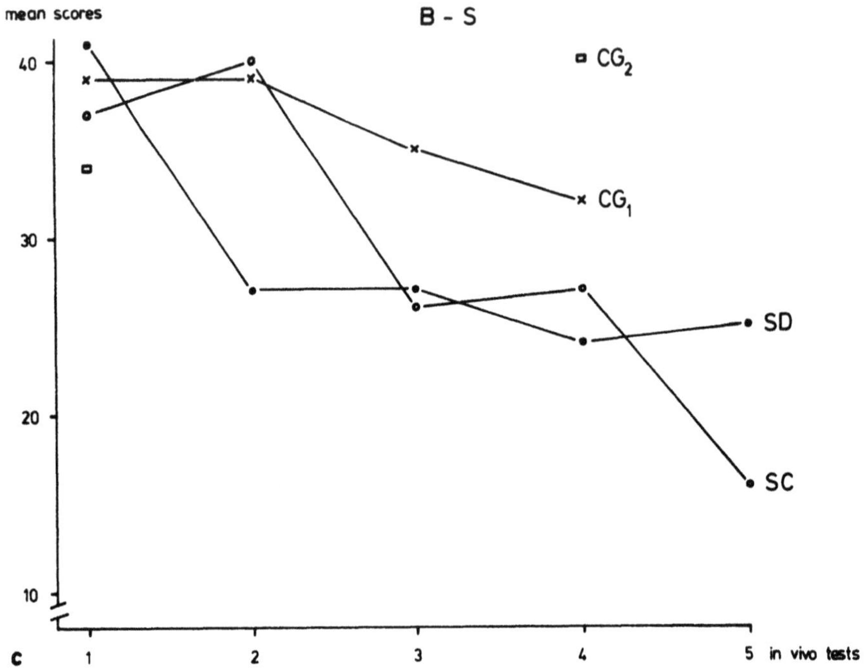

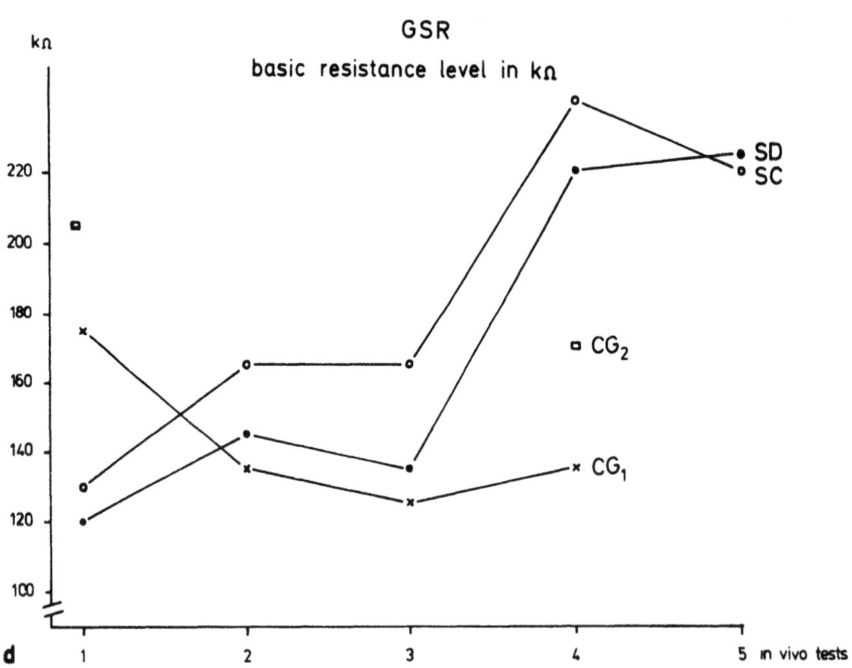

<u>b) Analysis of Variance and Trends</u>

In order to obtain a statistical test on changes and development during the course of therapy, one-way analyses of variance and trend analyses were done on the two subjective criteria (B-S, STATE) for behaviour observation and for average GSR (WINER, 1962). Taking the fifth <u>in-vivo</u>

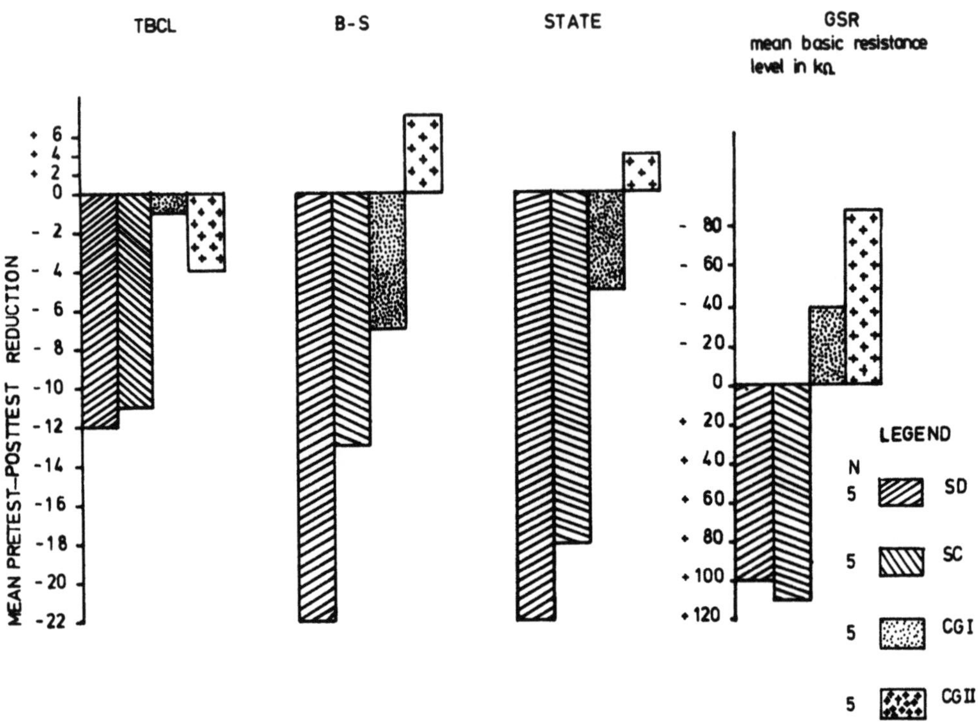

Fig. 3. Mean reduction on the various anxiety aspects from pre-treatment to post-treatment

Table 1. Changes in measurement results in the 1st to 4th <u>in-vivo</u> tests (Wilcoxon matched-pairs signed-ranks test; SIEGEL, 1956)

SD and SD Groups (N = 10)		CG_1 and CG_2 (N = 10)	
TBCL	:T = 5[b]	TBCL	:T = 19
B-S	:T = 2[c]	B-S	:T = 26
STATE	:T = 0[c]	STATE	:T = 12
GSR	:T = 7[a]	GSR	:T = 48

[a] p .025
[b] p .01
[c] p .005

test into consideration, the two therapy groups were additionally submitted to further variance and trend analyses. It was not possible to include Control Group I (CG I) in the fifth evaluation because they had already started therapy. Table 3 shows the results of our variance

Table 2. Changes in measurement results in the 1st to 5th *in-vivo* tests (Wilcoxon matched-pairs signed-ranks test; SIEGEL, 1956)

SD and SC Groups (N = 10)	
TBCL	:T = 6
B-S	:T = 1
STATE	:T = 0
GSR	:T = 0

[a] *p* .025
[b] *p* .005

and trend analyses. The desensitization group shows a clear linear trend in both questionnaires. The self-control training group shows a statistically significant result only in the State questionnaire. No significant changes could be found in the subjective tests for CG I. The behaviour survey shows the expected direction of trend only for the SD group. Analysis of variance of the data of the self-control group, as well as of CG I yielded no significant results (see Table 3). Analysis of autonomic reactions (average basic resistance in kΩ) shows a linear trend only for the desensitization group, and only including the fifth *in-vivo* test.

c) Analysis of significant deviations in development of the various aspects of anxiety (Wilcoxon-Wilcox test)

Several comparisons according to Wilcoxon-Wilcox (SACHS, 1972) showed a statistically significant variance in the subjectively experienced actual anxiety (STATE) for the desensitization group during the fourth measurement, that is, after therapy was completed. This variance increased further, as we found 7 months later in the follow-up (see Table 4). The self-control group showed a significant variance already during the third evaluation and this increased constantly up to the fifth evaluation (see Table 4). Behaviour survey showed a significant change only for the desensitization group during the third evaluation, i.e. after 75 % of therapy time had passed. It remained constant until after the later follow-up.

Analysis of autonomic reactions yielded a statistically significant variance for the desensitization group and this increased up to the later follow-up. The self-control training group, however, showed an essential change in anxiety response only at the follow-up 7 months later (see Table 4).

d) Analysis of variance in the other questionnaires (Wilcoxon test)

The trend of the evaluation data compared to the data at the end of the therapy program (see the experimental design) was checked nonparametrically. With the help of the Wilcoxon test for matched samples, we could prove a significant variance in the PRCS, TRAIT, and the speech anxiety questionnaire for both therapy groups (see Table 5). The

Table 3. Analysis of variance and trend of the three aspects of anxiety in the 1st to 4th tests and the 1st to 5th tests (WINER, 1962)

1st to 4th tests			
	SD Group	SC Group	CG I
TBCL	F = 5.84[a]	F = 1.25	F = .57
	F ratio = 15.02[b]		
STATE	F = 16.52[b]	F = 11.70[b]	F = .43
	F ratio = 43.26[b]	F ratio = 31.19[b]	
B-S	F = 4.65[a]	F = 2.57	F = .39
	F ratio = 12.13[b]		
PGR	F = 2.61	F = 1.57	F = 1.56

1st to 5th tests		
	SD Group	SC Group
TBCL	F = 4.97[b]	F = 1.91
	F ratio = 15.04[b]	F = 1.45
STATE	F = 24.06[b]	F = 7.19[b]
	F ratio = 91.37[b]	F ratio = 16.78[b]
B-S	F = 6.78[b]	F = 2.15
	F ratio = 24.23[b]	
GSR	F = 3.59[a]	F = 1.45
	F ratio = 11.67[b]	

[a] p .05
[b] p .01

follow-up 7 months later showed a further decrease in values for the therapy groups (see Table 6). Control groups CG I and CG II showed no significant changes in these tests (see Table 6).

Table 4. Critical differences in anxiety reduction from 1st to 2nd (A to B), 1st to 3rd (A to C), 1st to 4th (A to D) and 1st to 5th (A to E) tests (evaluated according to Wilcoxon-Wilcox, Lit. SACHS, 1972)

SD Group		SC Group	
TBCL			
from A to B :	2.5	from A to B :	6.5
" A " C :	9.5[a]	" A " C :	0.5
" A " D :	10.5[b]	" A " D :	8
" A " E :	10^{+}	" A " E :	6
STATE			
from A to B :	7	from A to B :	6.5
" A " C :	9	" A " C :	15[b]
" A " D :	15[b]	" A " D :	14.5[b]
" A " E :	19[b]	" A " E :	14[b]
GSR			
from A to B :	3.5	from A to B :	7
" A " C :	4	" A " C :	6
" A " D :	9.5[a]	" A " D :	7
" A " E :	13[b]	" A " E :	10[a]

[a] :crit.diff. = 9.4, p .05
[b] :crit.diff. = 10.5, p .01

Table 5. Changes in measurement results in the 1st to 4th *in-vivo* tests in regard to the test battery data (Wilcoxon matched-pairs signed-ranks test; SIEGEL, 1956)

	SD and SC Group	CG_1 and CG_2
PRCS	T = 3[a]	T = 21.5
TRAIT	T = 4.5[a]	T = 29
VELA	T = 10.5	T = 13
SOC.ANXIETY	T = 0[a]	T = 22

[a] p .025

Table 6. Overview on mean change in the test battery data in the 1st, 4th and 5th *in-vivo* tests

	SD Group	SC Group	CG I	CG II
PRSC	1st : 25	23	23	24
	4th : 20	19	24	24
	5th : 18	16		
TRAIT	1st : 54	53	40	53
	4th : 49	49	40	54
	5th : 48	46		
VELA	1st : 15	18	12	18
	4th : 13	16	28	19
	5th : 12	16		
SOC.ANX.	1st : 17	18	11	16
	4th : 13	15	11	17
	5th : 11	13		

VI. Discussion

Both therapy programs, SD and SC, resulted in a significant reduction in subjective, motoric, and autonomic anxiety. This decrease in fearfulness also showed a linear trend in all three aspects of anxiety for the SD group. Consequently, a steady reduction of subjective, motoric, and autonomic symptoms can be attained by consecutive treatment. The SC group showed a linear trend only in the subjective aspects. Repeated measurements showed lack of correspondence in the crucial variance of the subjective, motoric, and autonomic response modifications. Therapeutic results were found first in the subjective aspect, then in the motoric reactions and last in the autonomic response.

This lack of correspondence in response to treatment has been noted by other authors: LANG and LAZOVIK (1963), LANG (1968), HART (1966), DAVISON (1968), MILLER and NAWAS (1969). KRAPFL and NAWAS (1970) proved a discrepancy between subjective and motoric results in treatment of phobia. Indeed, contrary to our results, they attained a motoric modification before subjective relief was experienced. This deviation from our results could be due to the specific methods of behaviour evaluation. Whereas in the preceding studies, the avoidance test was utilized for evaluation of behaviour modification (approach to the previously feared object), our experiments were based on behaviour observation for any signs of motoric excitation directly in the anxiety-evoking situation, that is during a public speech. Thus a number of characteristics can be included in the survey, which are not considered in the avoidance test.

An example of discrepancy between autonomic and motoric results was given by LEITENBERG et al. (1971). In cases of successful phobia treatment with a positive reduction of avoidance response, the autonomic reactions (heart beat) either showed no change at all or showed change only after the reduction of motoric excitement.

This lack of correspondence of various anxiety characteristics only confirms the assumption that different methods apply to different aspects of anxiety. Consequently, evaluations should be made in the various sequences of motoric, subjective and physiological reactions. The success of therapy can be determined only when improvement is achieved in all 3 aspects of anxiety. It is evident, for example, that one reason for a relapse after completed treatment is the therapist's biased criteria of success. The probability of a relapse can be defined as the function of an insufficient reduction in the subjective, motoric or psychological aspects of anxiety response (TUNNER, 1972).

Self-control of physical excitation encountered with anxiety-provoking stimuli proved to be quite a successful method, as demonstrated in the SC therapy group, but, the basic mechanism of success is still unknown. All we can say is that the following characteristics of the therapy are plausible: Training the client to discriminate intensive anxiety stimuli should enable him to break the link in the chain of reactions leading to his fear at an early stage and to eliminate them by self-relaxation. The anxiety indicators are hereby defined as the physical reactions experienced in an anxiety-provoking environment. Immediate identification of the first signs of anxiety is the main requirement for coping with the situation in good time, in our example with the help of self-instruction and relaxation. Other techniques for coping with anxiety, such as those suggested by LAZARUS (1968) for the cognitive aspect, were also employed in the self-control training program. The fact that both of our therapy groups showed an initial anxiety reduction for the subjective variables can be accounted for by a cortical cognitive anxiety-overcoming process. Probably, the instructions and explanations given before treatment created ideal conditions for reduction of subjective anxiety characteristics. Examination of the therapeutic effects of instruction on desensitization supported this hypothesis (see OLIVEAU et al., 1969).

References

CLEVENGER, T., KING, T.R.: A factor analysis of the visible symptoms of stage fright. Speech Monographs 1961, p. 28.

DAVISON, G.C.: Systematic desensitization as a counter-conditioning process. J. Psychol. 73, 91-99 (1968).

DIXON, I.I., DE MONCHAUX, C., SANDLER, I.: Patterns of anxiety: an analysis of social anxiety. Brit. J. med. Psychol. 30, 107 (1937).

FERSTL, R.: Analyse des VELA-Fragebogens von Fahrenberg nach dem Modell von Rasch 1968. (Vervielfältigtes Manuskript: Max-Plack-Institut für Psychiatry, München 40, Kraepelinstraße 10.)

GOLDFRIED, M.R.: Systematic desensitization as training in self-control. J. consult. clin. Psychol. 37, 228-234 (1971).

GOLDFRIED, M.R., MERBAUM, M. (Eds.): Behavior Change through Self-Control. New York: Holt, Rinehart and Winston 1972, in press.

JACOBSON, E.: Anxiety and Tension Control. Philadelphia: Lippincott 1964.

KANFER, F.H.: Self-monitoring: Methodological limitations and clinical applications. J. consult. clin. Psychol. 35, 148-152 (1970).

KANFER, F.H., KAROLY, P.: Self-regulation and its clinical application: Some additional conceptualizations. In: JOHNSON, R.C., DOKECHI, P.R., MOWRER, O.H. (Eds.). Socialization: Development of Character and Conscience, p. 428-437. New York: Holt, Rinehart and Winston 1971.

LANG, P.: Fear reduction and fear behavior: Problems in treating a construct. In: SHLIEN, I.M. (Ed.). Res. Psychotherapy, Vol. 3, 90-102. Washington: American Psychological Association 1968.

LANG, P.J., LAZOVIK, A.D.: Experimental desensitization of a phobia. J. abnorm. soc. Psychol. 66, 519-525 (1963).

LAZARUS, R.S.: Emotions and adaptation: Conceptual and empirical relations. In: ARNOLD, W.I. (Ed.): Nebraska Symposium on Motivation. Lincoln: University of Nebraska Press 1968.

LEITENBERG, H., AGRAS, St., BUTZ, R., WINCZE, I.: Relationship between heart rate and behavioral change during the treatment of phobias. J. abnorm. soc. Psychol. 78, 59-68 (1971).

MILLER, H.R., NAWAS, M.M.: Control of aversive stimulus termination in systematic desensitization. Behav. Res. Ther. 7, 57-61 (1969).

OLIVEAU, D.C., AGRAS, St., LEITENBERG, H., MOORE, R.C., WRIGHT, D.E.: Systematic desensitization, therapeutically oriented instructions and selective positive reinforcement. Behav. Res. Ther. 7, 27-33 (1969).

PAUL, G.L.: Insight versus Desensitization in Psychotherapy. Stanford: Stanford University Press 1966.

PICHOT, P.: Quantifizierung der Angst. In: KIELHOLZ, P. (Ed.): Angst, p. 37-68. Bern: Huber 1967.

SACHS, L.: Statische Auswertungsmethoden, 3rd. Ed. Berlin-Heidelberg-New York: Springer 1971.

SIEGEL, S.: Nonparametric Statistics for Behavioral Science. New York: Wiley 1956.

SPIELBERGER, C.D.: Theory and research on anxiety. In: SPIELBERGER, C.D. (Ed.): Anxiety and Behavior, p. 3-20. New York, London: Academic Press 1966.

SUINN, R.M., RICHARDSON, F.: Anxiety management training: A nonspecific behavior therapy program for anxiety control. Behav. Ther. 2, 498-510 (1971).

TUNNER, W.: Zum Verlauf subjectiver, physiologischer und motorischer Reaktionen bei der Behandlung von Angststörungen durch systematische Desensibilisierung. Vortrag bei der Tagung experimentell arbeitender Psychologen, Regensburg 1972.

WINER, B.J.: Statistical Principles in Experimental Design. New York: McGraw-Hill 1962.

WOLPE, J.: Psychotherapy by Reciprocal Inhibition. Stanford: Stanford University Press 1958.

ZERSSEN, D.V., KOELLER, D.-M., REY, E.-R.: Die Befindlichkeits-Skala (B-S) - ein einfaches Instrument zur Objektivierung von Befindlichkeitsstörungen, insbesondere im Rahmen von Längsschnittuntersuchungen. Arzneimittel-Forsch. 20, 915-918 (1970).

Therapy for Smoking+

J.C. BRENGELMANN and E. SEDLMAYR

I. Acknowledgements

This experiment could not have been conducted without the help of a number of persons whose names cannot all be listed here. Particular thanks are due to the therapists, Renate de Jong, Roland Knebusch, Marina Kolb, Sibylle Kraemer, Sonnhild Schiöberg and Gerda Weck. Ronald Ramsay and Fred Kanfer helped in the training and discussions with the therapists. Gerhard Henrich, Norbert Mai, Dirk Revenstorff and Manfred Tettweiler were responsible for the statistical analyses. Finally Ellen Anderson, Friederike Wildhager and Gerlinde Winter gave much of their time for secretarial assistance.

Grateful acknowledgement is due to Uni-Chemie AG, Zürich, who generously supplied the lobeline and placebo capsules.

II. Justification of the Project

Smoking is a recognized health problem of major proportions. Attempts to reduce this problem need no particular justification, and studies on the modification of smoking behaviour are appearing at an increasing rate. OBER (1968) used operant, aversion and transactional treatment. At the end of a one-month follow-up period he found that the smoking rate was lower in all 3 treatment conditions than in a control group, but found no significant differences between the treatments. According to WHITMAN (1969), information on the harmful effects of smoking, aversion and self-control produced a significant reduction in smoking, but also in the control group. It was suggested that extratherapeutic variables were operating. WAGNER and BRAGG (1970) found significant differences between various kinds of treatment. A combination of systematic desensitization and covert sensitization proved superior throughout treatment.

Such inconsistencies in reports appear to be the rule if one follows the reviews by LICHTENSTEIN (1971) and MAUSNER (1971), who emphasize the general ineffectiveness of all kinds of therapies. BERNSTEIN (1969) comes to the conclusion that research in terms of design and method must be thoroughly upgraded and that a better theoretical understanding of the behavioural processes involved is needed if we are to develop effective treatment techniques.

+ The support of the project by the "Bundeszentrale für gesundheitliche Aufklärung" is gratefully acknowledged.

The present experiment was designed to eliminate some of the major points of criticism frequently levelled against the methodological weaknesses encountered in research on the modification of the smoking habit. (1) A number of different therapies are employed for comparison. (2) Long-term effects of treatment and maintenance of nonsmoking are investigated. Instead of the customary short-term before-and-after design, treatment effects are closely followed over a period of almost 5 months. Follow-up is going to extend to one year. (3) The dependent variable 'rate of smoking' is expressed in terms of the number of cigarettes consumed instead of the unsatisfactory change scores, frequently reported on a percentage basis. (4) A number of therapists are used and are rotated between treatment sessions. (5) Multiple baselines are used. (6) Several control groups are employed. (7) Motivational and volunteer effects are checked. (8) A defosit is used to restrain subject attrition.

III. Aims of the Experiment

The main aims of this experiment are: (1) to compare the relative effectiveness of various kinds of therapies, (2) to investigate the dynamics of maintenance of nonsmoking and of relapse, and (3) to assess the determinants of rate of smoking in terms of personality, socioeconomic variables and individual differences with regard to smoking behaviour and attitudes towards smoking.

The present report is limited to a period of investigation of about 5 months. Only a broad outline of results can be given here.

IV. Methodology

1. Subject Selection

In response to 11 small newspaper advertisements and notices posted on the boards of 44 firms, a total of 1100 persons showed interest in the treatment for smoking. These persons were informed that extensive testing would take place prior to treatment and that a sum of DM 100,- would have to be deposited for the entire duration of the experiment.

Of the 436 persons who appeared for testing and had kept daily records for a week of the number of cigarettes smoked, 416 were accepted for treatment. After the last therapeutic session, i.e. after just over 5 months, 354 clients had complied with the requirements, except for occasional missing data. This represents a drop-out rate of 15 %.

The two selection criteria employed were a minimum daily consumption of 20 cigarettes and absence of acute medical symptoms, except for complaints due to smoking. There were no limitations as to age or sex. A detailed description of the clients is given below.

2. Training of Therapists

There were 10 therapists in all: 6 who carried the main burden of conducting the psychological therapies, 2 substitute therapists, and a doctor and medical assistant who were responsible for the medical treatment. Half of the psychological therapists were newly graduated psychologists, the other half psychology students. Their acquaintance with behaviour therapy was minimal to modest. Apart from other preparations, the therapists attended a one-week training course before the beginning of the experiment. This was conducted by Dr. Ramsay of Amsterdam.

During the course of treatment a one-day discussion on therapeutic issues was held with Dr. Kanfer of Cincinnati. There were, of course, more or less informal discussions throughout therapy.

3. Therapies

The 9 treatments used are shown in Table 1. During 10 treatment and 3 baseline weeks the number of cigarettes smoked was recorded daily. The controls supplied their data by mail, and the only contact with the control group was before treatment when the Ss were tested in groups of more than 100 persons each. However, it was expected that the recording of cigarette consumption alone would reduce the rate of smoking, as this is one technique frequently used as a measure of self-control. Therefore, a second minimum-contact control group was used. These persons telephoned their baseline data before and after the treatment phase, and they will be asked again after a year, on completion of therapy. There was no other contact except to say that they were on a waiting list and were promised treatment at a later date. This group is not considered in the present analysis.

Placebo and lobeline pills were administerd following a double-blind procedure and in a decreasing fashion. Therapists and subjects (Ss) were not informed about the identity of the pills. The doctors were restricted to discussing problems of physical health, particularly those due to smoking, but they were instructed to refrain from exerting any undue suggestive influence as to the effectiveness of this kind of treatment. Incidentally, this was a general rule for all

Table 1. Treatments used in the smoking experiments

Treatment	N clients
Control	29
Placebo	26
Medical (lobeline)	27
Psychotherapy	40
Covert sensitization	45
Negative practise	48
Electric aversion	41
Self-control	46
Self-control + elec. aversion	52
Total N	354

treatments, with the exception of the control condition; they were presented as being of equal potential therapeutic efficacy.

While placebo was mainly intended to serve as a control for lobeline, Rogerian non-directive psychotherapy - in whatever fashion we were able to approximate this form of treatment - was used as a control for the behaviour therapies. The therapists provided no direct practical leads for combating smoking but clients proved to be very directive and inventive in dealing with their problem. Due to the particular laissez faire procedure used, they formed the closest group, exchanged vows of non-smoking, gave reminders by telephone and used other methods of control. Further, all psychological problems other than those due to smoking were discussed in a friendly and understanding, though non-directive atmosphere. During covert sensitization clients were relaxed, typical smoking behaviour was imagined and counterconditioned by means of two aversive stimuli: (*a*) feelings of sickness and nausea and (*b*) images of lung cancer due to smoking.

Negative practise required the clients to inhale at 10-sec intervals, signalled by the beat of a metronome. The procedure lasted for 30 min and was carried out in a small, tightly closed room. A number of clients were in fact sick.

For electric aversion the act of smoking was divided into a number of steps, ranging from reaching for a pack of cigarettes to actual smoking. These steps were contingently and non-contingently counterconditioned with 28 electric shocks per session according to a particular design.

For self-control, 37 items were constructed, intended to interfere with smoking, such as changing the make of cigarette, and delaying or omitting smoking at certain times or places. These items were presented in a hierarchic order of difficulty and had to be followed in standard fashion by all individuals.

Finally, self-control and electric aversion procedures were combined in one group. Aversion was added to self-control after the 6th treatment week. The expectation was that smokers would be relatively more dependent on the last few cigarettes, and that aversion would significantly contribute to breaking the habit.

The therapies were carried out in groups of about 8 clients. Therapy designs were variable but schedules were kept constant for individuals. The duration of the sessions also varied from about 20 to 45 minutes, depending on the requirements of each therapy. Care was taken to conduct each kind of therapy according to instructions in order to minimize the intrusion of unwanted therapeutic elements, particularly uncontrolled suggestive influence.

4. Predictors

A broadly based attempt was made to investigate possible determinants of smoking. For simplicity, only the major score categories are listed in Table 2. Some of the questionnaires were given several times in the course of the experiment, so that the total number of scores actually employed is well above 80. Further questionnaires concerning the motivation for treatment, as well as attitudes towards various aspects of treatment were also given but have not been analysed as yet.

The scales of smoking behaviour and attitudes towards smoking were specially assembled and analysed for the present purpose. Except for 'smoking personality', the various personality scores are derived from

Table 2. Score categories

Predictors	Number of scores or factors
Scale of smoking behaviour (183 items)	8
Scale of smoking attitudes (140 items)	5
Positive and negative achievement motivation	5
Positive and negative achievement anxiety	3
Extreme, unrealistic achievement orientation	4
Neuroticism	1
Extraversion	1
Smoking personality	4
Rigidity	3
Intelligence (Progressive Matrices)	1
Age	1
Sex	1
Socio-economic status	6
Subtotal	43
Smoking criteria	
Weekly number of cigarettes before and during therapy	13
Total	56

questionnaires developed in recent years. (Most of these scales await publication but specimens can be supplied.) They have been extensively employed in learning and achievement experiments, both in the laboratory and in the field. The neuroticism and extraversion scales are quite similar to the corresponding Eysenckian scales. 'Smoking personality' was constructed ad hoc in the form of an adjective check list: clients attributed positively and negatively toned adjectives to an assumed 'smoking personality'. Scores concerning the directionality and intensity of these attributes were derived.

The scores discussed above are either unrelated or correlate with each other at a fairly low level.

5. Smoking Criteria

For 13 weeks daily records were kept of the number of cigarettes consumed, and these were turned into 13 smoking scores, to which we will refer repeatedly.

6. Experimental Design

The general design of the experiment is shown in Fig. 1: 16 therapy sessions were carried out over a 21-week period. For 6 weeks there

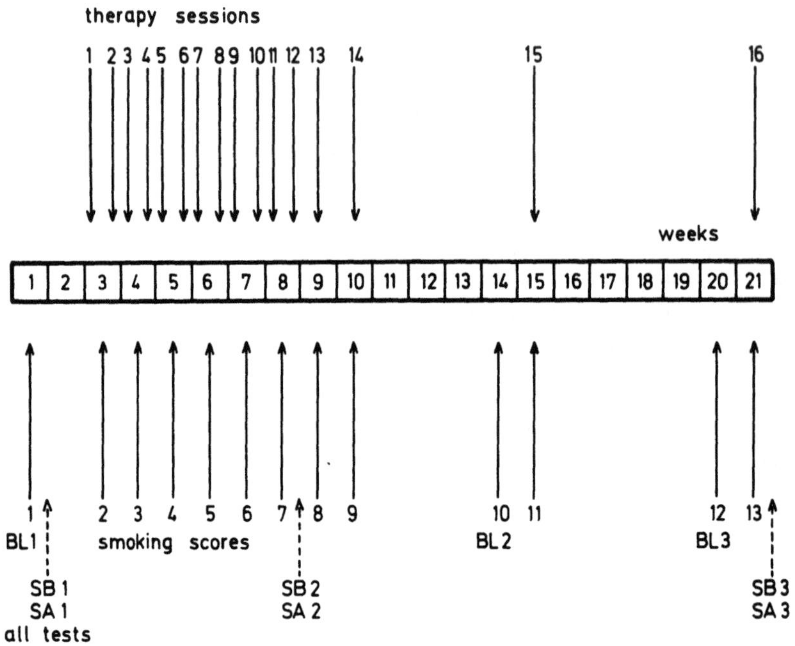

Fig. 1. Design of experiment. BL = baseline, SB = smoking behaviour, SA = smoking attitude

were 2 sessions a week, followed by 2 weekly (sessions 13, 14) and 2 monthly (sessions 15, 16) booster sessions.

The derivation of the 13 smoking scores is shown at the bottom. Ten of these were constructed for the weeks in which treatment took place. The remaining 3 represent baseline scores, one of which was collected before the start of treatment (BL 1), the other 2 being intermediate baselines (BL 2, 3) for the last 2 booster sessions.

It is further noted that, after collecting the first set of baseline data (BL 1), all persons fulfilling the requirements for therapy were invited to take the tests already described. Of these, the smoking behaviour (SB) and smoking attitude (SA) scales were given 3 times because they were expected to correlate more highly with changes in the smoking score than would the other scales.

7. Description of Subjects

The mean age of the Ss was 38.5 years (range from 17 to 70 years). There were 256 males and 99 females. Intelligence was somewhat above the general population mean, the Progressive Matrices raw score being 47.0 (SD = 9.6). Inspection of the personality and socio-economic scores reveals this group to be close to the normal average with regard to neuroticism and extraversion, and to be less extreme and dogmatic with regard to various attitudinal scores. Educational level and other criteria show this group to be socio-economically above the average of the general population mean.

The following 3 tables provide some insights into the motivational characteristics of our sample. Table 3 shows the main reasons for wanting to stop smoking.

Table 3. Reasons for wanting to stop smoking: N = 354

Reasons	% Ss
Health (fear of smoking disease, other current illnesses)	65.0
Financial	9.0
Attitudes (dependency, weakness of will, senselessness)	8.6
Social factors (partner non-smoker, social reproaches)	5.6
Other (sport activities, newspaper ads and reports)	11.8
	100.0

Health reasons account for about two thirds of all the reasons given. Beyond that, financial considerations, certain attitudes towards smoking, and the influence exerted by social partners account for most of the rest.

Table 4 shows the preferred means devised by the Ss themselves to end smoking.

A surprisingly large number of clients have turned to pharmaceutical therapy. Will power and the use of substitutes score relatively highly while only 10 % admit to ever having planned self-help procedures in any systematic fashion. Thus, the bulk of the population chooses or devises means of stopping smoking that are largely inefficient or if

Table 4. Preferred methods to end smoking as devised by the Ss themselves: N = 354

Means	% Ss
Medical therapy (drugs)	50.0
Will power, resoluteness, vows	19.6
Substitutes[a)] (e.g. sweets, chewing gum)	13.3
Planned gradual or abrupt stopping	10.0
Psychotherapy	2.2
Other (e.g. illness, vacation)	4.8
	99.9

a) By means of eating (69.6 %), drinking (11.8 %), more work or rest (9.8 %), and others (8.8 %).

sucessful, yield only short-lasting succes. About 61 % of all the Ss had tried more than one method.

Finally, Table 5 reveals the strength of motivation to stop smoking. It may be remembered that the clients had to pass through a comprehensive rigmarole of testing and other demands before they finally received treatment. A large number of weakly motivated persons may thus have dropped out already before treatment. Those actually entering treatment are highly motivated, as Table 5 indicates.

Table 5. Strength of motivation to stop smoking: N = 354

Strength of Motivation	% Ss
I have definitely decided and am sure to succeed	20.1
I have definitely decided and shall at least succeed somewhat	30.6
I shall honestly try but fear that I will not succeed completely	41.1
I shall try but my will is weak	7.9
I am curious to experience the therapy but am not really prepared to stop smoking	0.3
	100.0

Practically all the Ss appear to be honestly cooperative and half of the sample expect to succeed acceptably. Only 8 % have grave doubts as to success. These data have not as yet been correlated with actual smoking behaviour or therapeutic success, but they will be.

Of interest to some may be the life curve of smoking exhibited in Fig. 2.

This curve represents the number of cigarettes smoked daily during the entire lifetime and as noted in retrospect by all the clients whose mean age was 38.5 years (range 17 to 70). The curve is typical except that the peak is reached somewhat later than usual and that the intensity level thereafter drops relatively slowly, relative, that is, to the general population mean. The last 4 points of measurement comprise 87 % of the sample. For these, the variation with age in number of cigarettes smoked does not seem unduly great. This limits the possible effects that age may exert on smoking in this particular study.

8. Volunteer Characteristics

In a separate study by G. WECK (1972) 'normal' smokers selected at random from the general population were compared with our volunteer Ss. There were marked differences in attitude. Typical attitudes of the 'normals' are that smoking is a rather positive experience; that it is not as dangerous as it is frequently said to be; that the smoker is particularly well liked and that, in case of illness, the chances of recovery are good.

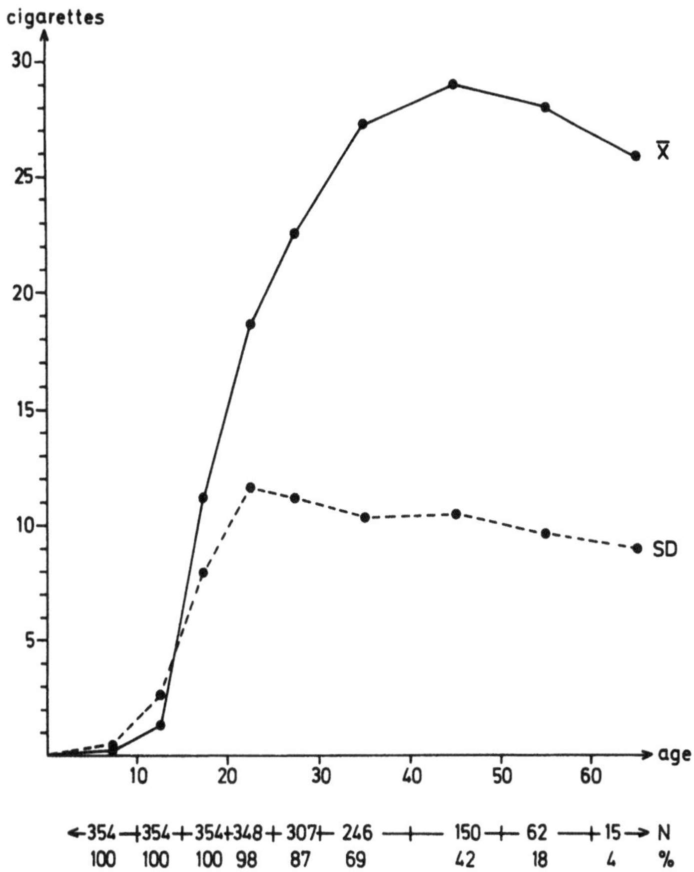

Fig. 2. Life curve of cigarette consumption

The volunteers in our experiment appear to be more apprehensive and uneasy. They admit to the dangers to health, to the dependency on the cigarette in stressful and social situations, they do not believe that the smoker is the 'good guy', or that the cigarette does indeed ease social relationships.

V. Results

Results are analysed in two main sections: rate of smoking and correlates of smoking.

1. Rate of Smoking

The complex design shows that the results may be analysed in a number of ways. We shall confine ourselves to 5 points: general and specific treatment effects, curve dynamics, standard deviations and individual differences. The means are shown in Fig. 3 separately for the 9 treatment groups. Because space is limited, results are discussed in broad terms only.

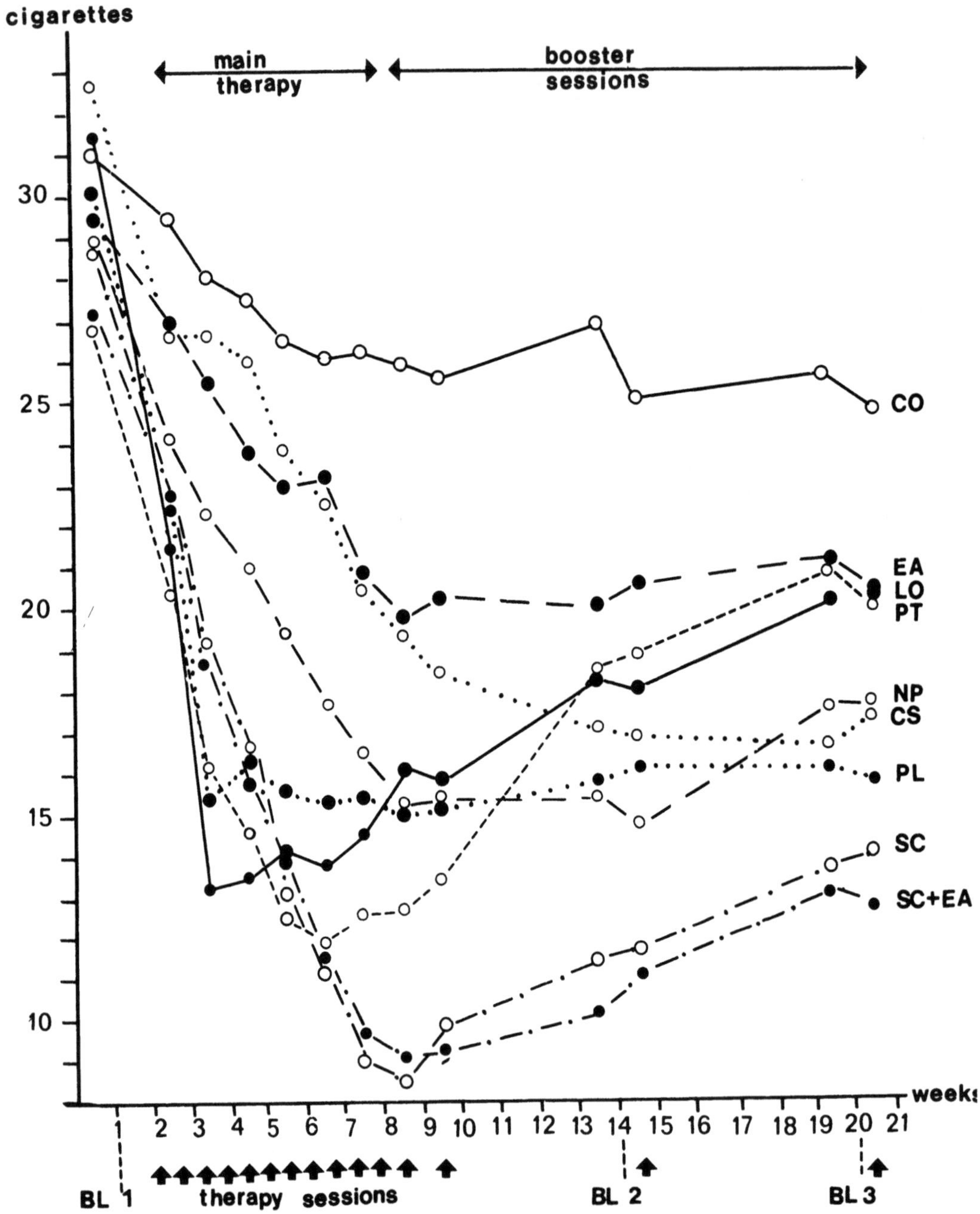

Fig. 3. Mean number of cigarettes smoked daily. CO = control group, CS = covert sensitization, EA = electric aversion, LO = lobeline, NP = negative practise, PL = placebo, PT = psychotherapy, SC = self-control

Fig. 3 provides the general impression (a) that the number of cigarettes smoked before the beginning of the experiment (BL 1) is greatly reduced during the time of the main therapy, (b) that this reduction is apparently greatest at about the end of the main therapy phase, and (c) that, in the overall picture, the rate of smoking gradually increases again over the following 3 months. The booster session of week 15 shows no appreciable effect, while that of week 21 shows some tendency to improvement, or at least to slowing down the rate of relapse. This would suggest that renewed treatment effort will be the more effective the greater the relapse.

Multivariate analysis showed the overall therapeutic change to be highly significant. For the present purpose, we confine ourselves to demonstrating the between-group F ratios pertaining to the 13 smoking scores (Table 6). These will reveal the general trend of significance as it develops during the course of therapy.

Before treatment (BL 1) the between-group differences are not significant. Thus, randomized allocation of clients to the therapies has produced the desired effect of equating the groups for rate of smoking. The significance of differences increases markedly until the end of the main therapy phase and decreases thereafter. The significance of differentiaion then closely follows the observations already made by mere inspection.

With regard to specific treatment effects, all groups are significantly different from the control group. A number of significant differences between treatments were obtained and these follow, by and large, the trends of means.

The 2 self-control groups are superior to and significantly different from all other forms of treatment. The 3 aversive therapies are significantly different from each other. They are clearly inferior to

Table 6. Differentiation of treatment groups at various time points of treatment by means of analysis of variance (DF = 8/346). Main therapy = 2 treatments per week. Booster = one single treatment

	Treatment week	Smoking score	F Ratio	Significance
Baseline 1	1	1	1.517	NS
	3	2	4.709	0.1 %
	4	3	8.492	0.1 %
Main	5	4	8.279	0.1 %
Therapy	6	5	8.937	0.1 %
	7	6	11.463	0.1 %
	8	7	10.411	0.1 %
Booster	9	8	8.748	0.1 %
Booster	10	9	6.967	0.1 %
Baseline 2	14	10	5.695	0.1 %
Booster	15	11	4.789	0.1 %
Baseline 3	20	12	3.698	0.1 %
Booster	21	13	3.175	1.0 %

NS = not significant

self-control and, at various time points, they are also significantly different from each other. Negative practise fares best, followed by covert sensitization and electric aversion.

The aspect of individual curve dynamics yields particularly interesting insights. Continuous recording of every cigarette smoked leads to gradual and long-drawn-out reduction. The effects of booster sessions 2 and 3 are noticeable. The remaining groups come out as follows. The two medical treatments (lobeline and placebo) show the most rapid initial gains, closely followed by psychotherapy. However, the efficacy of these therapies stops early, i.e. already during the main therapy phase and despite continued treatment. The relapse rate for the lobeline and psychotherapy groups is strikingly high.

All the behaviour therapy groups behave differently in this respect. Their rate of reduction in the number of cigarettes smoked continues to the end of the main therapy. From then on, the self-control groups show a distinct relapse while the 3 aversive treatment groups tend towards maintenance of behaviour. Nevertheless, the self-control therapies remain the most efficient.

Individual variation as measured by the standard deviation of the number of cigarettes smoked is referred to only briefly. The results are shown in Fig. 4.

Generally speaking, there is considerable variation in the treatment response of individuals which deserves further clarification in the light of the therapies used, as well as with regard to the characteristics of smoking behaviour and attitudes towards smoking. Inspection of Fig. 4 reveals a distinct tendency towards increase in standard deviation during the latter part of the experiment, while the behaviour of the curves is rather variable during the main therapy phase. Interestingly, with the exception of psychotherapy, standard deviation decreases with the success of therapy, as a comparison of Fig. 3 and 4 shows. This may indicate that successful therapies influence the smoking behaviour of people in general while less efficient therapies are more successful with some individuals and less successful with others. The lesson of this would be not to discard less successful therapies outright but to investigate the type of individual responding, and to use such therapies alone or in combination with other treatment forms in particular cases.

2. Correlates of Smoking

Results with regard to personality as measured by traditional personality questionnaires are not very satisfactory. Extraversion tends towards positive correlation, and various factors of achievement motivation, as well as rigidity, tend towards negative correlation with the rate of smoking. Neuroticism shows no significant relationship. Although some of the relationships are statistically significant, they are generally very low and are, for that reason, not further discussed in this context. This is also true for IQ and socio-economic factors.

The questionnaires concerning smoking behaviour and smoking attitudes (Table 2) were factor analysed and subjected to varimax rotation. The 183 items of smoking behaviour yielded 15 factors which covered 40 % of the variance. The first 8 factors were interpreted, and these covered more than 28 % of the variance. The 140 items concerning attitudes towards smoking yielded 15 factors for 50 % of the variance. The 5 factors retained explain about 33 % of the variance. The factors were named and correlated with the smoking scores, as shown in Table 7. The coefficients indicate optimal degrees of correlation as reached during

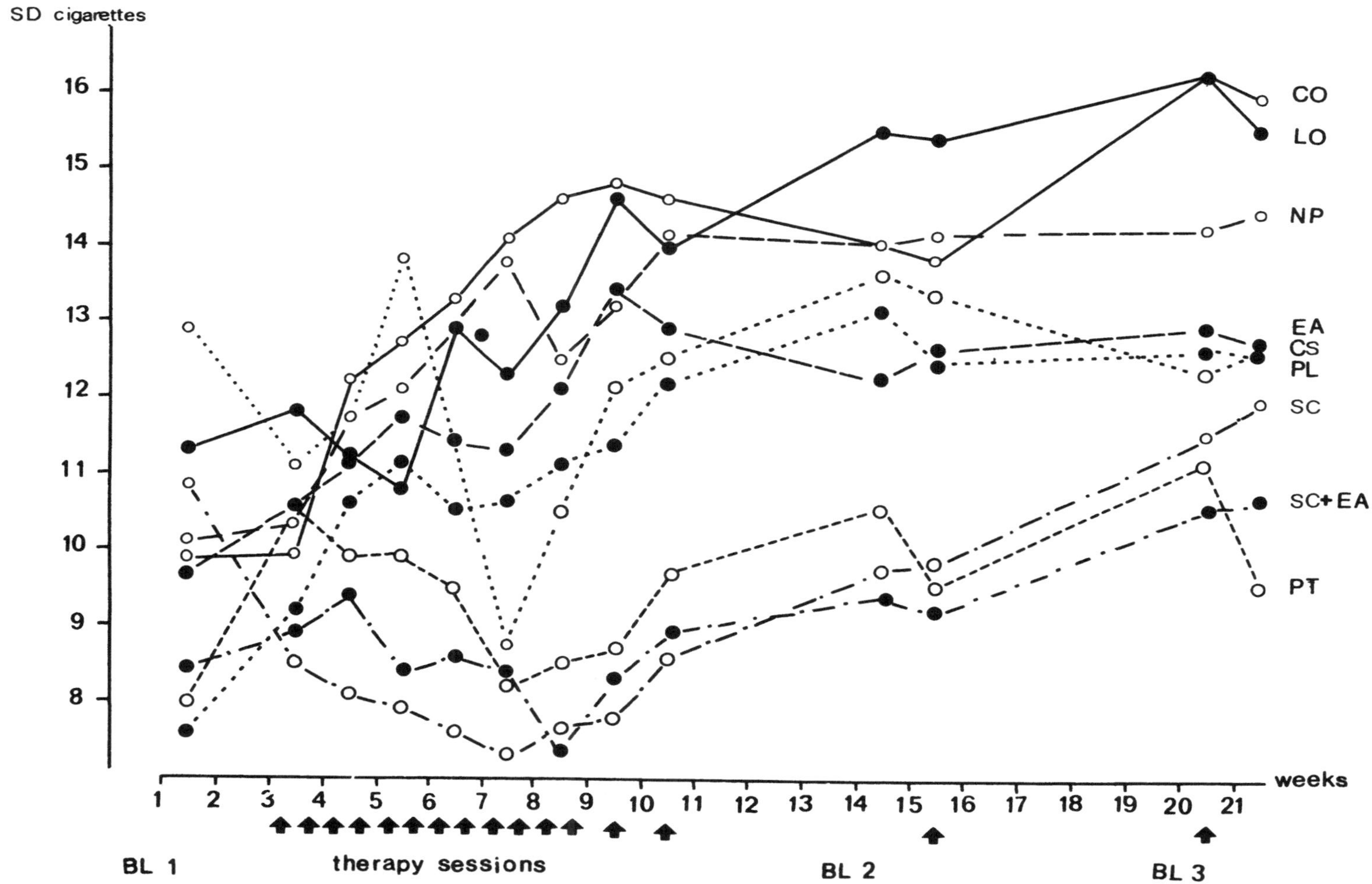

Fig. 4. Standard deviation of the number of cigarettes smoked daily. For abbreviations, see Fig. 3

the present experiment. (The degree of relationship is dependent on the time point of measurement, but this cannot be discussed here.)

To be emotionally dependent on smoking (1), to smoke compulsively (7), to stick to preferred makes and tastes (3), and to smoke anything that comes along (6) are the SB factors that correlate highest with rate of smoking. For the SA factors the belief that people smoke mostly because of stress (2) correlates highest with actual smoking. The two danger factors (SB 2, SA 1) also correlate positively with smoking, while to smoke irregularly (SB 8) and to be intolerant of smoking (SA 4) correlates negatively with smoking. The conclusion is that a number of behavioural and attitudinal factors correlate independently with smoking.

It is obvious that such factors may affect treatment response. Suppose one treatment group contained a number of persons highly emotionally dependent on cigarettes and another group did not, then the chances of successful therapy might be lowest for the first group. We therefore analysed the differences in SB factor scores between treatments and found no significant pre-treatment difference to speak of. However, the response to the SB factors varied significantly as a result of the degree of success that each therapy could secure for itself. These results will be reported separately.

VI. Discussion and Conclusions

All treatments, including the mere recording of cigarettes smoked (control group), yield a significant reduction in smoking. Individual treatment curves vary to an extreme degree.

Table 7. Factors of smoking behaviour and attitude towards smoking (20 items per factor with loadings ranging from 24 to 71)

Factor	Designation	Correlation with smoking
Smoking behaviour (SB)		
1	emotional dependency	0.53
2	danger to health	0.24
3	preference for make and taste	0.37
4	social assertiveness	0.11
5	leisure-time smoker	0.15
6	all-round smoker	0.34
7	compulsive smoker	0.51
8	irregular smoker	-0.22
Smoking attitudes (SA)		
1	smoking is dangerous	0.23
2	people smoke because of stress	0.47
3	smoking is not all that bad	0.11
4	intolerance (smoking to be curbed)	-0.20
5	imitation (people imitate smoking)	-0.05

Significant differences between these curves have been obtained. They are most economically described in terms of efficacy and time. On a longer-term basis, the self-control method clearly proved superior, followed by the aversive therapies as a group and, finally, by the other groups (psychotherapy, lobeline, control group). Further follow-up will show whether this constellation is maintained.

With regard to the onset of therapeutic efficacy, the fastest response is noted for biochemical treatment (lobeline, placebo) and for psychotherapy, while all the behaviour therapies develop more slowly. Two aspects need discussion here: firstly, that this fast initial effect is seen with very different kinds of treatment and, secondly, that this effect is short-lasting. Relapse occurs early despite continued treatment while, for the behaviour therapies, improvement continues at least for as long as treatment is given.

A number of factors unspecific with regard to the treatment given, but more preponderant in the non-behavioural than in the behavioural group of treatments, may be responsible for the foregoing result. Factors such as commitment to therapy, motivation to improve, certain forms of self-contracting, unspecific group experiences, the mechanics of coming to the treatment center, the experience of meeting new people and new ideas, the pleasure of interesting discussions, diverse other suggestible influences and/or differential expectancies with regard to medical, psychotherapeutic and behaviouristic therapies may account for the differences. We are not able to track down the effective components at the present time, but early relapse or cessation of improvement suggests that 'placebo' or other unspecific effects are massively involved in the non-behavioural treatment groups. The behavioural therapies are certainly less familiar, in part strange and even repellent to some, as may be the case with regard to electric aversion. This therapy indeed shows the slowest treatment response. All aversive measures are characterized by slowness of response. This may be the combined effect of low expectancy and reinforcement values for a relatively large number of persons, though by no means of all.

There is no point in discussing the fact that the effective treatment components are not known for any of the therapies, and that consequently, there can be no reasonable basis for comparison. This would be labouring the obvious. To investigate these treatment components is a necessary and surely rewarding task. It might yield better theoretical insight into the mechanics of therapies. On the other hand, it may be equally worthwhile to improve therapeutic efficacy by combining several forms of treatment, such as placebo with self-control coupled with covert sensitization (in that order). It would be interesting to see whether the non-smoking behaviour of former heavy smokers can be maintained under prolonged behavioural treatment conditions, whether smoking behaviour can be brought under complete control, whether the degree of relapse in this first experiment determines the treatment response of the same individuals in a subsequent experiment, or what the contingencies are for non-yielders to prolonged treatment.

The fact that teachable therapies such as self-control and covert sensitization are among the most efficient means of influencing smoking holds promise. It may be possible to offer such treatments to a large number of clients by teaching them how to become their own therapists. This could perhaps be achieved with a minimum amount of personal contact with the therapist.

VII. Summary

A sample of 350 persons who smoked at least 20 cigarettes a day were treated by means of self-control (self-control only, self-control coupled with electric aversion), aversion (electric aversion, negative practise, covert sensitization) and non-behaviouristic therapies (psychotherapy, lobeline, placebo). A no-treatment control group was used. During the main therapy phase 12 treatments were given in 6 weeks, followed by 4 booster sessions in another period of 13 weeks. Initially, there were strong positive treatment responses in the case of the non-behavioural techniques. These quickly subsided and considerable relapse occurred, even during the main therapy phase. In the long run the behavioural techniques proved superior, particularly self-control. Factors of smoking behaviour and attitudes towards smoking correlate differentially with rate of smoking.

References

BERNSTEIN, D.A.: Modification of smoking behavior: an evaluative review. Psychol. Bull. 71, 418-440 (1969).

LICHTENSTEIN, E.: Modification of smoking behavior: good designs - ineffective treatments. J. consult. clin. Psychol. 36, 163-166 (1971).

MAUSNER, B.: Some comments on the failure of behavior therapy as a technique for modifying cigarette smoking. J. consult. clin. Psychol. 36, 167-170 (1971).

OBER, D.C.: Modification of smoking behavior. J. consult. clin. Psychol. 32, 543-549 (1968).

WAGNER, M.K., BRAGG, R.A.: Comparing behavior modification approaches to habit decrement-smoking. J. consult. clin. Psychol. 34, 258-263 (1970).

WECK, GERDA: Die Veränderung von Einstellungen zum Rauchen bei der Rauchertherapie. Diploma of Psychology Thesis, 1972 (unpubl.).

WHITMAN, T.L.: Modification of chronic smoking behavior: a comparison of three approaches. Behav. Res. Ther. 7, 257-263 (1969).

Self-Control Techniques and Obesity

R.W. RAMSAY and J. JONGMANS

I. Introduction

In the literature of behaviour therapy more and more emphasis is being placed on self-control techniques. The aim of these techniques is to enhance the effectiveness of the therapy by actively involving the client in effecting changes, to speed the therapy by giving the client the means to continue without the therapist, and to give the client the tools to deal with the possible future development of maladaptive behaviour. The client in effect learns to be his own therapist. CAUTELA (1969) and KANFER and PHILLIPS (1970, Chap. 9) describe the concept of self-control, its advantages and possible disadvantages, and some of the techniques for applying self-control in systematic desensitization, thought-stopping, covert sensitization, assertive training, and operant procedures. BANDURA (1969, pp. 584-587) discusses the importance of symbolic control in self-regulating or self-control techniques. GOLDFRIED (1971) gives a good account of how systematic desensitization can be made more effective by including self-control. The purpose here is not to give a general review of the techniques, not to go into the theoretical discussions of PREMACK's (1959) principle or HOMME's (1965) further elaboration of the PREMACK principle. This account reports some practical applications of self-control and other techniques in two experiments dealing with the problem of obesity.

II. Obesity

SCHACHTER (1971) in a delightful article entitled "Some extraordinary facts about obese humans and rats" gives some theoretical and experimental findings on obesity. STUART (1971) states that at least one in every 5 Americans is overweight. From a survey of various studies, he concludes that "most obesities can be attributed to an excess of food intake beyond the demands of energy expenditure, and a major objective in treating obesity is a reduction in the amount of excess food consumed".

The problem is how to reduce the amount consumed. Obese people obviously cannot manage this by themselves; if they could, they would not be obese. Therefore they need help. STUNKARD and McLAREN-HUME (1959) observed "most obese persons will not stay in treatment of obesity. Of those who stay in treatment most will not lose weight and of those who lose weight, most will regain it". They go further and conclude that "the results of treatment for obesity are remarkably similar and remarkably poor". STUART (1971) surveys some of the most recent reports of therapy, and concludes that "behaviour therapy has offered greater promise of positive results than any other type of treatment". PENICK et al. (1971) come to a similar conclusion. Thus the dismal prospects for the obese person seem to be brightening, and this article deals with two experiments based on STUART's (1967) pioneering work, which provide further support for optimism.

III. Experiment I

In this experiment there were 5 groups: group A was taught the behavioural control techniques, group B, behavioural control plus additional information on good eating habits, group C was given covert sensitization, group D, non-therapy with therapist contact, and group E formed the control with no therapist contact.

1. Subjects

Subjects (Ss) were recruited by placing an advertisement in an university building, asking for volunteers for an experiment on slimming. Of 55 who originally applied, 6 dropped out due to sickness, lack of motivation and holidays. Of the remaining 49, 12 were men and 37 were women. They were mainly students, but there were also some housewives, secretaries and faculty members. They were randomly assigned to groups, 10 per group for A, B, C and E, and 9 in D. In the follow-up there were further drop-outs; numbers are given in the results.

2. Therapists

The 5 therapists (Ts) were all undergraduate students in psychology engaged in a group research project under the supervision of the senior author. They were trained in the relevant techniques but were not qualified or experienced therapists. Each T treated two Ss from each group, so that differences between groups could not be due to differences between therapists.

3. Group A

This group followed almost exactly STUART's (1967) behavioural control programme. This consists of a number of steps to be followed by the S, each step in itself easy to follow, but designed to disrupt the maladaptive habits of overeating, to make the S aware of his or her behaviour and to bring this behaviour under the S's own control. Details can be obtained from STUART's original article.

4. Group B

This group was similar to Group A in that the Ss received the behavioural control programme, but in addition they were given information concerning good eating habits. They received a pamphlet issued by a government department, which contains tables of calorific values for all types of food. This booklet was discussed with the Ss, and they were encouraged to alter their behaviour in accordance with what they learned. For example, fats contain about 900 calories per 100 grammes, so that peanuts and potato chips should be avoided. Low calorific value foods should as much as possible be substituted for high calorific value foods: eating an apple (± 40 calories) instead of a cream cake (± 450 calories) would give the same bulk. In this way, the Ss could regulate their food intake, without going on a rigid diet and without depriving themselves of food.

5. Group C

This group was given covert sensitization. During the first sitting the Ss were informed about the purpose of the experiment and were told that in many cases of overweight there is usually only trouble with certain types of food. For example, some people when confronted with a dish of peanuts will eat compulsively until the dish is empty. They then feel guilty and upset about not resisting the temptation to eat something which they know does their weight problem no good. The Ss were asked which foods they considered caused them trouble, and small hierarchies were constructed for a maximum of 3 foods. A hierarchy for chocolates might consist of: (1) walking along the street and looking in a shop window; (2) entering the shop and smelling the chocolates; (3) looking at the chocolates and ordering some; (4) taking a chocolate in the hand, looking at it, and being about to eat it.

The therapy, spread over 10 sittings, was as follows: the S was trained to relax for about 5 min at the beginning of the session, then asked to imagine an item from the hierarchy, and then suggestions were given of feeling sick. The suggestions were as vivid as possible, given for about 20 sec, and then the S was asked to imagine turning away, resisting the urge to eat, and feeling once again calm and relaxed. Most Ss during the first sitting or two gave no response to the suggestions and found the whole situation amusing. However, as therapy continued, they found that they were responding more, and with some Ss it was necessary to tone down the suggestions and to have a receptacle handy.

6. Group D

This was an attention-control group. The Ts were instructed to be non-directive, to encourage talk about the problem, but to give no instructions or suggestions: all had to come from the S. To minimize the Rosenthal effect the Ts were given to understand that this was true Rogerian therapy (an insult to Rogers, and our apologies) and that this form of therapy could be very effective. Some Ss took it seriously and devised quite adequate techniques, others talked the whole time about food, how much they enjoyed eating, exchanged recipes with the T, and gained weight during the therapy.

7. Group E

This was the non-contact control group. The Ss were asked for their weight at the beginning of the therapy and were then told that due to lack of therapists it would be impossible to treat them. They were contacted again at the end of the therapy period and for follow-up.

8. Duration of the Experiment

The therapy lasted 5 weeks. All Ss in the T-contact groups A to D were seen individually twice a week for 20 to 30 minutes. First and second follow-ups were conducted at 10 weeks and 24 weeks after the end of therapy.

9. Results

The follow-up figures of the results do not give accurate information about a particular therapy due to confusion. Many Ss were dissatisfied with their form of treatment, and the senior author was forced to give a lecture at the end of therapy to all who wanted to attend. In the follow-ups the Ss were asked if they had used the behaviour control techniques on a do-it-yourself basis, and two Ss from group D said that they had done so. The results are given below, including and excluding these Ss.

There were no significant differences in weight between the groups at the beginning of the experiment ($F = 1.37$; d.f. = 4 & 44; $p > .05$). The difference in weight between before and after therapy showed no significant differences between groups ($F = 1.50$; d.f. = 4 & 44; $p > .05$) but there was a highly significant difference due to the factor 'time' ($F = 81.07$; d.f. = 1 & 44; $p < .005$) and there was a highly significant 'groups X time' interaction ($F = 5.35$; d.f. = 4 & 44; $p < .005$).

The linear trend interaction of the 'groups X time' was also highly significant ($F = 4.08$; d.f. = 3 & 315; $p < .01$). Thus there was a difference between the groups in terms of the rate at which they lost weight. Scheffé's test for comparisons between groups gave significant differences for the behaviour therapy groups A, B and C vs. control groups D and E ($p < .05$).

Table 1. Average reduction in weight (in kg) at end of therapy (E), and at follow-up: F_1 10 weeks after therapy, and F_2 24 weeks after therapy. The number of Ss is given in brackets below the weight

Group	E	F_1	F_2
Group A	2.47	3.35	2.20
Behavioural control	(10)	(8)	(9)
Group B	2.07	2.54	4.50
Behavioural control	(10)	(10)	(9)
plus eating tips			
Group C	2.00	2.54	2.11
Covert sensitization	(10)	(9)	(9)
Group D	1.29	2.10	3.77
Therapist contact	(9)	(5)	(8)
control			1.99
			(6)
Group E	0.11	-0.40	-0.22
Control	(10)	(4)	(9)

Table 1 shows the average weight loss per group after therapy and at first and second follow-up. No statistical tests were done for these figures because of the different numbers in each group, and because, as mentioned earlier, the treatments are confused in the follow-up. The two Ss in group D had lost 19 and 17 1/2 lbs by the second follow-up. The second set of figures for group D in the last column give the mean for the group with these two Ss excluded.

IV. Experiment II

In this experiment there were 4 groups - a behavioural control group with T contact, a behavioural control group without T contact (by mail), a diet group, and a control group. The therapy was scheduled to last for 4 weeks with follow-ups approximately 6 weeks and 6 months after therapy.

1. Therapist

The T (H.J.) was a graduate student in psychology. Other than participation in the first experiment he had no experience in behaviour therapy.

2. Subjects

The Ss were recruited by placing notices in shops and laundromats in the city (Amsterdam) inviting anyone who was overweight to participate in an experiment on weight reduction. In all, 70 people responded by phone: housewives, office workers, business men, etc. Of these, 60 fulfilled the requirements of (a) being between 20 and 45 years of age; (b) being overweight+; and (c) being willing to sign a declaration that he or she was in good health. Of these 60 Ss, 42 were women and 18 were men. The average age was 27.6 years and the average overweight was 22 lbs (11 kg).

Seven classes of overweight persons were formed: class I was 1 to 6 lbs overweight, class II 6 to 10, and so on up to class VII (more than 30 lbs). Ss were assigned to these classes and from there randomly assigned to groups. This gave us 14 Ss per group with some reserves in the control group. In this way we had reasonably homogeneous groups. The results are calculated on the basis of 12 Ss per group and 10 per group in the final follow-up, due to drop-outs during the experiment.

3. Group A

This group received the same therapy as was given to group B in experiment I (behavioural control plus food tips). The therapy was individual, with 2 sessions per week, each of 20 to 30 min.

+ Our definition of "normal weight" was generous. For women normal was defined as the number of cm in height in excess of 1.05 m, expressed as kg; for men the number of cm in excess of 1.00 m, expressed as kg. For example, a man 1.83 m tall (6 ft) would be of normal weight at 83 kg (187 lbs). One Continental pound = 500 gm = 1.125 English or American lbs.

4. Group B

This group received the same therapy instructions as group A, but the only contact with the therapist was by mail. Twice a week the Ss received a short text on eating habits, the steps to be followed, and food tips. Included were food data sheets, a card for recording weight, and a stamped, addressed envelope for returning the weight card.

5. Group C

This group received a diet. Each week the Ss were given a text composed of information on food and calories, a government-approved diet made up by a qualified dietician, a weight card, and a stamped, addressed envelope. There were 4 of these texts covering the 4 weeks of therapy. In addition, the Ss met with the T once a week as a group to discuss the course contents and any difficulties. Group A met with T twice a week, this group once a week but the sessions lasted an hour, so that the time with T was about the same.

6. Group D

The Ss in this group were informed by mail that they could not be given therapy but their co-operation was requested in the sending in of the weight card at the end of 4 weeks.

7. Results

There were no significant differences between the groups in weight before therpay ($F = 1.57$; d.f. = 3 & 44; $n = 48$; $p > .05$). An analysis of variance of the weights at the beginning of therapy, at the end of therapy and at first and second follow-up, corrected for missing data in the second follow-up, gave highly significant differences over time ($F = 21.17$; d.f. = 3 & 132; $p < .005$) and for the interaction of groups over time ($F = 4.44$; d.f. = 9 & 132; $p < .01$). There was also a highly significant difference in the groups over time linear interaction ($F = 9.24$; d.f. = 3 & 132; $p < .005$).

When the drop-outs were excluded from the overall results and the differences between the starting weight and weight after therapy and at first and second follow-up were analysed, there was a highly significant difference between groups ($F = 14.63$; d.f. = 3 & 36; $p < .005$) but no significant interactions or linear trend. These results are shown in Fig. 1. It can be seen that the control group gained weight steadily during the 6-month period of measurement. The diet group (c) initially lost weight but were slowly regaining it. The behavioural control group with therapist contact (A) initially did best but relapsed slightly after treatment and then remained almost constant. The behavioural control group without therapist contact (B) were initially intermediate between groups A and C, but they continued to lose weight after therapy ended, and at second follow-up were at almost the same level as group A.

Taking just the results at F2, Dunett's test for comparisons with a control showed that all experimental groups were highly significantly different from the control, but according to Scheffé's test none of the experimental groups differed significantly from each other at F2.

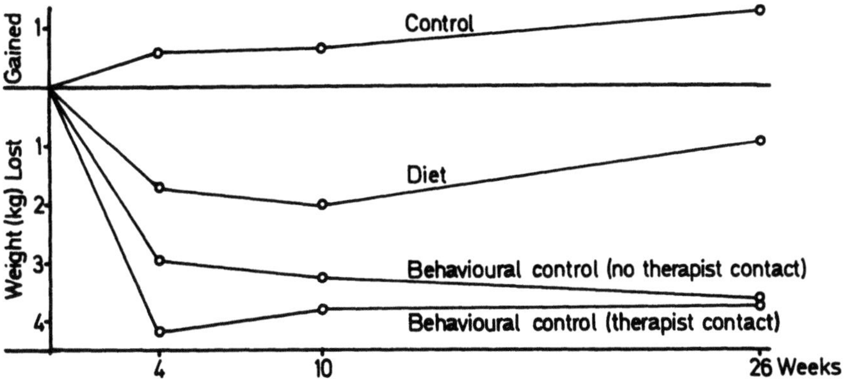

Fig. 1. Average weight change (in kg) for the different groups, at end of therapy (E), at first follow-up (F1), and at second follow-up (F2)

V. Discussion

In general it can be said that the experiments reported here have to a large extent replicated the good results STUART found with his behavioural control techniques. They also confirm the opinion of PENICK et al., that behavioural control is the best of a number of alternative programmes for the treatment of obesity. In both experiments the behavioural control groups did very well.

The most strikingly and encouraging results of the whole study were those of the non-T contact behavioural control. On follow-up after 6 months they were doing as well as the behavioural control group who had had contact with the therapist. This, of course, needs replication, but if such an effect can be obtained by preparing and sending out standard letters, it looks as though we have found something really worthwhile in the treatment of obesity.

The methods used with our Ss are not necessarily the most effective, and it would be worthwhile taking things further. Combinations of behavioural control and covert sensitization could possibly be more effective than either technique separately. Further, the therapy could be spread over a longer period of time, with gradual fade-out of the T. This might be expected to combine the good early results from group A and the later good results of group B in our experiment II. Contractual management could be tried, where an S deposits a sum of money with T at the beginning and gets it back only as targets are attained. Group instead on individual therapy would increase the number of Ss that could be treated per T, and the group interaction could be an added advantage. If the mass media were used, a large number of people could be treated for relatively little cost. It would be interesting to form a group composed of, for example, a housewife, a businessman, a secretary, a student, etc. that would give a good cross section of the population.

The weekly group meetings could be televised, and the TV audience at the end of each programme would be given a summary of the steps to be taken, on a do-it-yourself basis, and invited to take part. The audience could send their results in each week and get feedback from the TV as to how all Ss were doing. A good series with the stress laid on maintaining motivation, self-control and self-reinforcement, should make the large-scale treatment of obesity an enticing possibility. Would insurance companies, television corporations and clinical psychologists be interested in a co-operative endeavour?

VI. Summary

Self-control techniques appear to be gaining in importance to judge by the behaviour therapy literature, and in the two experiments described here these and other methods are used in the treatment of obesity. In the first experiment, behaviour therapy was superior to the therapist-contact and no-contact control groups, and self-control was the better of the behaviour therapy groups. In the second experiment, the diet group did slightly worse than the control on follow-up at 6 months, the therapist-contact self-control group did slightly better, and the self-control by mail did very well. Some suggestions are given for improving the behaviour therapy techniques for the treatment of obesity.

References

BANDURA, A.: Principles of Behaviour Modification. London: Holt, Rinehart & Winston 1969.
CAUTELA, J.R.: Behaviour therapy and self control: techniques and implications. In: FRANKS, C.M. (Ed.): Behavior Therapy: Appraisal and Status. New York: McGraw Hill 1969.
GOLDFRIED, M.R.: Systematic desensitization as training in self-control. J. consult. clin. Psychol. 37, 228-234 (1971).
HOMME, L.E.: Perspectives in psychology: XXIV. Control of coverants, the operants of the mind. Psychol. Rec. 15, 501-511 (1965).
KANFER, F.H., PHILLIPS, J.S.: Learning Foundations of Behavior Therapy. New York: Wiley 1970.
PENICK, S.B., FILION, R., FOX, S., STUNKARD, A.J.: Behavior modification in the treatment of obesity. Psychosom. Med. 33, 49-55 (1971).
PREMACK, D.: Toward empirical behavior laws: I. Positive reinforcement. Psychol. Rev. 66, 219-233 (1959).
SCHACHTER, S.: Some extraordinary facts about obese humans and rats. Amer. Psychologist 26, 129-144 (1971).
STUART, R.B.: Behavioral control of overeating. Behav. Res. Ther. 5, 357-365 (1967).
STUART, R.B.: A three-dimensional program for the treatment of obesity. Behav. Res. Ther. 9, 177-186 (1971).
STUNKARD, A.J., McLAREN-HUME, M.: The results of treatment for obesity. Arch. intern. Med. 103, 79-85 (1959).

The Effects of Monetary Rewards and Feedback on the Work Behaviour of Psychiatric Patients

B.E. STOFFELMAYR and L.G. WALKER

I. Summary

In an industrial therapy unit a treatment regime based on reinforcement principles was introduced on 5 January 1972. The unit is located outside the regional mental hospitals but administratively allied to them. It has places for up to 100 patients but the average occupancy is between 70 and 80. It is staffed by a manager with industrial experience, instructors and nurses. Patients are referred to the unit either because they have been hospitalized for a considerable period of time and therefore lack experience of industry, or because they have special difficulties in obtaining and holding down a job. The diagnostic distribution is schizophrenia 60 %, personality disorders 25 %, with 15 % made up of depression, mental deficiency and organic brain disorders.

Treatment is divided into 3 stages. Feedback and monetary rewards are the main tools of behaviour control employed; the effects of contingent social stimulation are being explored. Stage 1: Payment is contingent upon attendance and time spent at the bench. Stage 2: Treatment phase: payment is contingent on work speed and appropriate social behaviour. During this period patients are given frequent feedback. Stage 3: Patients receive full pay and are expected to maintain appropriate work without staff support and feedback.

Data are given on the effect of this treatment regime on patients' work and social behaviour and some of the problems associated with the assessment of the efficacy of the unit are discussed.

Industrial therapy has been part of psychiatric hospital treatment for a number of years. It is viewed either as a vehicle for therapy (BLACK, 1970), by which is meant some form of psychotherapy, as a place where patients can be occupied, or as an effort at rehabilitation. Although the literature regarding industrial rehabilitation is extensive, it is usually limited to discussions of techniques of management, siting of unit and number of staff, and rarely includes a description of the procedures by which an industrial therapy department can be transformed into a motivating environment. This is surprising, as it cannot be assumed that the provision of a workshop will automatically result in improvement in patients' behaviour. It has to be recognized that much therapy and rehabilitation for psychiatric patients has to provide not only the tools for the practice of a special skill but also motivation.

Both the literature and experienced clinicians suggest that the main handicaps of psychiatric patients, particularly chronic schizophrenic patients, in finding and holding down employment are: (1) low work speed (2) inappropriate social behaviour and (3) dependence on the hospital. This last aspect has been described as the main drawback of institutionalization (WING, 1962).

Several studies suggest that, even in chronic schizophrenic patients, speed of work can be increased through such procedures as social stimulation (WING and FREUDENBERG, 1961) and monetary rewards (SLETTEN et al., 1968; PFEFFER, 1953). In addition, a number of investigators have demonstrated that the work behaviour of chronic schizophrenic patients can be controlled through appropriate reinforcement procedures (JOHNSON et al., 1965; AYLLON and AZRIN, 1968). As yet, almost no reports on the introduction of motivating systems in large industrial therapy units have appeared in the literature. Indeed, judging from the King's Fund Report on Industrial Therapy, one wonders if information collected by researchers has infiltrated clinical practice at all.

The unit in which we and other staff are involved is a largish industrial therapy department. It is located outside the regional mental hospitals but is administratively allied to them. It has places for up to 100 patients, but the average occupancy is between 70 and 80 patients.

The permanent staff consists of a manager with industrial experience, three instructors and three nurses, driver/porter, secretary and maid. In addition, two psychiatrists and two psychologists visit the unit regularly. Only limited support is available from social workers.

Patients are referred to the unit either because they have been in the hospital for a considerable period of time and therefore lack experience of industry, or because they have special difficulties in obtaining and holding down a job. The diagnostic distribution is schizophrenia 60 %, personality disorders 25 %, with the rest made up of depression, mental deficieny and organic brain disorders. The almost complete absence of patients with neurotic disorders is noteworthy. The only officially diagnosed neurotics who have been at the unit are two patients who suffer from obsessional compulsive disorders.

Our attempts to transform this unit into a motivating environment have gone through several phases. The main consideration has always been that the system introduced should be manageable. The focus of treatment at the unit was and still is the increase of work speed and the learning of more appropriate social behaviour. The system initially adopted was one where patients were assessed weekly on a 5 point rating scale covering many aspects of social and work behaviour. The system we used was developed by CHEADLE et al. (1967); we added a few scales and related payment to assessment. Altogether patients were assessed on 18 scales and paid on 8. The main difficulties with this system were: (a) inter-rater reliability was low, (b) the 18 scales correlated highly, (c) the assessments did not relate to patients' behaviour but were influenced by staff likes and dislikes, (d) some patients were completely overlooked and never spoken to, and (e) there was no provision for systematic feedback.

A more systematic payment and reinforcement system was discussed, but several objections were raised. Foremost amongst these was the belief that the supervisory time required for systematic feedback would be too great, doubts were voiced as to the effectiveness of payment by results and several colleagues felt that an increase in work speed would result in a deterioration of social behaviour. In order to find out whether or not our patient population would be affected by a reinforcement procedure and whether a higher work speed would actually damage social behaviour, a 13-week experiment was conducted (NAPIER,

1971). This was a rather small study as it included only 8 patients, but it showed conclusively that (a) work speed increased dramatically (most of the patients trebled their performance) and (b) the amount of social interaction did not decrease when work was speeded up. The way was now open for the introduction of a new payment system. All that was needed was a psychiatrist or psychologist who could spend enough time at the unit to assist with it. Work on the new system finally started in October 1971 and it was introduced on 5 January 1972.

The new system which was introduced has 3 principal features:

1. Payment and praise (which we hope functions as a social reinforcer) are contingent upon work and social behaviour.
2. Feedback is an integral part of treatment; feedback is given 5 times a day when the work can be put on a piece rate and twice a day for unquantifiable jobs.
3. Payment is given for special problems. Initially, it was thought that patients who arrive late might be paid for coming on time, or that withdrawn patients might be paid for talking instead for working, etc. Patients are now assessed weekly on the E and F scale of Psychotic Inpatient Profile and the work is either counted or assessed twice daily.

Patients' stay at the unit is divided into three stages:

Stage 1 is an introductory period where patients are paid up to 50 p for attendance and up to 50 p for work. The payment for work is based on a rating of "effort". The main target behaviour for this stage is attendance at the unit.

Stage 2 is the main treatment phase. Patients are given frequent feedback and paid according to productivity and appropriate social behaviour. Up to ₤ 1.50 is available for payments relating to work and up to 49 p for payments relating to social behaviour. During this period some patients are also put on special programmes. Such programmes have been designed for 25 patients. The problems dealt with range from very low work speed, too much time spent away from the bench, not wearing dentures or glasses, and excessive body odours, to temper tantrums, fighting and unwillingness to follow instructions. Programmes were planned for many more than 25 patients but a number of patients improved miraculously once a clearcut programme was decided on.

Stage 3: patients are moved to this stage when they have obtained full pay in Stage 2. The goal now is for the patients to learn to monitor and control their own work speed and to tolerate industrial discipline.

The idea behind this schedule is that most of our patients will not work on production lines but rather in unskilled jobs where they are responsible for their own work speed. During this period patients are paid a flat rate of ₤ 1.99. Although they do not receive feedback, records are kept of their work behaviour and social behaviour. If a patient's performance drops for two successive weeks, he is returned to Stage 2.

The main problem with the system as it is running at present is that not all jobs are on a piece rate, because it is difficult to obtain large contracts in Aberdeen. Furthermore, the assessment of social behaviour by means of a rating scale is unsatisfactory; it does not allow precise feedback and staff are still not fully trained.

Despite all its shortcomings the system appears to work. Money has taken on an importance far beyond its purchasing power. Patients challenge staff even if they have lost only 1 p. Visitors who come repeatedly into the unit feel it now has a genuine factory atmosphere. As regards the effect of the system on the patients' behaviour, we would like to present a functional analysis of the treatment regime based on extensive data about the relationship between intra- and extra-therapy behaviour. This last point is of particular interest, as a pilot study of 13 patients showed that responsiveness to treatment does not relate to good adjustment outside (WALKER et al., 1972), those who responded best being the ones with the most restricted social behaviour outside the unit. However, up to now we have been occupied with the introduction and monitoring of the payment and assessment system. The only systematic experimentation has been concerned with the effect of social reinforcement.

The most meaningful data we have regarding the functioning of the unit concern the productivity of a changing carton team (Fig. 1). Carton-making is an easily quantifiable job and data have been collected since long before the introduction of the new system. The number of people working on cartons varies from 10 to 30, and the better workers are moved on to unquantifiable, i.e. more complex jobs. The increases in productivity shown in Fig. 1 are genuine insofar as they cannot be attributed to either practice or the introduction of better workers to the carton team. A major increase in productivity occurred before the new system was put into operation, about the time we decided to go ahead with the new system, and again in December, when the system was given a trial run. During this trial run the system was put into operation as described except that payment was not contingent. The increases may not look very large but it has to be recognized that the difference between 30 and 40 cartons is one of working at a comfortable speed and one of working pretty fast. One can speculate as to the reason why the increases occurred during the run-up to the new system, but what is of importance is that the level of productivity was maintained. Even if a Hawthorne effect might account for the increases, it cannot explain the maintenance of productivity (STOFFELMAYR and WALKER, 1972).

Fig. 2 shows the mean production level of a changing group of patients who had been working on jobs where payment is related to staff ratings. Because the graph shows the mean productivity of a changing group, individual increases are concealed. However, 't-test' for matched pairs show that, while individuals did not improve during the baseline period, they did so after the introduction of contingent payment and feedback. Reliability checks show that this improvement is not due either to rater inconsistency or a tendency to rate more leniently.

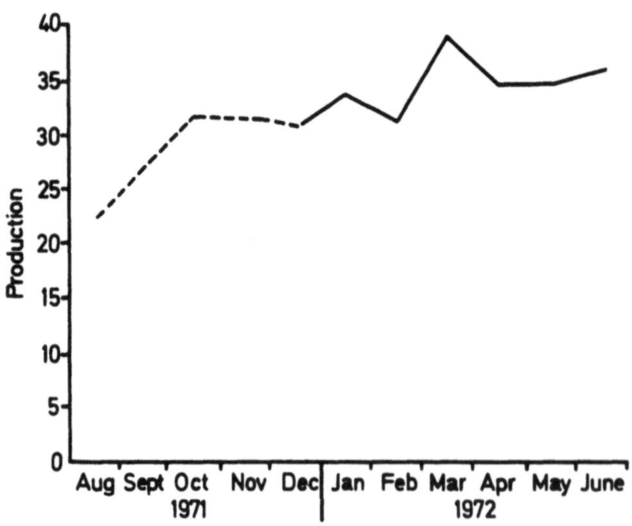

Fig. 1. Production level of a changing carton team

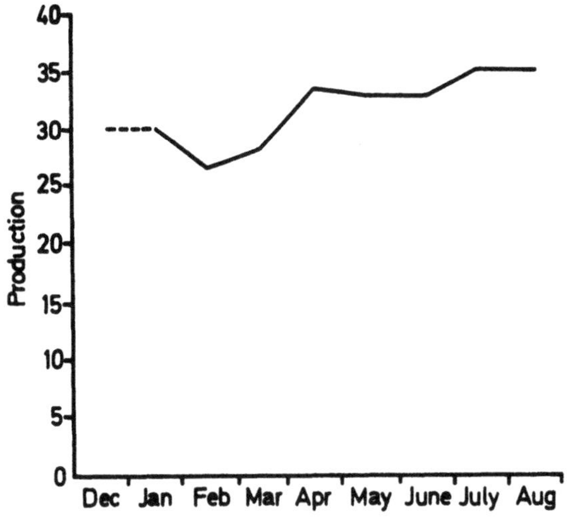

Fig. 2. Average production level per month of all patients on work assessments

The second focus of treatment is social skill (Fig. 3). The system we are operating is primitive inasmuch as we are relying on a rating scale, so that feedback, which is given weekly, is not as specific as one would wish. The kinds of statements staff make are: "You don't talk to anyone." "You never join a group." "You are too slow." "You don't take care of yourself." Nevertheless, a massive change can be observed over the time the system has been in operation. We have, of course, considered that the curve in Fig. 3 may be only an artefact, but the examination of individual records and frequent reliability checks suggest that the changes are real. It is highly unlikely that the weekly feedback can account for all the changes observed. Probably staff now pay attention to and attempt to modify varieties of behaviour which they previously ignored. In addition, thanks to the feedback system, staff now interact with all the patients in the unit.

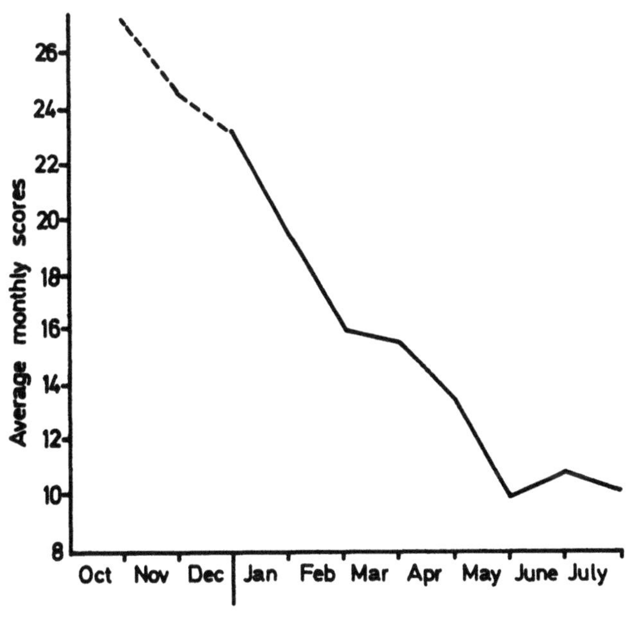

Fig. 3. Monthly averages of seclusiveness and retardation scores for all rehabilitees

We are still concerned with the effect of higher productivity on patients' social behaviour. For this reason, data were collected during November 1971 and August 1972.

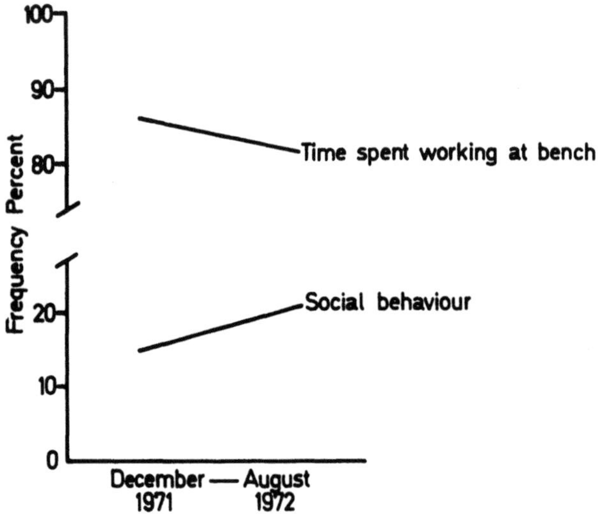

Fig. 4. Observational data on social behaviour and time spent working at bench

As Fig. 4 shows, an increase in productivity did not adversely affect social behaviour, and there was a significant increase in the amount of social interaction between patients in August as compared to November. Actual time spent working at the bench had not changed, therefore higher output cannot be accounted for in terms of longer periods of time spent working.

The question remains: Is the system worthwhile? The object of the unit is to rehabilitate patients, therefore any decision as to effectiveness of treatment has to be made in relation to the discharge figures. The data given in Fig. 5 are not up-to-date. They show a gradual increase in the number of patients discharged from the unit between 1969 and 1972, i.e. before the introduction of the new system. An interesting aspect is that more patients were discharged during the winter than during the summer. This is contrary to expectations based on the seasonal unemployment figures for the region.

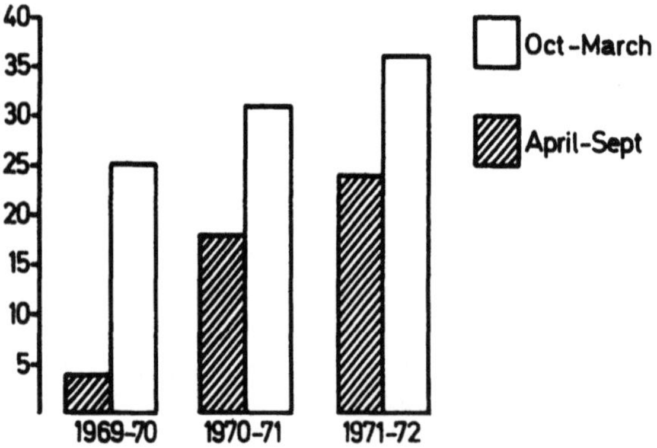

Fig. 5. Number of discharges

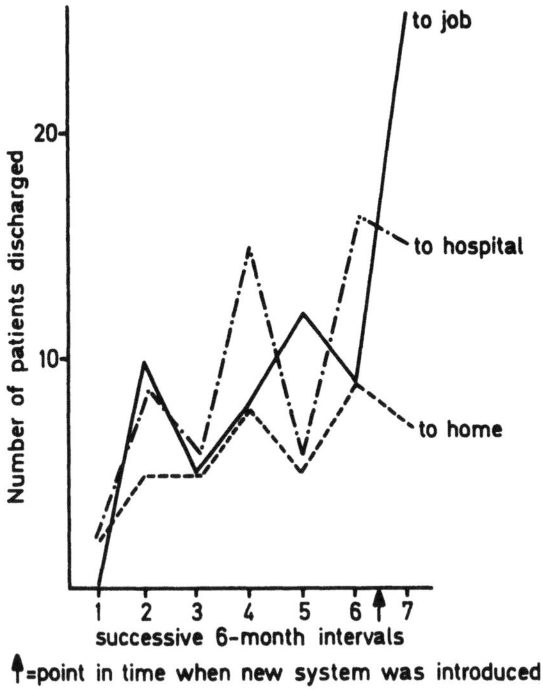

Fig. 6. Discharges to home, job and hospital before and after introduction of the new system

Fig. 6 shows what happened to patients upon discharge. Successes were patients who obtained employment in the community, failures patients who had to return to hospital, and those who were discharged home are regarded as intermediate. It can be seen that a dramatic increase in the number of successfully discharged patients occurred during the 6-month period since the new system has been in operation.

We think that the data presented show that, despite all its shortcomings, the enterprise in which we are engaged is worthwhile. However, further research into the operation of the system is necessary. From a practical point of view the priorities are (1) a more clear-cut specification of appropriate social behaviour, (2) better staff training and (3) further development of a system which not only allows the modification of behaviour in the unit but also has the effect that patients leave the unit, obtain and keep a job.

Our ongoing research is concerned with the analysis of the effective ingredients of the treatment regime and an investigation of the relationship between intra- and extra-therapy behaviour.

References

AYLLON, T., AZRIN, N.H.: The token economy. New York: Appleton Century Crofts 1968.

BLACK, B.J.: Industrial Therapy for the Mentally Ill. New York: Grune and Stratton 1970.

CHEADLE, A.J., CUSHING, D., DREW, C.D.A., MORGAN, R.: The measurement of work performance of psychiatric patients. Brit. J. Psychiat. 113, 841-846 (1967).

JOHNSON, R.F., HAUGHTON, E., LAFAVE, H.G.: Behaviour therapy - use in a sheltered workshop. Dis. nerv. Syst. 26, 350-354 (1965).

NAPIER, B.S.: A comparison of the effects of group and individual reinforcement conditions on the behaviour of male psychotic patients. Unpublished B. Sc. Thesis, University of Aberdeen 1971.
O'CONNOR, N., HERON, A., CARSTAIRS, G.M.: Work performance of chronic schizophrenics. Occupational Psychol. 30, 150-164 (1956).
PEFFER, P.A.: Money, A rehabilitation incentive for mental patients. Amer. J. Psychiat. 110, 84-92 (1953).
SLETTEN, I.W., HUGHES, D.D., LAMONT, J., OGNJANOV, V.: Work performance in psychiatric patients. Dis. nerv. Syst. 29, 261-264 (1968).
STOFFELMAYR, B.E., WALKER, L.G.: The researcher effect. Unpublished manuscript. Department of Mental Health, University of Aberdeen 1972.
TOPPING, G.G., O'CONNOR, N.: The response of chronic schizophrenics to incentives. Brit. J. med. Psychol. 33, 211-214 (1960).
WALKER, L.G., ADAMSON, F.P.C., ALEXANDER, D.A., STOFFELMAYR, B.E.: The relationship between increase in production level in response to contingent staff approval in a psychiatric rehabilitation unit and social interaction outwith the unit. Unpublished manuscript, Department of Mental Health, University of Aberdeen 1972.
WING, J.K.: Institutionalism in mental hospitals. Brit. J. soc. clin. Psychol. 1, 38 (1962).
WING, J.K., FREUDNEBERG, R.K.: The response of severely ill chronic schizophrenic patients to social stimulation. Amer. J. Psychiat. 118, 311-322 (1961).

V. Some Physiological Aspects of Behaviour Modification

The Relationship between Psychological and Psychophysiological Measures of Sexual Response+

P.J. GRAHAM, J.J.M. HARBISON, H. McALLISTER and J.T. QUINN

Two main techniques have been employed in the assessment of sexual orientation: psychometric and psychophysiological. Changes in penile erection have been shown to be the "the most highly reliable and discriminating" indices of sexual arousal (ZUCKERMAN, 1971). In a recent article BANCROFT (1971) illustrated how penile plethysmography can be used (a) in the assessment of sexual problems (b) as a measure of change during treatment and (c) as part of the treatment procedure itself. We have elsewhere discussed the use of psychological methods of assessment in sexual disorders in a similar fashion (HARBISON et al., 1973).

It is important to examine whether psychometric measures correlate with psychophysiological indices of sexual orientation and interest. BANCROFT (1971) used the semantic differential alongside psychophysiological assessment. He found a low significant correlation between change in erectile response and change in attitudes. LEE-EVANS (1971), working in collaboration with us, found significant correlations between the Sexual Orientation Method of FELDMAN et al. (1966) and psychophysiological measures of sexual orientation. The present study compares the penile response of 35 homosexual patients with scores on the Sexual Orientation Method and on a semantic differential.

I. Subjects

All subjects in this study were male homosexuals who had been referred to the Department of Mental Health. All were volunteers. In addition to being homosexual, 3 of the 35 were transexuals.

II. Procedure

1. Assessment of Psychophysiological Response

The procedure followed was similar to that described by LEE-EVANS in 1971. A standard series of slides of nude or semi-nude pin-ups (half

+ This research was carried out as part of an M.R.C.-supported project (M.R.C. G970/340/C) under the general direction of Professor J.G. GIBSON. Four of us (JTQ, H McA, JJMH and PJG) constitute a research team. No seniority of authorship is implied by the order of names on this paper.

male and half female) was presented to each subject, who was instructed to look at each picture as it was presented and to think of "whatever it prompted him to think of", but to keep his attention on the picture throughout its presentation. The slides were presented in a balanced order. There was a minimum inter-stimulus interval of one minute. Penile responses were monitored with a mercury-in-rubber strain gauge similar to that described by BANCROFT et al. (1966) and were recorded on a Devices M8 Polygraph.

In an earlier study, LEE-EVANS (1970) indicated that the most useful measure of sexual orientation is the greatest adjusted amplitude of response within a 60-sec stimulus exposure (i.e., the greatest positive change less any negative deflection in a 60-sec period). For each subject, a psychophysiological orientation score was derived, based on comparisons between each subject's response to the two different classes of stimuli, i.e. male or female slides, and comparisons were made using the Mann-Whitney U-test. (The Mann-Whitney U scores derived for each subject were expressed in a range of 0 to 100, where 0 indicates maximum homosexual preference, 100 maximum heterosexual preference, and a score of 50 no obvious sexual preference.)

2. Sexual Orientation Method (SOM)

This test is widely known and will not be discussed here. Five scores were derived, a heterosexual orientation score, a homosexual orientation score, a heterosexual inconsistency score, a homosexual inconsistency score, and a homosexual preference score, the latter derived by subtracting the heterosexual from the homosexual score. LEE-EVANS (1971) found maximum correlation between the homosexual preference score and the psychophysiological measure.

3. Semantic Differential Test

Twelve bipolar adjectival scales were used to measure the 3 factors of evaluation, potency and activity. The 12 scales used to measure these 3 factors were based on the cross-culturally derived semantic differentials of JANSEN and SMOLENAARS (1967).

Four psychological constructs were measured on each of the 3 factors; two of the concepts dealt with homosexual behaviour (kissing and sexual intercourse with a man) and the other two with similar heterosexual concepts. The attitudinal scores derived from each of the heterosexual concepts were added to produce total heterosexual evaluation, potency and activity scores, and 3 similar scores were derived for homosexual concepts. Finally, a similar homosexual preference score for each of the 3 factors was derived by subtracting the heterosexual from the homosexual score. Thus, 9 attitudinal measures were derived.

All attitudinal measures were completed either on the same day or as close as possible to the day when the psychophysiological test was completed. The 15 scores were then intercorrelated by product moment correlation, and a principal-component analysis and varimax rotation carried out.

III. Results

1. The Relationship between Psychophysiological and Psychological Measures of Sexual Orientation

Table 1 shows that significant correlations (p 0.05) exist between the psychophysiological preference score and the heterosexual score of the

SOM. A significant correlation was also obtained between the penile response score and the homosexual preference score. No significant correlations exist between semantic differential scores and penile plethysmographic responses.

2. The Relationship between Semantic Differential and SOM Scores

A number of semantic differential and SOM scores are highly correlated. The highest correlations occur between all sets of homosexual preference measures, on both SOM and semantic differential evaluative, activity and potency scales. The SOM preference score is also significantly related to heterosexual evaluative and potency measures, but not to the equivalent homosexual scores.

3. Varimax Rotation of Principal Components of the Correlation Table

This analysis produced 3 principal components which accounted for almost 70 % of the variance. Table 2 shows these three factors and the loadings of the 15 psychophysiological and attitudinal variables on each factor. It can be seen that factor 1 (which accounts for over 30 % of the variance) appears to be a "semantic differential". Differential scores have loadings of 0.5 or above on this factor, and none of the SOM or psychophysiological scores exceeds 0.30. Factor 2 (which accounts for 19.5 % of the variance) is a factor with high loadings from the psychophysiological response, and 4 out of the 5 SOM scores. The only SOM score which is not highly loaded on factor 2 is the heterosexual inconsistency score. Interestingly enough, the homosexual inconsistency score has a loading of 0.67 on this score. Factor 3, accounting for 20 % of the variance, is mixed and appears to have loadings from the heterosexual measures. For example, the heterosexual SOM score loads 0.59 on the factor, and the 3 heterosexual semantic differential scores load respectively 0.56, 0.72 and 0.75 on this factor.

IV. Discussion

The results indicate that significant relationships exist between SOM scores and the measure of psychophysiological sexual orientation. No significant relationship was found between semantic differential measures and psychophysiological index. These findings are all the more striking since a high correlation exists between the two attitudinal measures.

The varimax analysis clarifies the relationship between the 3 measures of sexual orientation. Two clearly distinguishable components of orientation emerge, the first of which appears to be derived almost entirely from the semantic differential scores, and the second from the combination of penile and SOM orientation measures. Thus it appears that the semantic differential and the Sexual Orientation Method measure rather separate aspects of sexual attitude, and that the SOM measure is more closely linked to physiological arousal. Nevertheless, the semantic differential score is an important component of sexual attitude and contributes to over 30 % of the variance. Further work is urgently required to refine our understanding of the relationship between these various measures of sexual orientation and arousal. A practical conclusion from the work reported here is that it is perhaps unsafe to use either the semantic differential or the SOM measure alone in the assessment of homosexual patients for monitoring progress in their treatment.

Table 1. Intercorrelation of psychophysiological response (1) SOM score (2-4) and semantic differential scores (5-13)

	Penile Orient.	Het	Hom	Hom Pref	E	P	A	E	P	A	E	P	A
	1	2	3	4	5	6	7	8	9	10	11	12	13
1	1.0	0.34[a]	-0.32	-0.40[a]	0.06	0.20	0.06	0.21	0.0	0.01	0.10	0.14	-0.09
2		1.0	-0.37[a]	-0.84[b]	0.68[b]	0.53[b]	0.42[a]	-0.22	-0.16	-0.27	-0.53[b]	-0.44[b]	-0.48[b]
3			1.0	0.82[b]	-0.42[a]	-0.29	0.01	0.16	0.16	0.19	0.34[a]	0.28	0.13
4				1.0	-0.67[b]	-0.50[b]	-0.26	0.24	0.19	0.28	0.53[b]	0.44[b]	0.38[a]
5					1.0	0.79[b]	0.41[a]	-0.41[a]	-0.34[a]	-0.52[b]	-0.82[b]	-0.75[b]	-0.66[b]
6						1.0	0.49[b]	-0.21	-0.21	-0.29	-0.58[b]	-0.79[b]	-0.55[b]
7							1.0	-0.08	-0.20	-0.10	-0.25	-0.39[a]	-0.70[b]
8								1.0	0.66[b]	0.53[b]	0.85[b]	0.56[b]	0.44[a]
9									1.0	0.51[b]	0.60[b]	0.75[b]	0.56[b]
10										1.0	0.63[b]	0.52[b]	0.72[b]
11											1.0	0.77[b]	0.65[b]
12												1.0	0.64[b]
13													1.0

[a] P 0.05
[b] P 0.01

Table 2. Psychophysiological (1) SOM (2-6) and semantic differential (7-15) variables

Measure	Factor 1 (30 % Variance)	Factor 2 (19.5 % Variance)	Factor 3 (20 % Variance)
1	0.22	0.65	0.16
2	-0.23	0.55	0.59
3	-0.10	0.06	-0.64
4	0.19	-0.85	0.04
5	-0.20	0.67	-0.35
6	0.26	-0.84	-0.35
7	-0.59	0.40	0.56
8	-0.36	0.28	0.72
9	-0.15	-0.02	0.75
10	0.87	0.06	0.04
11	0.82	-0.03	0.03
12	0.77	-0.12	-0.04
13	0.88	-0.19	-0.30
14	0.75	-0.21	-0.43
15	0.65	-0.07	-0.55

References

BANCROFT, J.: The application of psychophysiological measures to the assessment and modification of sexual behaviour. Behav. Res. Ther. 9, 119-130 (1971).

BANCROFT, H., JONES, H.G., PULLAN, B.P.: A simple transducer for measuring penile reactions. Behav. Res. Ther. 4, 239-241 (1966).

FELDMAN, M.P., MacCULLOCH, M.J., NELLOR, V., PINSCHOF, J.M.: The sexual orientation method. Behav. Res. Ther. 4, 289-299 (1966).

HARBISON, J.J.M., GRAHAM, P. JOAN, QUINN, J.T., McALLISTER, H.: Psychological assessment of sexual dysfunction. In: BRENGLEMANN, J.C., TURNER, W., (Eds.). Behaviour Therapy. München: 1973.

JANSEN, M.J. SMOLENAARS, A.J.: A short report on an interculturally standardized semantic differential. Acta psychol. 26, 209-215 (1967).

LEE-EVANS, M.: Male homosexuality: A review and exploratory study. Unpublished M. Sc. Thesis, Queen's University of Belfast 1970.

LEE-EVANS, M.: Penile plethysmographic assessment of sexual orientation. Paper read at Third Conference Behaviour Modification, Wexford/Ireland 1971.

ZUCKERMAN, M.: Psychological measures of sexual arousal in the human. Psychol. Bull. 75, 297-329 (1971).

Changes in Cardiac Rate Effected by Operant Reinforcement Contingencies

E.W. THORNTON

The problem of whether responses of the autonomic nervous system can be brought under the control of operant contingencies has been tackled in a vigorous and often ingenious manner in many eminent laboratories. A number of species have been used as experimental subjects: NEIL MILLER (1969) and his associates chose the rat, ABRAHAM BLACK, the dog (1967), whilst recently GARY SCHWARTZ (1972) and BERNHARD ENGEL (1972) used monkeys and humans.

The wide range of subjects represents the different emphases that have been placed on the problem. Thus, the focus has been variously on psychological learning theory, the control of cardiovascular and autonomic function, or the etiology and treatment of such problems as psychosomatic hypertension. It is this wide field of interest that has stimulated the large amount of experimental data that has accumulated over the last 5 years. This explosion of studies is remarkable when one considers that the theoretical problem was explicitly formulated by two-process theorists as early as the 1920's and 1930's. For example, SKINNER (1938) stated: "glands and smooth muscles do not normally produce the kinds of consequences involved in operant reinforcement."

It was unfortunate that theorizing outstripped experimental investigation at that time. However, it is not improbable that those early theorists were aware of the problem that has plagued some of the more recent experiments: whether the autonomic response is mediated by a change in some other response. This controversial point was highlighted by KENDON SMITH (1954, 1964), who demonstrated that both overt and covert skeletal activity could mediate learnt changes in cardiac response.

New interest in the operant conditioning of autonomic responses was aroused by the study of TROWILL (1967). He seemed to overcome the problem of mediation by shaping changes in the heart rate of rats deeply paralysed by a curariform drug. A considerable number of studies (MILLER, 1969; THORNTON and VAN TOLLER, 1973) have confirmed and extended TROWILL's finding. I have been particularly interested in the neurological basis of such learning. The work of STEELE RUSSELL (1971), utilizing the technique of spreading depression, has convincingly shown that operant learning of skeletal responses requires an intact cerebral cortex. Since it has been shown (BURGOYNE et al., 1967) that such spreading depression has no effect on the acquisition of a classic conditioned heart-rate response, it seemed useful to determine the effects of this functional decortication on the ability to shape cardiac changes in the curarized rat.

I. Method

An escape/avoidance schedule was used, with a fixed 0.1-sec pulse of shock of 0.5 mA as the aversive stimulus. A bidirectional design was employed in which half the rats avoided or escaped from shock by increases in heart rate to a criterion level, and half by decreases in rate. A shaping procedure was used such that, if the animal was consistently avoiding shock, criterion levels were successively changed by approximately 2 %.

The method of determining whether the heart rate of the rat was above (or below) a criterion level involved a circuit which determined whether a sample number of heart beats occurred in a faster (or slower) time than predicted for a steady heart rate at a given criterion level. Samples were taken over intervals ranging from 1.7 to 2.3 sec.

Operant trials were signalled with a 60-W lamp. If, on any operant trial, the criterion level was attained within 5 sec, the light went out and no shock was delivered. However, if the criterion level had not been attained within 5 sec, a shock pulse was delivered. Similar shock pulses were delivered if successive samples of heart rate indicated that criterion level had not been reached. Thus, pulsed shock was delivered at the end of each sample until the criterion level was attained, at which point the light went out and the trial terminated. Throughout training, the last trial in every block was an operant test trial, in which the light came on for 5 sec but the criterion circuit was inactive. This enabled the heart rate to be determined in the presence of the operant stimulus, without contamination by light termination or shock presentation. A 5-sec blank trial was incorporated into the training schedule. During this blank trial, no stimulus was presented but the number of heart beats was recorded.

The operant training schedule comprised 8 blocks of 30 trials, 10 operant and 20 blank trials. The end of each block of trials was marked by a single operant test trial. Trials were presented at a fixed intertrial interval of 20 sec. Within any block, each trial occurred in a predetermined random manner which was consistent throughout each block of training and was identical for all animals.

During heart-rate training procedures the animals were placed in a sound-attenuating chamber, fitted with a 60-W lamp which served as a discriminative stimulus. Shock was applied via two wires wrapped around the tail. Electrodes for recording heart rate were stainless steel needles inserted subdermally on either side of the thorax. The indifferent electrode was a hypodermic needle inserted into the peritoneal cavity. A connection from this to the outside of the chamber by polyethylene tubing allowed additional doses of the drug to be administered during training. The EKG output was electronically formed such that only the QRS wave of the signal operated the criterion and counter circuitry.

Throughout the experiment, artificial ventilation was maintained by a small-animal respirator connected to the animal inside the chamber via tubing and a snout mask. The technique has been described in detail by HAHN (1970) and THORNTON and VAN TOLLER (1973). To produce functional decortication by bilateral spreading depression (CSD), a chronic preparation was attached to the skull in a simple operative procedure, as described by SCHNEIDER and BEHAR (1964).

II. Procedure

Four days after the operative procedures attaching the cannula to the skull, CSD was initiated by application to the dural surfaces of filter paper soaked in the solution of potassium chloride. Immediately after initiating CSD the rat was injected with 0.6 mg/kg of d-tubocurarine chloride. In preliminary studies it had been found that this dose completely suppressed EMG activity from the gastrocnemius muscle, if supplemented with equivalent doses injected each hour through the indifferent electrode. When the rat became flaccid and showed signs of respiratory failure, it was fitted into the face mask. Artificial ventilation was applied at 70 cycle min at a peak pressure of 14 cm of water. The temperature of the enclosure was maintained at approximately 30° C. Electrodes for recording heart rate were inserted under xylocaine anaesthesia. After the shock electrodes were attached, the chamber was closed. A period of 30 min was allowed for the heart rate to stabilize and to enable selection of an initial criterion level that would be attained in about 40 % of the sampling periods.

If, during training, the animal successfully avoided shock on 4 consecutive operant trials, the criterion level was made more difficult (by approximately 2 %). If a combined total of more than 20 shocks was received on any two consecutive trials, the criterion level was reduced by an equivalent amount.

Fifteen hooded rats were used as experimental subjects. Data from one animal were lost because of an apparatus failure.

III. Results

There were no differences in the baseline heart rates of animals shaped for increases or decreases at the end of the 30-min adaption period ($t = 1.11$, $df = 13$). There were also no differences in the heart rates during operant test and blank trials throughout training for any animal. The results were therefore analysed in terms of the 8 blocks of operant test trials.

The percentage change in heart rate for each animal between the first and last block of training trials is presented in Table 1. The data indicate no relationship between the specific operant schedule used and the changes obtained. The group mean changes in heart rate over the training period for each group of animals are presented in Fig. 1. An analysis of variance of the data used to compile Fig. 1 revealed no significant interaction between heart-rate changes over blocks of trials. The analysis consequently confirmed the absence of any significant differential effect of the operant schedules on the heart-rate responses of animals in the two groups.

No differential change in heart rate occurred despite a significant difference in the mean number of shocks received by the two groups per block of operant trials ($t = 3.2$, $df = 13$; $p > .01$).

IV. Experiment 2

The effect of the same operant contingencies on control, sham-operated animals was entirely different. Ten animals were used, 5 being shaped

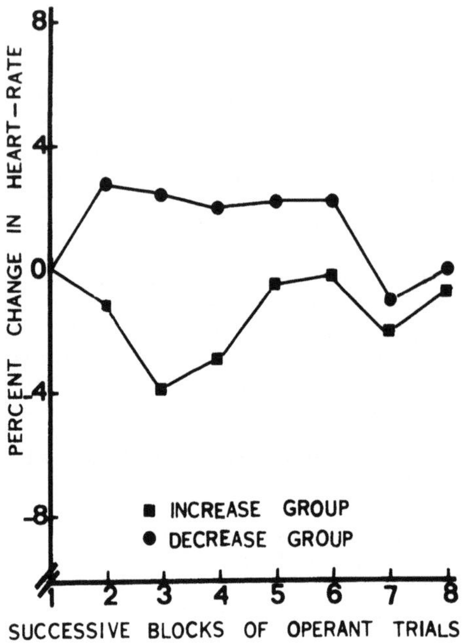

Fig. 1. Mean hart-rate changes for each group of functionally decorticate animals over successive blocks of operant trials

for heart-rate increases and 5 for decreases. As with the decorticate animals there were no differences in the baseline heart rates of the two groups after the 30-min adaption period (t = 1.01, dif = 8), nor was there a separation of heart-rate changes between operant test and blank trials.

The mean heart-rate changes of the increase and decrease groups over the 8 blocks of training trials are presented in Fig. 2. The figure

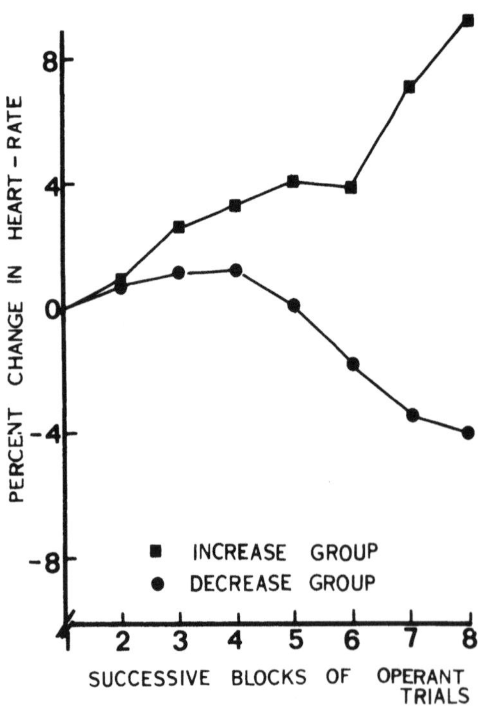

Fig. 2. Mean hart-rate changes for each group of sham-operant animals over successive blocks of operant trials

Table 1. Percentage in heart rate during training of functionally decorticate and sham-operated rats shaped for increases or decreases in rate

	Functionally Decorticate Animals	Sham-Operated Animals
Increases	2.1	10.3
	11.5	-1.5
	0	17.7
	-5.5	3.3
	-1.7	17.8
	-1.5	
	-6.9	
	-1.6	
Decreases	4.3	5.3
	-7.4	-6.4
	4.9	-1.5
	-1.5	-12.4
	0	-5
	2	
	-1.4	

Negative numbers indicate a decrease in rate.

shows how the expected divergence in heart rate between the two groups emerged as training proceeded. The percentage change in the heart rate of each animal over the training period is presented in Table 1.

An analysis of variance of the heart-rate changes of animals in each group over the 8 blocks of trials revealed a significant interaction ($F = 3.229$, $p > .01$). The percentage difference in heart-rate change between animals shaped for increases and decreases in rate was significant ($t = 2.8$, $df = 8$; $p > .05$).

As with the decorticate animals, there was a significant difference in the same direction in the mean number of shocks received per block of operant trials ($t = 5.35$, $df = 8$; $p > .001$). From this, it would seem reasonable to conclude that the differences in heart rate between the two groups in this second experiment were not a function of differences in this parameter of shock frequency.

The results of these experiments support the proposition that operant conditioning is dependent on the cerebral cortex.

V. Discussion

I would like now to examine the importance of the above type of experiment and to point out some of the practical and theoretical issues involved in operant conditioning of cardiac and cardiovascular changes in humans.

There are numerous studies in which attempts have been made to condition cardiac changes in humans by using operant techniques. These studies have been strongly criticized, and KATKIN and MURRAY (1968) in a literature review suggested that a distinction must be made between controlling e.g. blood pressure and conditioning it. Though clearly not unaware of the problems, they suggested that the issue could be resolved only by the use of conscious, curarized humans. TEPLITZ (1971) tried to assess the suitability of operant techniques as a research tool for explaining the etiology and determining therapy in essential hypertension. Though his paper directed attention to certain issues - for example, he emphasized the danger of generalizing from the ability of operant conditioning to effect decreases in normal levels of blood pressure to the lowering of chronic high levels - he too was very concerned about the problem of mediation. He suggested that, because of the subtleties of humans in changing respiration and muscle tone: "these should be minimised if we are to demonstrate operant conditioning of ANS responses in humans, and are to find suitable therapies." Presumably, the preceding authors are dubious of the value of studies like that of BENSON et al. (1971), which have claimed to demonstrate operant decreases in blood pressure in patients with essential hypertension.

Rather than clarifying the issue, the attempt to distinguish between control and conditioning may have created confusion. ENGEL (1972) is clearly of this opinion and has pointed out that the distinction is less real than apparent, for control responses may themselves be dependent on previous learning. The argument for separation is even more tenuous if it is based on an awareness of the means of control. Many responses can be controlled or learnt in the absence of awareness of the reasons for improvement.

These arguments are not meant to imply that the problem of mediation is nonexistent. The problem is best seen as one of experimental attempts to distinguish between somatic and cardiac control mechanisms rather than as one of theoretical semantics.

It may appear that experiments with curarized animals of the type I have described provide the conditions necessary to resolve the issue. Unfortunately, these studies deal only with the problem of mediation of changes in autonomic responses by <u>peripheral</u> skeletal responses. It could still be argued - and has been by BLACK (1967) - that cardiac response changes may be mediated by <u>central</u> motor responses.

It is interesting for the psychologist to consider here the work of the physiologist on cardiovascular and cardiac dynamics. In particular, the authoritative work of RUSHMER (1961) has provided ample evidence for feedback of cardiac changes to the CNS, the suggested prerequisite for operant conditioning. This information contrasts with the views of early theorists such as SKINNER, who clearly implied that the autonomic nervous system was a purely efferent system. RUSHMER's work also indicates a considerable overlap of cortical areas controlling cardiac and motor responses. This evidence suggests that the theoretical premise of two-process theories is weak and that a solution to the problem of experimentally separating cardiac and skeletal response control is likely to prove elusive.

This conclusion is not based solely on neurophysiological evidence but is supported by other work, notably that of OBRIST and associates (1970), which argues the case for the close integration of cardiac and motor response changes. It is worth noting that close integration of the two systems makes adaptive biological sense, since complete independence of either system would be disastrous.

The experiment I have described does not permit any definite conclusions regarding mediation. It is interesting in that it suggests that operant heart-rate changes in the curarized rat depend on cortical processes, but it does not show whether such changes are mediated by motor cerebral control mechanisms. The results merely tell us more about the level of control involved. Hence, although we have pushed the issue formulated by the two-process theorists into problems of cerebral processes, we have not resolved it.

In conclusion, if we are interested in the practical aspects of operant therapies for autonomic response activity, perhaps we should ask whether the theoretical problem of mediation is confusing the issue. Is it important that autonomic response changes may be mediated by covert somatic changes? The evidence of ALEXANDER (1950), which has shown increased muscle tone in hypertensives, adds yet more force to the question.

At the present time, it would seem that the clinician would do better to ignore the problem of mediation and concentrate on aspects more familiar to the learning therapist. These are many, but first of all we need to determine the most effective schedules of reinforcement. We need to determine whether external feedback of response change is required and, if so, of what type. Replications of BENSON et al.'s 1971 study are required, with additional data on the duration of the effects of the therapy and its transference from the laboratory, now made possible by the use of telemetry. The investigation of such problems would bring greater profit and more useful data than diligent searches for "unknown" covert mediating responses.

References

ALEXANDER, F.: Psychosomatic Medicine. Its Principles and Applications. New York: Norton 1950.

BENSON, H., SHAPIRO, D., TURSKY, B., SCHWARTZ, G.E.: Decreased systolic blood pressure through operant conditioning techniques in patients with essential hypertension. Science 173, 740-742 (1971).

BLACK, A.H.: Operant conditioning of heart rate under curare. Technical Report No. 12. Department of Psychology, McMaster University 1967.

BURGOYNE, L., POTE, R., FREEDMAN, N.: Conditioned cardiac acceleration under cortical depression. Psychonomic Science 9, 417-418 (1967).

ENGEL, B.T.: Operant conditioning of cardiac function; A status report. Psychophysiology 9, 161-177 (1972).

HAHN, W.W.: Apparatus and technique for work with the curarised rat. Psychophysiology 7, 283-286 (1970).

KATKIN, E.S.. MURRAY, E.N.: Instrumental conditioning of autonomically mediated behaviour. Psychol. Bull. 70, 52-68 (1968).

MILLER, N.E.: Psychosomatic effects of specific types of training. Ann. N.Y. Acad. Sci. 159, 1025-1041 (1969).

OBRIST, P.A., WEBB, R.A., SUTTERER, J.R., HOWARD, J.L.: The cardiac somatic relationship: Some reformulation. Psychophysiology 6, 569-585 (1970).

RUSHMER, R.F.: Cardiovascular Dynamics. Philadelphia: Saunders 1961.

SCHNEIDER, A.M., BEHAR, M.: A chronic preparation for spreading cortical depression. J. exp. Anal. Behav. 7, 350 (1964).

SCHWARTZ, G.E.: Voluntary control of human cardiovascular integration and differentiation feedback and reward. Science 175, 90-92 (1972).

SKINNER, B.F.: The Behaviour of Organisms: An Experimental Analysis. New York: Appleton Century Crofts 1938.
SMITH, K.: Conditioning as an artifact. Psychol. Rev. 61, 217-225 (1954).
SMITH, K.: Curare drugs and total paralysis. Psychol. Rev. 71, 77-79 (1964).
STEELE RUSSELL, I.: Neurological basis of complex learning. Brit. med. Bull. 27, 278-285 (1971).
TEPLITZ, T.A.: Operant conditioning of blood pressure: A critical review of some psychosomatic considerations. Commun. behav. Biol. 6, 197-202 (1971).
THORNTON, E.W., VAN TOLLER, C.: Effect of immunosympathectomy on operant heart-rate conditioning in the curarised rat. Physiology and Behaviour. In Press, January 1973.
TROWILL, J.A.: Instrumental conditioning of the heart-rate in the curarised rat. J. comp. physiol. Psychol. 63, 7-11 (1967).

Physiological Correlates of the Extinction of an Avoidance Response Under Three Conditions of Activation

R. FERSTL, C. BECKER-CARUS and S. KRAEMER

Avoidance is a characteristic component of neurotic behaviour. The phobic patient avoiding anxiety-evoking situations, as well as the obsessive patient who seeks to avoid aversive consequences by his ritual behaviour, are both trying to avoid unpleasant events. These patients typically show high resistance to extinction, obviously due to the self-reinforcing system of avoidance behaviour. A great deal of work has been done on this subject in animal studies (e.g. SIDMAN, 1966), but the literature on human avoidance behaviour is limited.

In a series of experiments studying the influence of the activation level on the extinction of different conditioned phenomena, we tried to establish some of the physiological correlates of avoidance behaviour. Our primary purpose was to answer the question whether any characteristic elements can be found in the physiological records that correspond to learning and extinction. A further aim was to record the subjective certainty of the separate reactions and to investigate its variation over a whole period of conditioning and extinction. We know from our earlier experiments that, the more the subject (S) is activated, the more the conditioned GSR reaction is inhibited in its extinction. We therefore set out to see whether the same result could be obtained for avoidance behaviour. Our hypothesis was supported by an article by IWAKAMI (1970), reporting the effects of muscular relaxation on the acquisition and extinction of a conditioned avoidance response. To obtain more explicit information on the effects of single-stimulus conditions, we planned a sequential analysis of the physiological data at the time when a CS (critical situation) or a CS plus S_D (discriminative stimulus) were presented.

Fifteen Ss were divided into 3 groups. In the activation condition group the Ss were told between the conditioning and extinction phase that they would now feel small electric shocks from the EEG electrodes. Subjects in the second group were trained in muscular relaxation before the experiment and were instructed to relax during the extinction phase. The third group served as controls. With the exception of the different activation conditions, the experiment was the same for all Ss.

Three different tones (350, 500, 800 cps) were presented in a randomized order. The duration was 10 sec for each tone and the inter-trial interval varied from 15 to 25 sec. At the end of each tone an electric shock was delivered to the S's right hand. In randomly chosen presentations of the latter two tones a short, high sound of 1 sec duration (1700 cps) could be heard; this served as the S_D. Only after this S_D did Ss have the possibility to avoid the electric shock by pressing a lever.

The task was complicated by a CS-dependent choice-reaction task on one of two levers. Altogether Ss heard three tones (CSs), but only during the latter two and in the presence of S_D could electric shock be avoided (Fig. 1). Beside the lever-pressing reactions, the Ss were asked to estimate their subjective certainty on a scale from 1 to 5, where 1 stood for a low and 5 for a high certainty.

The tones, which were always followed by an electric shock during acquisition, were intended to serve as models for the critical situations (CS without S_D) in the extinction phase. The Ss were expected to recognize the changed experimental conditions, because in the extinction phase no electric shock was delivered in any case. There were 59 acquisition and 71 extinction trials.

During the whole experiment, reactions and physioligical data were recorded on a Schwarzer polygraph and simultaneously recorded digitally at intervals of 4 msec on magnetic tape. In the final form of the experiment two EEG channels (temporal, occipital - left and right) were recorded as well as the EKG, EMG and the GSR. Fig. 2 shows an example of a polygraph record. The stimuli were presented from an analog tape-recorder. The experimental setup is shown in Fig. 3.

Besides the lever-pressing reaction for the learning and extinction criteria, we analysed mainly the EKG and GSR. The frequency of the EKG was analysed on a PDP/8 L computer. We chose the following intervals for the analysis: from 4 sec before to the onset of CS, and from 4 to 8, 8 to 12 and 12 to 16 sec after the onset of CS. The first served as baseline. The second interval should contain all the changes, relevant to the onset of CS (e.g. orienting response). In the next interval (4 to 8 sec) we expected changes in frequency connected with the

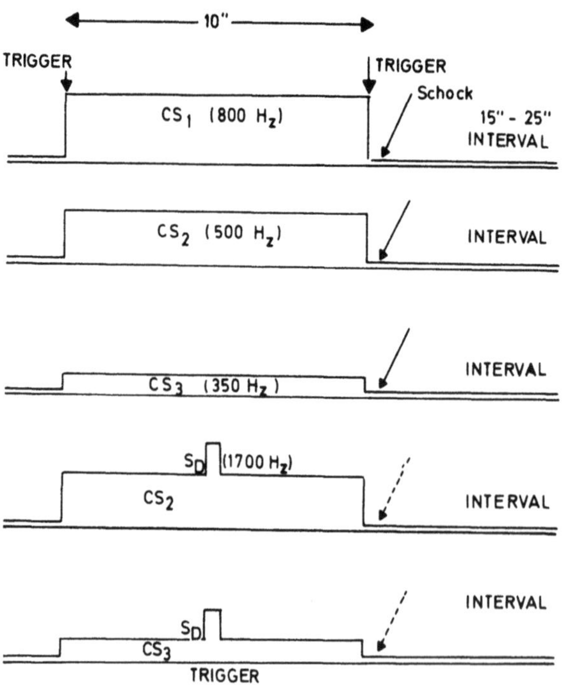

Aquisition	Extinction
20	24
10	14
12	14
9	9
8	10
59	71

Fig. 1. The five experimental conditions and number of trials for the acquisition and the extinction phase

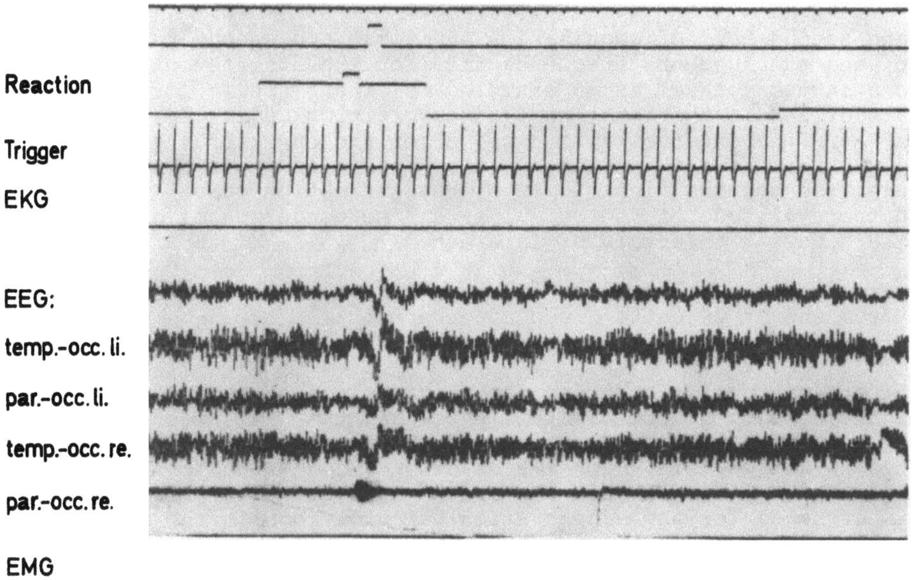

Fig. 2. Example of a polygraph record

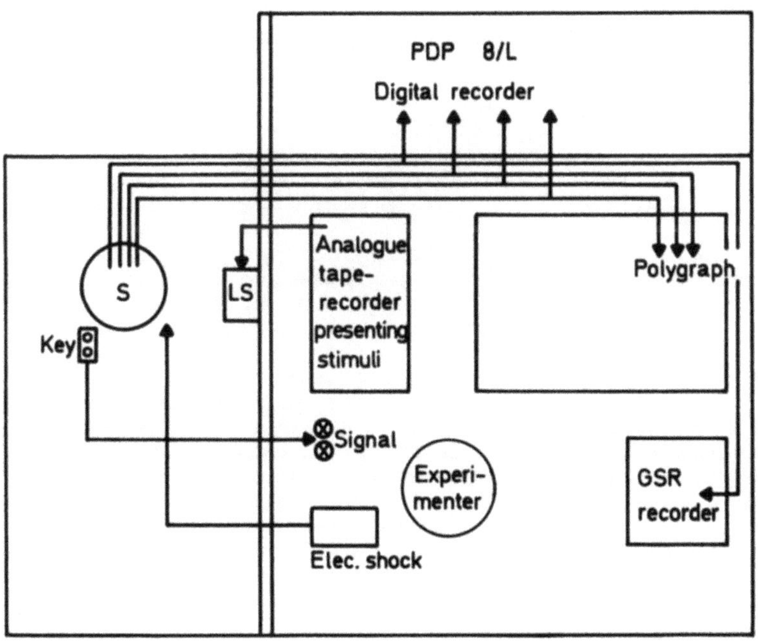

Fig. 3. Experimental setup

expectation and/or actual appearance of S_D. In the time from 8 to 12 sec after the onset of CS we expected EKG correlates corresponding to the expectation of shock and/or actual shock. The fifth interval should show similar data to the baseline interval. Since it is impossible to demonstrate systematic changes from a single trial, we used the technique of summation: we divided the total experiment into 4 phases (first and second half of acquisition and first and second half of extinction) and averaged the frequency data for the 5 different stimulus conditions in each phase. As an example, we cite a result for the main heart rate of a S in the first half of acquisition under the condition CS_2 plus S_D in the interval 4 to 8 sec after the onset of the CS. As regards GSR, besides the spontaneous fluctuation in the first 5 min of the acquisition and the first 5 min of the extinction phase, we determined the amplitude of the stimulus- and response-specific potentials. There were 3 intervals of interest:

1) time from onset to the end of CS
2) time from end of CS until 5 sec afterwards
3) time from end of S_D to end of CS.

In the first interval we expected orienting responses and in the second interval the effects of the electric shock and the S's expectation. The third interval (from end of S_D to end of CS) should show potentials correlated to the certainty for the reaction and the tension of expectation before the end of the CS. As in the analysis of the EKG, the data were averaged for the single-stimulus conditions in the 4 phases of the experiment.

I. Results

Thirteen of the 15 Ss reached the learning criterion of 8 consecutive correct reactions before the extinction phase. Only 4 out of the 15 Ss reached the extinction criterion (no more lever pressing); this was realized in the first half of the extinction phase. Two of these 4 Ss had been relaxed at the beginning of that phase, another belonged to the activated experimental group, and the fourth was from the neutral group. This result ruled out our hypothesis, that extinction is facilitated by a low level of activation. It also supported existing evidence that the extinction of avoidance behaviour in humans is very difficult.

Fig. 4 shows the course of subjective certainty for the reactions of all Ss. In the second half of the acquisition phase one can see that, after a short period of uncertainty at the beginning of the experiment, all subjects reached a high level of certainty which was maintained throughout. From the analysis of the EKG one can see that in all groups the pulse frequency declined from the beginning to the end of the experiment. Analyses of variances and trends indicated a significant linear trend for all CS and CS + S_D conditions (Fig. 5). A comparison of the baseline interval with the last interval showed no significant difference at any experimental phase. Therefore it was possible to take these two intervals as baseline points of reference for the other intervals. Intervals 2, 3 and 4 were each compared to these data. The second and fourth intervals showed no consistent changes. In the third interval (4 - 8 sec after onset of CS) at the beginning of which S_D could also occur, we consistently found characteristic results (Fig. 6). During acquisition and the first half of extinction a marked deceleration of heart rate can be seen under the conditions CS_1, CS_2 and CS_3 without S_D. When S_D appeared, the opposite result could be seen, i.e. acceleration of heart rate. This was true also for the 4 Ss who extinguished their avoidance behaviour in the first half of the extinction phase. In their case the physiological effect followed the behavioural extinction in the second half of the extinction phase: in this half the reaction pattern of the extinguishing Ss exhibited a change of frequency (deceleration) only in the presence of a S_D, while the nonextinguishing Ss showed no change in acceleration in the presence of a S_D and deceleration during the CS.

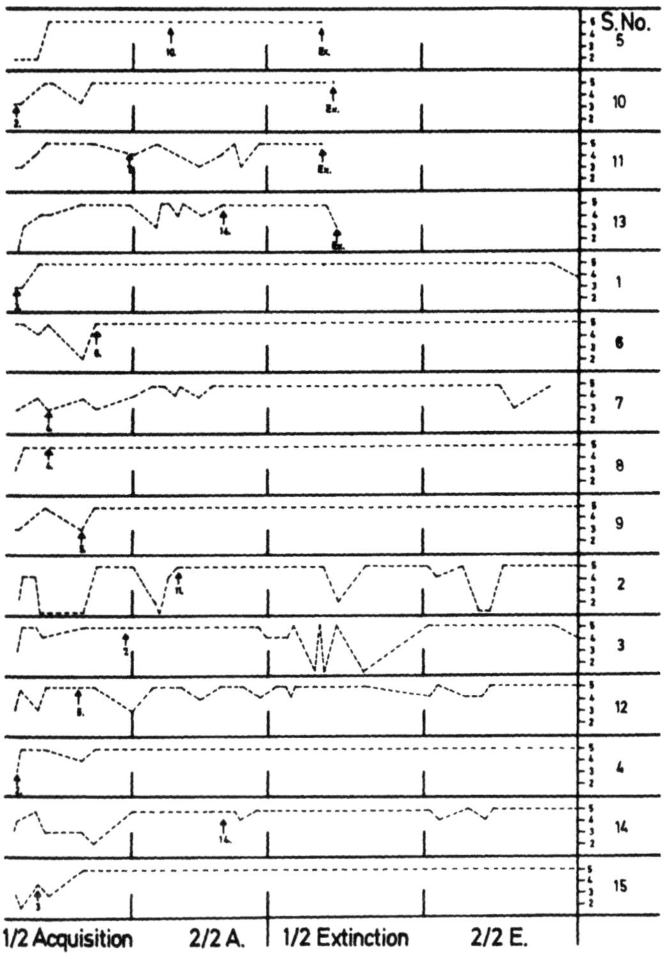

Fig. 4 Course of subjective certainty in the 15 subjects

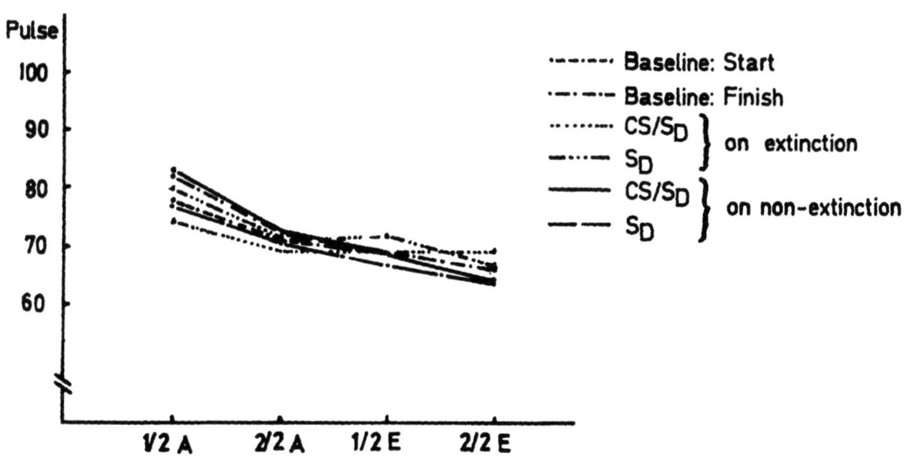

Fig. 5. Decrease in the mean heart rate in the 5 intervals of the EKG analysis from the beginning to the end of the experiment

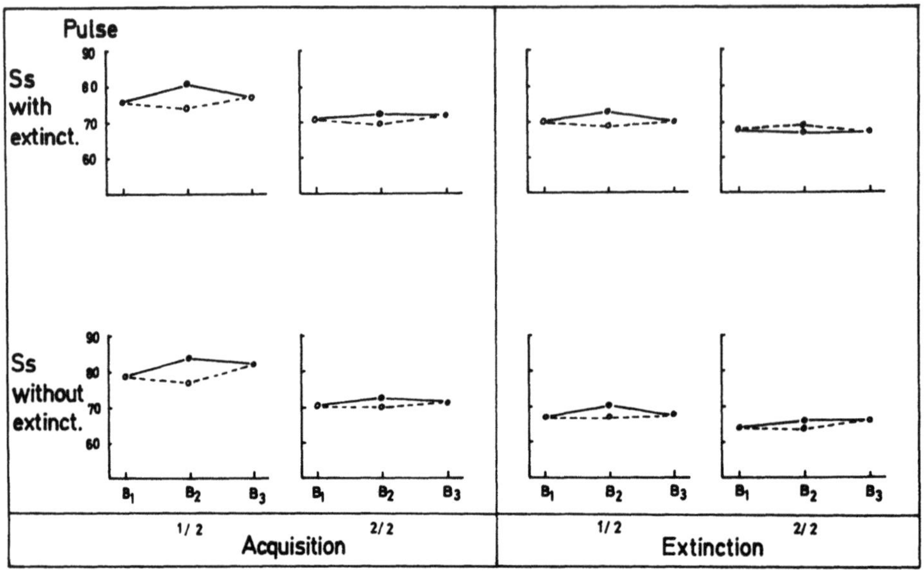

Fig. 6 Mean heart rate in 3 intervals of the EKG analysis: B_1 baseline before the onset of a CS; B_2 critical interval from 4 to 8 sec after the onset of the CS; B_3 12 to 16 sec after the onset of the CS. Full lines show changes in heart rate in presence of S_D; dotted lines show changes in absence of S_D

For technical reasons analysis of the GSR was possible for only 12 of the 15 Ss. As described above, the analysis was done separately for the 4 phases of the experiment. In all 3 experimental groups, the spontaneous fluctuation in the first 5 min of acquisition and extinction showed no correlation with EMG activity, and no group showed any systematic trend in any phase. It was impossible to determine a significant difference between activated, normal and deactivated Ss. For the 5 stimulus conditions no significant difference could be found in GSR activity during CS. In the 5-sec interval after the end of the CS, 7 Ss showed the characteristics typical of the classic conditioned GSR, namely, expectancy potentials for the electric shock in the extinction phase, where no shock was applied. They did not extinguish behaviourally either. This reflects the continuation of an anxiety reaction and the avoidance behaviour associated with it.

In the interval between the end of S_D and the end of CS we expected GSR potentials to be correlated to the emotional response before the reaction. We found, that nonextinguishing Ss had very high GSR potentials in this interval, while extinguishing Ss showed steady or decreasing ones. Fig. 7 shows the change in the potential amplitude for two extinguishing (dotted lines) and two nonextinguishing Ss (full lines).

II. Discussion

It is clear from the EKG analysis that the presentation of a CS without S_D leads to deactivation. The decelaration of the heart rate indicates that the organism is physioligically preparing itself to assimilate

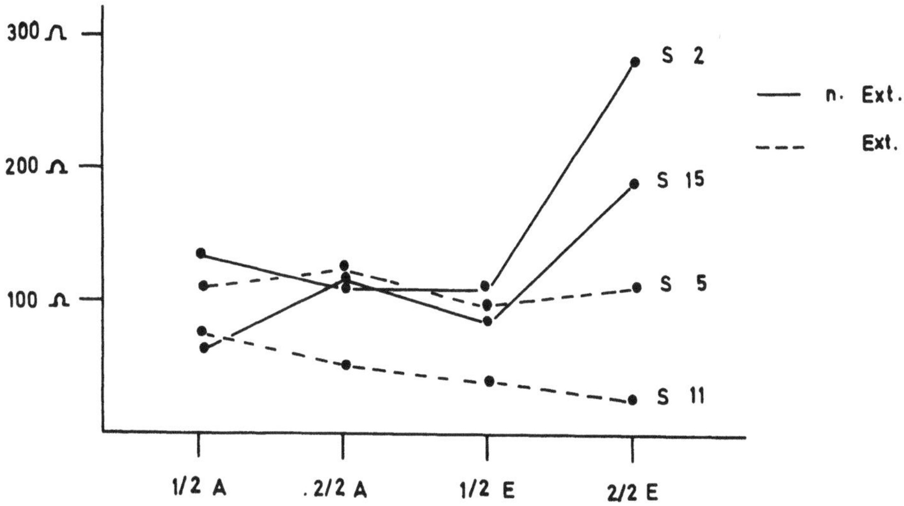

Fig. 7. Changes in GSR potential amplitude in the period from the end of a S_D to the end of a CS for two subjects with extinction (dotted lines) and two without (full lines)

the electric shock. Ss who did not extinguish showed this reaction from the beginning to the end of the experiment. After extinction, 4 Ss no longer showed deceleration in the presence of CS; thus, they no longer expected an electric shock. It is interesting that physiological extinction was obtained only in the second half of the extinction phase.

Acceleration of heart rate after S_D can be interpreted in two ways: (1) as due to activation correlated with the uncertainty of the decision task and (2) as due to general activation following S_D, which maintains the S_D-contingent acceleration even after the correct response has been learned. As long as the Ss did not extinguish, no habituation could be obtained. This result is supported by the finding in the analysis of the GSR. There the S_D-contingent potentials as well as the S_D-contingent heart-rate acceleration were observed over the whole experiment. Only in Ss who extinguished did the GSR potentials decrease in amplitude and the heart rate cease to change.

The 3 experimental groups did not differ in their activation level during extinction because all Ss had been relatively deactivated. This was due to the fact that it is necessary to have deactivated Ss to ensure relatively disturbance-free physiological recordings. The experimental variation of the activation level was restricted accordingly. As the results show, correlates can be found in the EKG and GSR during learning and extinction of an avoidance reaction. It would be interesting if these results could be generalized to the avoidance behaviour of neurotic patients, for example phobic ones. Regarding the strong resistance to extinction, there is some evidence from other studies to show that the physiological response, like the behavioural response, continues even when there are no longer aversive consequences to be avoided. Additionally, subjective certainty inhibits extinction. If it were found that the same types of behavioural and physiological indices were exhibited by neurotics, we would be better able to define measures of anxiety.

References

IWAKAMI, EILEEN E.: The effects of muscle relaxation on the acquisition and extinction of a conditioned avoidance response. Diss. Abstr. Internat. 1970, 30(7-B).

SIDMAN, M.: In: HONIG, W.K. (Ed.): Operant Behaviour: Areas of Research and Application, p. 448-498. New York: 1966.

Clinical Observations Regarding the Use of Elektromyographic Feedback with Chronically Anxious Patients

G. JOHNSON, M. RASKIN, J. RONDESTVEDT, R. LONGABAUGH and F. CHRISWELL

The prospect that internal physiological states, and possibly their subjective correlates, can be systematically and voluntarily controlled through biofeedback and conditioning techniques has resurrected widespread interest in Yoga, Zen and Jacobsen's Progressive Relaxation, as well as Schultz and Luthe's autogenic training. In addition to these techniques, the encouraging reports from behaviour therapists practising systematic desensitization have indicated the significance of deep muscle relaxation as a major therapeutic technique with anxious patients.

An estimated 5 % of the population of the United States suffers from chronic anxiety; 50 % or more of these patients are not relieved by either insight psychotherapy (MILES et al., 1951; RASKIN et al., 1972) or behavioural therapy (LAZARUS, 1963; GELDER, 1969). Although the use of drugs in the treatment of chronic anxiety is widespread, anti-anxiety medication is not entirely satisfactory in maintaining symptomatic relief, and there are often undesirable side-effects.

In 1969 BUDZYNSKI and STOYVA described the development and use of an instrument for producing deep muscle relaxation by means of an analogue information feedback (BUDZYNSKI and STOYVA, 1969). An advantage of this system is that it gives both patient and therapist objective information regarding the degree of muscle relaxation. BUDZYNSKI points out that one important aspect of operant conditioning is that the individual receives immediate information about the events he is attempting to modify. Since some chronically anxious patients may never have experienced deep muscle relaxation, or are unable to distinguish between levels of muscle tension, this instrument is an important device in relaxation training. It has been shown that individuals can achieve muscular relaxation more quickly with feedback training than with no feedback or with irrelevant feedback (BUDZYNSKI and STOYVA, 1969).

Because of these clinical reports, a program of deep muscle relaxation for chronically anxious patients was initiated via feedback training. BUDZYNSKI and co-workers have demonstrated the utility of feedback-induced muscle relaxation in augmenting desensitization (BUDZYNSKI and STOYVA, 1969). However, the primary focus of our program was to train the patient to control anxiety by using deep muscle relaxation and to determine whether these techniques would be helpful in allowing the patient to control his anxiety outside the laboratory. The purpose of this paper is to present our experience in teaching feedback-induced muscle relaxation to chronically anxious patients.

I. Method

1. Subjects

The 23 subjects we studied were outpatients at the Langley Porter Neuropsychiatric Institute. They were generally college-educated young adults who had had symptoms of chronic anxiety for at least 2 years prior to participating in this project. Patients with a diagnosis of chronic brain syndrome, psychosis, or evidence of current major medical problems were excluded. Each subject participated voluntarily. Approximately one third of the subjects had been taking Librium (40 to 80 mg per day) prior to the relaxation training, but had remained symptomatic. These subjects continued with the same level of medication throughout the program.

2. Procedure

The subjects were interviewed by trained therapists to validate the diagnosis of chronic anxiety and screen out inappropriate referrals. They were given a Self-Report Mood check list to complete. This included items adapted from the Hamilton Anxiety Rating Scale and the Bendig Anxiety Scale. This instrument is described in a previous publication (RASKIN et al., 1972). This check list was used weekly to assess "current anxiety levels." A baseline of anxiety was taken on a weekly basis for 2 months prior to the training program using the same check list. Subjects were shown the laboratory and the electromyographic (EMG) equipment and given an explanation of how the instrument functioned. If the subjects suffered from insomnia, headaches or other somatic complaints, they were asked to maintain a record of the frequency and degree of discomfort. For example, 7 subjects with tension headaches were asked to record the frequency and intensity of their headaches using the system described by BUDZYNSKI et al. (1971).

The training instrument was developed and described by BUDZYNSKI and STOYVA. The system provides a pre-amplifier, a main control panel and speaker. The main control panel has a gain setting which permits the pitch of the tone to be manually regulated. In addition there is a device for controlling the volume of the tone; measurement of EMG activity can be divided into time sequences, such as 64 sec of measurement and 20 sec between sequences. The numerical average of EMG activity was displayed visually after each sequence.

Prior to each session, the electrical noise level in the room was measured and subsequently subtracted from the subject's EMG activity levels to obtain a true measure. The subject was asked to lie on a couch. His forehead was cleaned with acetone, the placement sites for the electrodes were scraped to remove dead skin, electrode jell was rubbed on these sites, jell was put into the electrodes, and the electrodes were taped to the forehead. The frontalis muscle was selected because it is a very difficult muscle to relax voluntarily. It was believed that, if subjects could learn to relax this muscle voluntarily, there would then be some generalization of muscular relaxation throughout the body.

Prior to each training session the subjects were asked to rate their current subjective level of tension on a scale from 0-10, with zero meaning completely relaxed and 10 representing panic. Their pulse was taken and then the relaxation training began. After the feedback tone was set at a level which the subjects reported to be comfortable they were instructed to close their eyes and relax as deeply as possible. The room was darkened and the experimenter was present at all times.

The experimenter recorded the average EMG activity after each 64-sec trial. Each training session consisted of 15 trials. During the trials the experimenter noted the occurrence of body movement, coughing, etc. Such movements can suddenly increase the tone and EMG scores. After each session the subjects again rated their subjective tension and their pulses were taken. These training sessions were conducted on 3 to 5 days a week for each subject. The subjects were also asked to practice at home daily.

When the subjects' EMG level averaged less than 2.5 µV for 25 min in repeated sessions they were rated as able to maintain profound frontalis muscle relaxation. We then interspersed sessions without feedback to be sure that the patients could relax deeply on their own. Lastly, subjects were taught to relax with their eyes open in a sitting position.

II. Results and Comments

All the subjects in the study learned to maintain low levels of frontalis activity, and in most instances this was accomplished by subjective tranquillity. Two of the 23 subjects, an alcoholic and a barbiturate addict, did not complete the study. The loss of these subjects was related to their inability to follow a prescribed regimen rather than an inability to lower EMG activity.

During a few training sessions some subjects reported experiencing brief periods of relaxation which were followed by increased anxiety. These experiences were reflected by their EMG activity, which indicated decreased muscular tension followed by a dramatic increase in EMG activity. These subjects described anxiety related to the feeling of "letting themselves go." The presence of the experimenter proved to be helpful in these and other situations. The gain setting could be adjusted and the volume of the tone could be adjusted; the subject's responses could be hand-shaped by these manipulations to tailor the session to the individual subject. The experimenter was also available to explain various phenomena that might puzzle or worry the subject, such as the anxiety which followed brief episodes of relaxation.

In addition to subjective tranquillity, we found other changes within the session. For example, during profound relaxation subjects manifested improvement when nausea or tension headaches had been a problem at the start of a session. The success of some of the subjects in alleviating tension headaches is similar to that reported by BUDZYNSKI et al. (1971). One subject also learned to control his perspiration. At times he would begin to feel hot and perspire in the middle of a session. This produced scores unusually high, even for this anxious subject. The episodes of sweating were precipitated at times by heavy clothing or high subjective anxiety. Initially the experimenter would interrupt the session, disconnect the electrodes, wipe the patient's forehead and start again. The subject learned to prevent these interruptions by imagining that his forehead felt cool.

We were successful in teaching our patients to control previously intolerable situational anxiety. The following is an example of a subject who attained success using the relaxation techniques. A young college-educated male, who had previously been in psychotherapy for 2 years and was on medication prior to and during the study, had been unable to attend conferences at work, drive in congested traffic, drive across bridges, or drive too far from home alone. He could not go into crowded restaurants or sit in a cinema. These situations produced severe, immobilizing anxiety. While in relaxation training, he began to do all of these things. When he felt an impending anxiety attack, he would use the techniques he had been taught in the laboratory.

Although there was a low, non-statistically significant correlation between subjective reports of tension and EMG scores, there were also instances of major discrepancies. Most of the subjects who reported high subjective tension despite low EMG activity were using Librium. These experiences are similar to the findings in a review by LADER and MATHEWS (1971).

Unfortunately, there are very few controlled studies related to the problem of relaxation and anxiety. We are currently initiating such a controlled-outcome study. The experiences of this project indicate that relaxation training can be useful, particularly in situational anxiety, a state which is often uncontrolled despite medication.

References

BUDZYNSKI, T.H., STOYVA, J.M.: An instrument for producing relaxation by means of analog information feedback. J. appl. behav. Anal. 2, 231-237 (1969).

BUDZYNSKI, T.H., STOYVA, S., ADLER, C.: Feedback-induced relaxation: application to tension headaches. J. Behav. Ther. exp. Psychol. Res. 15, 479-486 (1971).

GELDER, M.: Behaviour therapy for anxiety states. Brit. med. J. 1969I, 691-694.

LADER, M.N., MATHEWS, A.M.: Electromyographic studies of tension. J. psychosom. Res. 15, 479-486 (1971).

LAZARUS, A.A.: The results of behaviour therapy in 126 cases of severe neurosis. Behav. Res. Ther. 1, 69-79 (1963).

MILES, H.H.W., BARABEE, E.L., FINESINGER, J.E.: Evaluation of psychotherapy with a follow-up of 62 cases of anxiety neurosis. Psychosom. Med. 13, 83-105 (1951).

RASKIN, M., RONDESTVEDT, J.W., JOHNSON, G.: Anxiety in young adults: a prognostic study. J. nerv. ment. Dis. 154, (April) (1972).

RASKIN, M., RONDESTVEDT, J.W., JOHNSON, G.: Anxiety in young adults: a prognostic study. J. nerv. ment. Dis. 154, 229-237 (1972).

VI. The Implementation of Behaviour Modification in the Environment

Interaction Patterns in Clinical Behaviour Therapy

D. SCHWARZ and M. GERLINGHOFF

I. Introduction

"While we are convinced of the efficiency of behaviour therapy for the patient as a single individual, we are missing any hint on interpersonal effects in the dramatic improvement of the patient." So wrote WATZLAWICK (1969) in his book on human communication.

Indeed, in clinical behaviour therapy with adults interaction processes are taken very rarely into consideration. This is surprising, as in the last decade much work was done on ethology and social psychology. The reason for this neglect may lie in the historical development of behaviour therapy.

Reinforcers that proved useful in animal experiments, e.g. food, were transferred to behaviour modification techniques with good results, as we know, especially in children and psychotics. But despite our knowledge of the reinforcing effects of social signals in higher animals, a contingent use of social reinforcers has rarely been made in clinical behaviour therapy.

Perhaps I should amend this to "in clinical behaviour therapy with adults", because there are very impressive results on mother-child interaction as well as on marital therapy with outpatients. Also there has been much interest in patient-therapist relations, e.g. KRASNER's (1962) "The therapist as a reinforcing machine."

The aim of our paper is to focus attention on the control and contingent use of natural partners as social reinforcers in clinical behaviour therapy. In recent years we have treated many patients in whom effective treatment was only made possible by management of social reinforcers. The criteria for admission in these patients did not differ from those for other patients, i.e. degree of disturbance and failure of long-term outpatient treatment. These patients' symptoms at the first impression gave no hint of a disturbed interaction.

Let me first give a brief theoretical framework. Interpersonal relations are important in evocation and maintenance of behaviour disorders. A simple schedule may differentiate three types of interaction patterns:

1. The patient manipulates his partner by his symptoms. The symptom serves as a medium for communication.
2. The patient is manipulated by his partner. His symptoms are maintained by the behaviour of his partner.
3. The relations between the partners could be described, as JACKSON

(   ) has done, as a pathological homoeostasis. In such a case, often both partners display clinical symptoms.

In clinical behaviour therapy social signals and social reinforcement mechanisms between the patient and his partner can often be managed much better than in outpatient therapy. Some of the factors which are effective in therapeutic management of social reinforcement are:

1. Deprivation. (Separation of the partners reveals a growing need for the social reinforcement dispensed by the partner.)
2. Systematic delay between contacts. This may influence the reaction on social reinforcement.
3. Changing the punctuation of behaviour sequences.
4. Changing the context and therefore introducing the possibility of new means of communication instead of the symptoms.

We are now going to concretize these theoretical remarks by some case reports and to demonstrate some problems which may arise in practice.

II. Introduction of Treatment

The indication for partner therapy is not given by the symptoms which prompted admission. Impaired interaction patterns may be important in psychosomatic symptoms, phobias, drug abuse and other deviations, not to mention sexual difficulties. Often it takes time to recognize that successful therapy is not possible without reference to the troubled interaction with the partner:

Case History

A 35-year-old married woman was admitted because of alcoholism. There were some conflicts with her husband, but we found no contingent relationship with her drinking problem. After chemical aversion therapy, the patient improved and remained abstinent for the next year. One year later she was re-admitted because of deep depression. Now she intended to get divorced. Marriage difficulties had worsened in spite - or should we say because - of her improvement the year before. At this time we started simultaneous treatment of both partners, directed only toward the difficulties in their relationship. Depression improved and there was no relapse during the following years.

If an interaction disturbance is identified, it is often difficult to motivate both the patient and his partner to accept appropriate therapy. Difficulties are created not only, as expected, by the resistance of the partner but also by the patient himself. This is the case where the symptoms of the patient are strongly rewarded by the partner, or where communication between partners has dwindled to the extent that it can only be maintained by talking about the symptoms.

III. Different Roles

There are different roles the patient or his partner can play during therapy. Often it is possible to use the partner as a cotherapist. In this case it is necessary to train the partner as a reinforcement dispenser. It may be useful to forbid all contact between the patient and his partner for some time. During this time the patient gets reinforcement from the therapist and the nursing staff. The partner is gradually introduced as cotherapist and at the same time the therapist as social reinforcer is faded out. Very often the situation is highly complex and a pathological balance has developed between the partners. Treating only the patient would change this balance and produce new behaviour disturbances in the patient or his partner.

Case History

A 34-year-old married woman was admitted because of severe sleep disturbances. At first she was reluctant to enter the hospital, but her husband, himself a doctor, insisted on her admission after which she improved rapidly. At the same time her husband began to suffer from nervous symptoms, insisted on visiting her more often, and asked for her discharge. In order to test the stability of her improvement, we agreed to a longer visit by the husband; the day after this the patient was much worse. Her husband on the other hand seemed to feel better and again agreed to longer treatment of his wife. As we did not arrange partner therapy in this case, we observed a similar change of intentions twice more.

A situation like the preceding case leads, so to speak, to the ideal kind of partner therapy, whereas a single treatment necessarily causes disturbances in the partner. A third constellation occurs rather seldom: the situation in which the patient who enters the hospital is less disturbed than his partner. Treatment here is very difficult as it presumes an exchange of roles, the patient being the cotherapist while his partner becomes the patient.

IV. Methods of Treatment

There is no fundamental difference between the methods used in inpatient and outpatient treatment. The sooner the disturbance can be considered as unidirectional, the earlier can both partners be given treatment. Most patients admitted to the hospital have widely generalized the social stimuli causing the disturbance. Short contacts between the partners may revive the whole pathological process and any therapeutic gain will be lost. In such cases only inpatient treatment offers the opportunity to modify and control the interaction processes.

Case History

A 48-year-old married woman 3 years before admission had suffered a psychotic depression. Her husband and her 17-year-old daughter took more interest in her at that time than ever before. When she improved, her relatives again took up their own activities. The patient began to show many hypochondriac symptoms, and in the following years she was rewarded more and more by her relatives when talking about her symptoms. After admission to hospital we interrupted all contacts between the patient and her partners. On the ward she was reinforced only when she did not talk about her symptoms; she quickly improved. One week later we permitted the husband to visit the patient and next day she felt much worse. We then started a training programme with her husband: he was advised to react only to desired behaviour and to ignore all utterances concerning the symptoms. The visits were limited in the beginning to 10 to 20 minutes. During the first visit the therapist remained in the room. The patient showed continual improvement on being reinforced by her husband only for desirable activities.

If contacts with the partner have a strong rewarding effect, it is possible to use a token system, in which contacts are contingent on decreasing pathology or increasing frequency of desired behaviour. The more generalized the pathological interaction pattern, the more rigid the system. I will try to summarize the course of such a treatment:

1. Immediately after admission the therapist interviews both partners, which serves to identify the main interaction patterns.
2. Contact between partners is interrupted for up to two weeks. In most cases this extends not only to visits but also to contact by letter or telephone. During this time the partner is free to question the therapist as much as he likes about the well-being of the patient.
3. During the time of interrupted contact between partners the therapist arranges separate interviews with each partner. These interviews serve to work out further interaction patterns and to reveal special tensions in interacting with the partner. It is then possible to start a systematic desensitization against irritating behaviour or utterances by the partner.
4. In separate talks each partner is prepared for the contact. Instructions are given to avoid special subjects, or how to react to certain behaviour patterns of the partner.
5. The first visit is limited to 10 to 20 min, during which time the therapist is present. He takes no part in the interaction but he can signal undesired reactions by a previously agreed sign. If things get too bad, he can interrupt the visit. After the visit the therapist discusses the difficulties observed with each partner separately and tries to develop alternative reactions.
6. The partners can now meet without the therapist being present. Sometimes it is useful to check the interaction by audio- or videotape.
7. In the further course of treatment the frequency of meeting can be determined by the partners themselves, but each contact is discussed with the therapist. Sometimes it is useful gradually to replace intact interaction by a process of shaping.

The more behaviour deviations there are present in both partners, the more important it is that each partner will be rewarded by the other in the various steps of therapy.

Case History

A 28-year-old married woman suffered from agoraphobia. During the preceding years she had developed extreme dependency behaviour and annoyed her husband by frequent phone calls during working hours. For her part, she suffered from lack of sexual interest by her husband. Her partner complained that it was impossible to have reasonable talks with his wife as he had before. Now she usually talked only about her difficulties, even at parties. Each partner received different instructions: the patient had to inform herself on special subjects supposed to be of interest to her husband before meeting him and was told not to mention her symptoms during talks. The husband was advised to avoid reproaches and to be kind and loving to his wife, whatever his real feelings. Frequency of meeting depended on the way in which each partner had carried out the instructions.

In such cases neither partner would be able to function as a cotherapist without being rewarded himself. Each partner must receive positive reinforcement during contacts if he is to be able to reinforce the desired behaviour of his partner.

V. Problems in Clinical Partner Therapy

Sometimes clinical treatment is interrupted prematurely. This can be due to the patient as well as his partner. Briefly, we could say that in such cases we had failed to create the correct balance between reward and demand for the patient or his partner: for example, we may have failed to recognize the disturbances in the partner, or have asked the partner to work as cotherapist before he was sufficiently trained.

Case History

A 31-year-old woman was admitted to hospital because of tranquillizer abuse. Although she had relapsed repeatedly, her husband had never drawn any conclusions. After she had taken all his money out of the bank without informing him, he talked of divorce, but he soon changed his mind although his wife did not respect his conditions to change her behaviour. When we suggested to make his visits contingent on the behaviour of the patient, he agreed. However, when his wife threatened to divorce if he did not take her home immediately, he ignored psychiatric advice and asked for his wife's discharge.

Sometimes treatment is interrupted because the partner regards the therapist as a competitor. This can easily happen if the therapist does not talk to the partner.

Other factors which can hamper successful therapy are lack of time, or the patient's home being too distant, so that new interaction patterns cannot be established sufficiently well. In some cases treatment of both partnes is insufficient because the aims of therapy may clash with interests of other persons, who were not or could not be taken into therapy themselves.

Case History

A 32-year-old man was treated because of social phobias. Treatment of his symptoms was at first successful and led to an improvement in the interaction with his wife. But these same improvements caused difficulties with the patient's mother, who lived in the same house. Apparently she had gained much reward from the dependency of her son, who often visited her when he had trouble with his wife. Fortunately, in this case, the patient was stable enough to withstand her threatening him with psychogenic heart attacks. In other patients this could easily cause a relapse.

VI. Terminating Clinical Therapy

Various factors must be taken into account in deciding to terminate clinical treatment:

1. kind and degree of the symptoms in the patient and his partner;
2. state of training of the patient or his partner as reinforcement dispenser;
3. external conditions such as the need to find a new job or home.

The stress of real life cannot be simulated sufficiently well under clinical conditions. Discharged too abruptly, the patient will relapse and a new course of therapy will be much more difficult. Therefore the patient is sent home for short periods, first for some hours, later for a day, overnight, or for a weekend. While discharging him stepwise, it is possible to recognize new difficulties connected with home conditions and to work these out. After final discharge, the patient should be seen in an outpatient setting, depending on the interaction pattern, separately or together with his partner. Such a setting should be arranged in the beginning once or twice a week, then at longer intervals. Checklists of self-control may be effective sometimes, using a token system based on social reinforcement and controlled either by the therapist or by the patient's partner.

VII. Summary

Social interaction, especially interaction between natural partners, is considered the most potent reinforcer in adult patients. In clinical behaviour therapy it is possible to control this reinforcer and to make it contingent on desired behaviour. Depending on the structure of the interaction, the partner can play the role of cotherapist as well as copatient. Treatment of a wide range of behaviour disturbances will be more effective, and relapses can be avoided if interaction patterns are taken into account. Clinical experience has been encouraging. It should have stimulated the integration of the results of practical behaviour therapy into social psychology more than it has done up till now.

References

JACKSON, D.D.: "The Question of Family Homeostasis", Psychiatric Quaterly Suppl. 31, 79 (1957).

KRASNER, L.: The psychotherapist as a social reinforcement machine. In: H.H. Strupp & L. Lubovsky (Eds.) Research in Psychotherapy. Vol. II, Washington DC APA, 1962.

WATZLAWICK, P. et al.: Menschliche Kommunikation, Hans Huber Verlag Bern, Stuttgart, Wien 1969.

The Application of the Principles of Behaviour Modification to Social Work Agencies in the South West Lancashire Area

P.J. NOLAN

This paper deals with the modification of adolescent and adult deviant behaviour by community-based social workers. It deals with two types of cases; (1) patients who have had an in-patient psychiatric admission or who have been attending an out-patient clinic; (2) those not referred to a psychiatric agency. The agencies involved are:

1. the South West Lancashire Probation Service
2. the Liverpool Family Service Unit
3. the Liverpool Social Services Department.

It is common for each of these agencies to refer people to hospital who are then discharged to the care of the appropriate social agency. In view of this, it seemed essential that cases treated in the hospital by a behaviour modification approach be consistently managed after discharge. The mobility of the social agencies and their ability to observe the behaviour of their clients in the natural environment means that they are in a better position to attempt certain types of behaviour modification than anyone in the hospital setting. I discuss here this aspect of attempting to modify behaviour in the natural environment.

More specifically, I discuss an attempt to use a behaviour-modification approach to social casework - cases that would otherwise have been referred to a psychiatric agency are dealt with by a social worker using some form of behavioural engineering. The model followed is that described by THARPE and WETZEL (1969).

Notwithstanding the criticism of the medical model of deviance and the aggravating factors involved in hospital admission implicit in much of the work discussed here, there are certain cases that are dealt with by social workers after the client has been admitted to hospital. In such cases the role of the social worker is twofold; (1) he acts as ancillary therapist when the patient is discharged, using techniques similar to those employed by the hospital-based therapist, and (2) he works closely with the family and trains them in an ancillary therapeutic role. A similar procedure is employed with out-patient referrals. Quite a number of patients are referred for some form of behavioural engineering, and it is not desirable that this should stop merely because the patient is discharged from hospital. When a social worker has a case referred by a therapist who is using a behavioural approach, it is essential that the social worker understand the principles and techniques being used and act in accordance with them. Inconsistency of approach may well be harmful. Take, for example, a patient being given assertive training within the hospital setting. As much orthodox social work involves the 'helping' role of the social worker, it is common for social workers to arrange the lives of their clients in a practical way in the sphere of employment, accommodation and interpersonal events. For a social worker to approach a case in this way may well be incompatible with the approach of the therapist giving the assertive training.

We realised that social work agencies could do far more in the natural environment than we at the hospital, and we were keen to enlist their expertise in this field. The social workers were invited to attend training sessions or lectures in behaviour modification in the Social Work Department, the Psychology Department and the Nurses Training School of the hospital. The object was to attempt to stimulate interest and to teach the basic principles involved in the approach. Social workers and psychologists from the hospital also visited the appropriate social work agency and discussed the case with them in terms of a behaviour modification approach. Where appropriate, the social worker to be involved in the community would be invited to participate in discussions at the hospital. Reading lists and article references, along with offprints of articles where possible, were presented to social workers who wished to learn more. Much attention was paid to follow-up, and close contact was maintained with the social work agency by means of visits, progress reports and meetings involving the patient, Social Services social worker and hospital social worker.

A wide range of presenting problem behaviour was treated and referred in this way, using a variety of clinical techniques in the Psychology Department and a programme of contingency management, often including a contract, in the natural environment. The presenting problems that proved to make up the bulk of the material included gambling, a host of phobic behaviours, sexual problems and a general class of marital or family disharmony.

In this way the social work agencies were introduced to, and encouraged to take an interest in, a behavioural approach to social casework. Given this interest, I felt it would be extremely interesting to test the possibility of using a behavioural approach to social casework so as to eliminate the necessity of referral to the hospital at all. The plan was to train social workers in the techniques of behavioural modification so they could deal with cases without referral to a psychiatrist. For the purposes of this research my role was that of educator and not of social worker employed by a hospital. There was no question of cases being referred to me because I was a "psychiatric social worker".

The relapse rate of psychiatric patients when they return to their natural environment is obvious to all staff of psychiatric hospitals. It appears that to remove an individual from his environment and place him in one of our large psychiatric hospitals is not always a successful form of treatment. In many cases a programme disrupts the individual's social relationships and may lead to a disorganisation in social behaviour. It is possible that, in the treatment of certain types of presenting problems, the most serious handicap is the concept of "mental illness". The literature on the "myth of mental illness" is vast and I do not intend to review it here. Most readers will be aware of the work of SZASZ (1961) and the analysis of BANDURA (1969), and it is on this type of model that the hypothesis is based. In simple terms, it is felt that while it is undeniable that some behaviour may be caused by physical disorder, it is irresponsible to assume that all or even most behaviour arises from similar causes. Mental illness, if seen as a branch of deviance, may be analysed as a sociological phenomenon, and when it is analysed in this way the problems look different. Many so-called psychiatric symptoms involve considerable amounts of social judgement, these judgments being evaluative rather than actual qualities of the behaviour. Any behaviour which is labelled as pathologic involves the standards of those who make the judgments, the social context in which the behaviour is exhibited and observed, and the nature of the behaviour and the characteristics of the person seen to be the deviator. The obvious problems posed are in terms of varying cultures and subculteres, as psychopathology appears to be inferred from the degree of deviance from a societal norm which defines how people are expected to behave at different times and at different places. Also, as BANDURA points out, it is important to remember that deviations which have been seen to benefit society are tolerated and praised, while deviations which are not beneficial are punished. To be a good patient in a large psychiatric hospital means to go along with the regime. Placed in a regime which demands dependent behaviour, the patient finds it very hard to emit responses of assertion and independence.

Such an analysis has implications for the treatment of behaviour which presents as deviant behaviour and strongly suggests that some alternative to the medical model should be investigated. The medical diad PSYCHIATRIST-PATIENT has for some time been the predominant model in this field. THARPE and WETZEL suggested that it was dependency upon professionalism which had in large measure been responsible for many of the adverse effects of treatment given in this way. They hypothesized that the natural environment contained tremendous therapeutic potential, if this potential could be harnessed and arranged in some way. The principles of learning theory led to the following hypotheses:

1. Undesirable behaviour may be weakened by not rewarding it.
2. Desirable behaviour may be strengthened by following it with reward.
3. Reinforcers may be described as those consequences of behaviour which strengthen or weaken it as they are presented or withdrawn.

THARPE and WETZEL added two more:

4. The most powerful reinforcers lie within the natural environment of an individual and are embedded within the social sphere.
5. These reinforcers are controlled by people bearing natural relationships to each other, and these people are seldom professionals.

As an alternative to the medical diad, THARPE and WETZEL used a four-part referral system:

a) SUPERVISOR	A person with specialized knowledge of behavioural techniques
b) BEHAVIOUR ANALYST	Persons instructed in learning theory by the supervisor
c) MEDIATOR	People with power to reinforce who consult with the behaviour analyst
d) TARGET	The person with the problem.

In an attempt to use this model, it was decided to arrange a formal course with one of the social work agencies, putting myself in the position of supervisor and the social workers in the position of behaviour analysts. There are important differences between the model and our trial. The work of THARPE and WETZEL took place in Tucson, Arizona. The site was chosen because there was a paucity of existing social and mental health facilities, and it was felt that it was going to be easy to establish new and quite different services there. The area in which my work took place already had numerous such facilities, well established by tradition. Thus, I was forced to attempt to set up a novel referral system within an existing one. The behaviour analysts of THARPE and WETZEL were graduates, chosen specifically for their lack of training in sociology, psychology or psychiatry. In this way it was hoped to train them in behaviour modification techniques without contamination by previous learning experiences. Our behaviour analysts were established social workers, many of whom had considerable service experience.

I felt that it would be most useful to choose one social work agency for this more specialized piece of work. The service chosen was the Probation Service, for a host of reasons, including many practical considerations. The Social Services Department was in the process of reorganisation in an attempt to offer a generic service, and seemed too much involved with the problems of this reorganisation. The Family Service Unit seemed a more viable proposition, not being troubled by reorganisation nor restricted by statutory duties; unfortunately, because of the small staff and intensity of their casework, the practical factors of arranging the teaching sessions and meetings proved insurmountable. The Probation Service in the area was very stable and under the direction of a progressive and enthusiastic Assistant Principal. Criticism of the behavioural approach always appeared to be constructive and, as most officers adopted a very practical approach to their casework, they were attracted to the practical aspects of much of the contingency-management approach to behavioural engineering in social casework.

The officers to be trained as behaviour analysts were chosen from nine offices of the South West Lancashire Probation and After Care Service. This group met over a period of 6 months every other week for 1 1/2 to 2 hours. The first six sessions consisted mainly of teaching, and the last six were involved with discussion and practical problems of case management, officers presenting cases that they were dealing with using the techniques that they had learnt.

In the introductory session the probation officers were introduced to the basic concepts of the model, i.e. that reinforcement for a client is controlled by the people to whom he or she is naturally related. It was explained to them that, once this approach is accepted, the task of social casework becomes an attempt to reorganize the patterns of reinforcement control exercised by the people in the environment of the individual. The task is to specify the desired pattern of reorganized control and to modify the behaviour of the people bearing natural relationships so that they will reorganize it for the ultimate benefit of the client. The direct-contact individual, that is, the person exercising control, is very seldom a professional. It is hypothesized that a considerable amount of therapeutic potential lies within the range of natural relationships.

The next session involved some definitions essential in understanding a behavioural approach to social casework. The most important point made was that behaviour must be defined accurately, i.e. what a person is seen to be doing, and must be recorded precisely; it was important not to attempt to infer anything from the behaviour as this would involve guesswork. JEHU (1967) and KRUMBOLTH (1965) provided the basis for two sessions in which we looked at the relevance of behaviour modification research to the interview situation.

After this basic information, the probation officers were introduced to the further concepts of using a behavioural approach that would involve the family of their client. Along with the illustrations of THARPE and WETZEL, I found it useful to refer to an article by LIBERMAN (1970a), which proved to be of value in discussing approaches to behavioural casework, The probation officers at fieldwork level were now in a position to start engineering behavioural change. They were in direct contact with their client, or target, and were involved in recording baseline frequencies of behaviour before change was instituted. They were responsible for instigating the techniques to bring about change, and also to assess the effectiveness of the intervention.

One of the most important roles the probation officers filled was that of educator of the mediator. In certain of our cases the probation officer was both behaviour analyst and mediator. Many young adolescents on probation have no family, or significant other companions, and the relationship with the probation officer may be the only meaningful, and highly reinforcing, one. Most often, however, the mediator will not be a professionsal, but the parents of an adolescent, or the husband or wife of a client. The link between the probation officers as behaviour analysts and the mediators was threefold: (1) the probation officer considered which person in the natural environment would be the most effective mediator; (2) the probation officer had to discuss suitable reinforcers with his chosen mediator; (3) the probation officer had to discuss with his chosen mediator the feasibility of dispensing these reinforcers in a suitable contingent manner. The management of a case by behaviour analyst and mediator depended on the individual problem.

The probation officers were also given some tuition in alternative models of certain aspects of deviant behaviour and their implications for casework, e.g. classical conditioning, operant conditioning, shaping and imitative learning. It was considered important that they should look at learning theory interpretations of the aetiology of deviant behaviour. For illustrative purposes we used the topic of social drug abuse and examined this topic in terms of behaviour contingencies, based on arguments along the lines of those of Howard Becker and the paper "Promoting Adaptive Behaviour" in KRUMBOLTZ (1965). It was emphasized that learning theory hypotheses of the aetiology of deviant behaviour present different approaches to the changing of that behaviour. The final pieces of teaching material were SARASON and GANZER (1969) and Chapter 3 of JEHU (1972).

The following sessions of the group centred upon case discussion, incorporating the problems the probation officers experienced in attempting to use the approach.

Discussion at the end of the 6-month period provided useful feedback from the group as to the value of our project. It was felt by all that the work had been valuable but it was stressed that what we had discussed was often good 'orthodox' casework. I think this point is well taken in that much of the behavioural approach to casework presents in the same way as other forms of casework, but with a different interpretive model. A great deal of the psychodynamic model can be explained in terms of behavioural contingencies (e.g. LIBERMAN, 1970b). Nonetheless, the probation officers seemed to think that a behavioural approach gave them a more rational footing on which to base their casework. They also realized that such an approach was important because it helped them to decide how progress had come about in a case and facilitated a more rigorous assessment of the effectiveness of their casework. They also found the approach helpful in that they got a fuller picture of the home circumstances, because they were attempting to use people in the home as therapeutic agents.

The probation officers seemed to be using the approach to deal with a large number of their cases, and one of them was in the process of setting up a group, using role playing and modelling techniques somewhat along the lines of SARASON and GANZER (1969). It is hoped that the group will continue to use these methods and that interest will not die out with the disbanding of the formal group. At present, arrangements are being made to provide information on behaviour modification to other social work agencies in the area, and it is hoped that members of our group who are still interested can be used as speakers or lecturers.

References

BANDURA, A.: Principles of Behavior Modification, New York: Holt, Rinehart, Winton 1969.

JEHU, D.: Learning Theory and Social Work. London: Routledge and Kegan Paul 1967.

JEHU, D.: Behavior Modification in Social Work. New York: Wiley Interscience 1972.

KRUMBOLTZ, J.D. (Ed.): Revolution in Counseling: Implications of Behavioral Science. Boston: Houghton, Mifflin Co. 1965.

LIBERMAN, R.: Behavioral approaches to family and couple therapy. Amer. J. Orthopsychiat. 40 (1) (1970a).

LIBERMAN, R.: A behavioral approach to group dynamics. Behav. Ther. 1 (2) (1970b).

SARASON, I.G., GANZER, V.J.: Developing inappropriate social behaviors of juvenile delinquents. In: KRUMBOLTZ, J.D., THORESEN, C.E. (Eds.): Behavioral Counseling: Cases and Techniques. New York: Holt, Rinehart and Winston 1969.

SZASZ, T.S.: The Myth fo Mental Illness: Foundations of a Theory of Personal Conduct. New York: Harper 1961.

THARPE, R.G., WETZEL, R.: Behavior Modification in the Natural Environment. New York-London: Academic Press 1969.

Behaviour Modification in a Therapeutic Community

M. HALLIDAY, D.H.G. HOPKINS and B. SCHULTZE

This paper describes the operation of a behaviour modification programme in a hospital which is known particularly for its work as a therapeutic community. This may suggest to some the operation of medical and nursing policies that are fundamentally opposed to the aims and practices of behaviour modification. Therapeutic communities place great emphasis on concepts and principles such as the value of open communication, shared leadership, decision-making by consensus, patient leadership and self-determination, and use is made of crisis situations and feedback information to facilitate the process of social learning. Many of these principles lend themselves to the operation of a behaviour modification programme and facilitate its working. In our view, some of the work done in conventional therapeutic community settings is in fact behaviour modification, using group pressure as the agent for changing behaviour and a system of rewards and punishments in the form of verbal responses or a silence to signify approval or dis-approval to facilitate learning. Other patients participating in the group process quickly perceive what the therapist considers "right", "good" or acceptable behaviour and learn to discriminate it from what is "wrong", "bad" or unacceptable behaviour.

A token economy system is perhaps too open a recognition of this factor of therapy for the taste of some, and at a recent conference of therapeutic communities held at Dingleton Hospital accusations of reducing humans to the level of rats were levelled by a few, when Glenkinnon ward, which operates a behaviour modification programme for 35 moderately mentally handicapped patients, came up for discussion.

Dingleton Hospital, situated in the Scottish Borders, provides a comprehensive service for the Counties of Berwick, Roxburgh and Selkirk and part of Peebles. The population of this area is 100,000 and the hospital has 418 beds, the majority of them occupied by psychogeriatric patients. We do <u>not</u> have responsibility for the area services in subnormality, however, and the majority of the retarded came to us for special reasons. Most have been in Dingleton for several years and are still there, because there is no satisfactorily sheltered accommodation in the community.

The behaviour modification programme was agreed to by the hospital community and initiated about 4 years ago, following a proposal made by a visiting American psychologist who stayed to see it through its first year of operation. Previously, the ward was considered a problem area, and the staff were demoralized.

Central to the operation of the hospital is the daily community council meeting through which all communications pass; the meeting ratifies all decisions influencing the working of the hospital. Wards and working areas of the hospital are represented in community council. Information, therefore, can be disseminated throughout the hospital on a day-to-day basis and decisions, once made by the council, are agreed to and accepted by the hospital as a whole. An area which fails to cooperate cannot later plead ignorance, and such an area can be and usually is challenged, thereby making programmes effective and consistent in their application throughout the different areas of the hospital.

The second feature of work at Dingleton Hospital to be borne in mind is the high degree of development of community links. It is policy always to involve the family in the treatment situation when possible. The family is seen, operationally speaking, as a microcosm of the hospital so that an attempt is made to introduce to the family the principles of open communication, shared leadership, decision-making by consensus and the use of feedback information. Use is made of crisis situations for growth and learning, which often involves studying the family *in situ* during domiciliary visits.

The operation of a behaviour modification programme in a therapeutic community - and perhaps some of the advantages of such a setting - are apparent in the case history of a hyperactive retarded girl who suffers from petit mal and psychomotor seizures and who was aged 15 at the time of referral. She is the oldest of four children, all of whom are bright and in no way handicapped. Her parents are intelligent, able people, who are concerned about their daughter's future and happiness. She was born after a normal full-term delivery, weighing 7 1/4 pounds. She thrived, and sat at 7 months, stood at 11 months and walked at 19 months. Her language development was delayed. At 2 years of age she fell downstairs, and a little while later she hit her head against a car windscreen, sustaining a fracture. She was in the hospital for a few days and was thought to have made a good recovery. About 6 weeks later, she had an episode of unconsciousness lasting several hours, and her parents think this was followed by a fit. These events occured in the first part of her third year. At 3 1/2 years, the parents became aware of behaviour difficulties, consisting of severe restlessness and impulsiveness and temper tantrums. Her behaviour became repetitive and language development remained poor. She was investigated at the Great Ormond Street Sick Children's Hospital, and an EEG showed a mild diffuse abnormality. There were no abnormal neurological signs and a diagnosis of a "probable psychosis" was made. Because of increasing behaviour disorders, repetitive ritualistic behaviour and an inability to acquire educational skills, she entered the Camphill Rudolf Steiner School at 8 years of age. There she remained until 15 years of age, during which time she developed skills in household and kitchen work and was noted to have improved steadily until puberty, following which progress decreased and she became more obviously epileptic and insecure in her behaviour. She remained overactive and she perseverated in her speech and behaviour. At 15 years, she was referred, with severe hyperkinesia, to a child psychiatrist, and it was said to be "impossible to contain her in a room with another person". She was only quietened briefly in certain situations in the family when she felt in a secure situation, but one in which she nevertheless exercised a good deal of control of the family by her unbearable hyperactive, ritualistic behaviour. Mother considered that the 3 younger children lacked proper attention because of Ruth's behaviour. Father was frankly despairing to the point that he frequently referred to taking the child's life as the only way out and the kindest thing to do in the circumstances.

Subsequent investigations have suggested that the region of greatest damage is over the right temporal region. Educational tests showed that for many things Ruth is functioning at a level somewhere between 2 1/2 and 5 years, and on numbers she reached approximately a 6-year score.

Ruth was referred to us in December 1970 by her General Practitioner because her parents could no longer tolerate her behaviour at home. She had left Rudolf Steiner Camphill Village Trust School 6 months previously. Attempts to place her in training centres had failed due to her very disturbed behaviour.

Dr. Hopkins and myself visited the home on the initial assessment. Conversation was very difficult as Ruth continually interrupted by attempting to drag her mother away and clinging to her breast. When she did not succeed, she turned to her father trying to divert his attention to her. She caused further interruptions by placing uncovered jam pots on the head of each person, followed by maniacal laughter. Her parents were clearly desperate and did not know what to do. Father hoped for a magic drug that would control Ruth to prevent her eventually being a vegetable in some institution. Mother, understandably enough, wanted immediate relief from the situation at home even if it meant Ruth's admission to hospital.

We required time to consider the type of treatment Ruth should be offered in Dingleton and in the meantime she was prescribed chlorpromazine (50 mg 3 times a day). One of our anxieties centred around the possible aggressive reactions of other handicapped patients in Glenkinnon ward if we admitted Ruth. We invited the parents to visit to see the ward and to talk about our and their fears for Ruth in order to enlist their cooperation. We agreed it would be wiser for Ruth to attend 3 days a week as a day-patient initially, and to extend this to 5 days a week she became more integrated into the ward culture.

Her behaviour was extremely disturbed, due in part to frequent changes of staff, a pattern which she still displays to a lesser extent during changes in her environment. The situation became intolerable and it was clearly not a learning situation for Ruth. She was admitted full time after a crisis group involving staff and parents. An attempt was made to control her disturbed behaviour with drugs, and this caused considerable anxiety to the parents who attempted to control the treatment. The parents, at our request, agreed not to visit for 3 weeks as we felt they influenced the course of treatment to everyone's detriment. Previously Ruth had slept in a single room but we now placed her in the 15-bedded dormitory. Her behaviour continued to cause a considerable amount of anxiety for staff and patients. Her continued repetitive chatter in a penetrating voice such as: "Lady I've got you", "You have a delicious bottom" and "Man, I'am making your back warm", and her attempts to put her hand down the neck of one's garments, provoked anger in some and howls of laughter from others, successfully making her the centre of attraction. When rejected, she would spit and swear and give one of her maniacal laughs. She was an incredible tease, putting objects on people's heads, or throwing them out of the window to cause annoyance, and telling her to stop only led to more outrageous and excitable behaviour. She also ran away frequently the first week, causing concern as she had no road sense.

For behaviour that could not be ignored under a behaviour modification programme, for example, running away, we set strict controls on where she could go, that is only within hospital grounds. It was clearly explained to Ruth that if she left the hospital grounds, she would lose a future weekend at home. She tried this out once, then learned that we meant what we said. We patiently explained why the weekend was refused.

Whenever she was provocative to other patients, we explained to them in the ward group how much better it was to ignore her. Once the ward had learned to ignore her inappropriate behaviour and she failed in her attempts to gain attention there, she moved into other areas of the hospital to provoke the kitchen and dining-hall staff, the painters, porters and reception staff. We attempted to deal with each crisis individually and also at hospital meetings, explaining the need to ignore inappropriate behaviour as this was necessary to her treatment programme. We arranged a case conference of those who were regularly persecuted by Ruth's behaviour. We gave a brief history and explained her programme, which we proposed should be based on a token economy system. She would earn tokens which would earn time at home while working with the main dining-hall group. Time at home was the only incentive we could find. We had previously discussed this with the parents who agreed, though they were apprehensive that she might not be able to buy enough time at home. There was, however, general agreement in the conference that the programme should be initiated. People were invited to discuss their problems concerning Ruth and we explained how these might be handled in each situation, which helped with some of the antogonistic feelings. We invited people to contact the ward whenever they felt anxious in relation to Ruth's behaviour.

The parents were doubtful of Ruth's ability to learn in such a programme, and so a number of family groups were held. These groups comprised Ruth's parents, a work therapist from the main dining-hall, the psychiatrist and the ward staff. We discussed the parents' continuing anxiety about Ruth's medication. When she was at home, they were inclined to give her less medication than the prescribed amount, and we stressed the necessity of her receiving a consistent dosage. We had in fact reduced the dose of chlorpromazine from 175 mg daily to 100 mg daily. She was also receiving drugs for petit mal seizures.

Ruth's disturbed behaviour after returning from weekends at home continued to be a cause of concern to the staff. We agreed in a family group that Barbara, an interested student nurse on the ward, should accompany Ruth on her next weekend to assess the family situation at home. Barbara's observations were that a lot of Ruth's behaviour was understandable within the family's pattern of behaviour, for example, her stereotyped phrase, "Lady I've got you" evoked the response from her mother "I've got you too" which, although inappropriately used, was a language of affection. Moreover, she used such phrases to her parents only when they were paying attention to the other children, so Ruth used them in competition. Her parents encouraged her dependence, for example, by helping her to buckle her sandals. This would not be considered therapeutic on the ward. Barbara also discussed with the parents their doubts about Ruth's medication, explaining the effects of each drug.

On Barbara's second weekend visit, she discovered that Ruth's parents reinforced many responses we were attempting to extinguish, leading to a situation of intermittent reinforcement of undesirable responses and making them almost impossible to extinguish. In general, Ruth's father's attitude to our work was one of "change my daughter at Dingleton, but whatever you do, don't make her unhappy". He was sceptical of her comprehension and her ability to learn. Armed with Barbara's information about the home situation, we followed this up with another family group in which we stressed the necessity of a consistent learning situation for Ruth. Ruth's father questioned our use of controls and expressed doubts about her ability to develop further. We invited them to see videotape of Ruth at work, in the ward situation and in groups, to show them how her behaviour could change. We also invited them to spend time on the ward each week to see Ruth's progress and with a view to promoting consistency.

Initially, we had difficulty finding an incentive for Ruth. We started off by using money tokens, only to discover they had no meaning for her.

The only incentive we could find was time at home. We used small green plastic tokens, each worth 15 mins at home. These she could earn for appearance, personal hygiene, coming for her medication on time, going to work on time and working throughout the designated work period. She also received tokens for activities such as sewing and cooking. After a few months there was a considerable improvement and Ruth became well integrated into the ward and work area. She developed new skills, such as helping to count plates that she put on the tables. Her bizzare ritualistic phrases appeared less frequently. She became a valued worker. She was able to sit through an hour-long community council meeting. Our videotapes show Ruth initially disrupting each verbal group by spitting, mauling people and wandering around. We introduced tokens for appropriate group behaviour. She could earn a token for coming to the group on time, remaining in the group and responding appropriately. She was less disturbed and we were able to discontinue the Largactil.

In March this year, one year after admission, she began to show interest in the money tokens which the other patients earned, and she asked for money to go to the canteen. After discussion, we decided Ruth should earn brass money tokens as well as green time-at-home tokens. We used the money tokens as an added reinforcement in the work area to increase her performance, bringing her to the level of the other patients. The tokens were used to help Ruth stay in her work area throughout the work period. During slack periods, she was inclined to wander off causing disruption to the work of others who had to fetch her. Money tokens have now become of more value to her than the green tokens. Being able to cash these tokens at the bank at night and to spend the money on herself in the canteen is a modest but significant improvement. Previously she had been described as "an absolute pest" in the canteen for demanding whole boxes of apples to "take home to Mummy", and she appeared to have no social sense whatever and no sense of the value of money.

Her relationships are now more mature and spontaneously friendly. She converses and argues instead of screeching and having temper tantrums. She still used her ritualistic phrases but less frequently. One can now talk to her about her inappropriate behaviour, and she listens and usually responds appropriately. She seems to have more self-awareness and she dresses more like a young adolscent than a small child. Her ability to cooperate led her to diet successfully, so that she is less self-conscious about being fat and her health has improved. Her concern for her appearance is increasing.

Summary

Dingleton Hospital, which is run as a therapeutic community, has evolved a unique social and administrative structure. This report describes how such a structure can operate to further a behaviour modification programme in a ward of 35 mentally handicapped patients. Daily meetings of a community council in which all wards and areas of the hospital are represented provide communication channels which can be used to make a consistent programme operate in the ward, at work and in the dining hall.

The paper also describes how consistency of approach can be maintained into the family, as illustrated by the case of a disturbed autistic adolescent who regularly exhibited disturbed behaviour following weekends at home. Improvement followed.

VII. Analysis and Evaluation of Behaviour Modification

A Mathematical Model for the Analysis of Therapies

D. REVENSTORFF

I. Introduction

Checking of therapeutic efficacy may be carried out at several levels of sophistication. The most elementary check is to demonstrate significance of change. This can be done in a simple before-and-after design. Apart from the problem of spontaneous remission, even here some intricate statistical problems appear (cf. HARRIS, 1962). A more comprehensive picture of therapeutic effects is provided by repeated observations of a client's behaviour as therapy continues. Data from this kind of extended design constitute a time series. Again significance tests for change are in order. Moreover, the time course itself can be analysed with respect to rate of change, turning points, asymptotes and other features of shape. To acquire some descriptive shorthand of the change, curve fitting may be applied. The whole time series then is summarized as an exponential decay, a logarithmic curve or a parabola. Very common is the use of polynomials, which fit virtually everything if a proper degree is taken. Besides description of the data, such curve fitting sometimes has significance for the formulation of a theory to explain the change, e.g. Hull's exponential acquisition curve of habit strength. It is only in connection with a theory that the use of a fitted curve for prediction by extrapolation appears to be reasonable. But the often used orthogonal polynomials (in analysis of variance) seldom have any theoretical justification. Furthermore, the statistical tests involved assume independence of data at successive times, which is not true of most organismic behaviour sequences.

II. Markov Models for Therapeutic Processes

For these reasons another type of data description, called data generating models, is more appealing than curve fitting. Here a process whose mathematical properties are well known is assumed to have generated the actual data. Such models are miniature theories which may be delineated in terms of postulates concerning the behaving organism. They are often formulated in a probabilistic fashion, which seems to be more adequate for organismic behaviour than a deterministic function (parabola) with an ad hoc added error. Some of them explicitly take into account sequential dependencies. (For a discussion of both types of models see GOTTMANN et al., 1969.)

A widely used model of this kind is a Markow process, which has been recommended for the area of mental health by HERTEL, 1972. (For other applications cf. SUPPERS and ATKINSON, 1960; ATKINSON et al., 1965.)

Its usefulness for the analysis of therapeutic change is explored in a simple example. For this purpose, people are classified as either mentally healthy (H) or ill (I): 67 % (u_{01}) are considered healthy and 33 % (u_{02}) ill in a normal population. A natural variation is postulated, causing a flow from one state to the other. This natural variation is expressed in a transition matrix (P), that contains the conditional probabilities of staying healthy (p_{11}), changing to illness (p_{12}), changing to health (p_{21}) and staying ill (p_{22}). The percentage of people healthy and ill after such a transition (u_{11}, u_{12}) may easily be calculated+ and further extrapolation is achieved by performing a string of such transitions (Table 1). A transition can be thought to take place within a year of treatment, or in a single therapeutic session or whatever else makes sense. From this model a time course is derived by stating the proportions of people healthy after successive transitions.

The same procedure may be applied to a probability vector describing a patient population, for instance, 75 % ill and 25 % healthy. Now the model provides prediction of spontaneous remission. These proportions may be empirically verified by the actual data from patient and untreated control groups (chi^2 statistics) (Table 1, left).

A similar transition matrix can be devised to characterize transitions under therapeutic impact. The time course that results from its application to the patient population provides a forecast of therapeutic effects, which may again be compared to empirical data to check the model (Table 1, right).

Table 1. Changes predicted by two oversimplified Markov models for a spontaneous remission and a therapeutic process. (Above: two examples of transition matrices. Below: U_0, U_1 ... successive proportions of healthy and ill)

p(H/H)	p(H/I)
p(I/H)	p(I/I)

	80%	20%	80%	20%
	40%	60%	60%	40%
U_0	25%	75%	25%	75%
U_1	50%	50%	65%	35%
U_2	60%	40%	73%	27%
U_3	64%	36%	75%	25%
U_4	66%	34%		
U	67%	33%	25%	75%
	healthy	ill	healthy	ill
	"Natural variation"		"Modest therapeutic effort"	

+ $u_{11} = u_{01}\,p_{11} + u_{02}\,p_{21}$; $u_{12} = u_{01}\,p_{12} + u_{02}\,p_{22}$

III. Some Properties of Markov Processes

A basic property of many Markov models+ is that after a number of transitions a steady distribution of people over the states is finally reached, which is the same irrespective of the initial distribution from which the process started. This asymptotic distribution constitutes the upper limit of potential therapeutic success. Further, the average number of transitions necessary to move from one state (e.g. ill) to another (healthy) may be computed.

The simple version of a 2:2 transition matrix is readily generalized to more than two states, and a variety of special features can be incorporated, such as periodic returns to a certain state (periodicity) or states from which there is no escape (absorbing states). Further, the transition matrix may change as time goes by (nonhomogeneity with respect to time). In many learning applications, however, homogeneous Markov models have done a good job (cf. ATKINSON et al., 1965).

The kind of Markov model discussed so far implies that current behaviour is wholly determined by the behaviour of "yesterday" (the last trial or whatever time interval is used), except for an unpredictable random component. This may prove inadequate, when behaviour is influenced by long-term memory events. The last 2, 3 etc. trials must then be taken into account to explain current behaviour. Appropriate variations of the model may be devised in such cases and are called Markov models of order two, three etc. respectively.

For empirical behaviour sequences the fit of such a model may be checked by statistical tests of such properties as homogeneity with respect to time or homogeneity of different data generators (individuals), order of the process, its periodicity and absorbing states (see e.g. HOEL, 1954; ANDERSON and GOODMAN, 1957). A number of these tests have been combined in a computer program by HALPERIN and LISSITZ (1971).

To date, applications of Markov models to the mental health area are few. HERTEL (1972) outlines their potential usefulness for the analysis of changes in the patients' condition. BROWNSBERGER (1965) studies simulations of the sort depicted in Table 1. He compared outcomes of spontaneous remission models with therapeutic models. He demonstrated that even under the assumption of remarkable therapeutic efficacy, large samples of patients must be observed over several years to yield significant results. RODDA et al. (1972) applied Markov models to the change of depression and anxiety.

IV. Correlational Analysis of Markov Processes

If the states of a system are discrete points along the dependent variable in a therapeutic experiment - e.g. number of cigarettes smoked - then a transition matrix becomes much like a bivariate scatter plot relating the behaviour at the two times++. The larger probabilities will be found in the diagonal if there is no systematic change and in the supradiagonal, if there is a decrease in the behaviour studied. Such a scatter plot is shown in Table 2.

+ True for all so-called nonperiodic, irreducible Markov processes.

++ The usual correlation scatter displays the joint probabilities of the marginal variables, while the Markov matrix contains conditional probabilities. The rows of the Markov matrix must be reversed in order to make the relationship to the correlation scatter apparent.

Table 2. Hypothetical transition matrix for cigarette consumption from before [x(t)] to after [x(+1)] a therapeutic session

x(t) no. of cigarettes								
30						50 %	50 %	
25					40 %	40 %	20 %	
20				40 %	40 %	20 %		
15			40 %	40 %	20 %			
10		40 %	40 %	20 %				
5	40 %	40 %	20 %					
0	80 %	20 %						
	0	5	10	15	20	25	30	x(t+1)

In any case, the Markov matrix is conveniently summarized by the Pearson correlation coefficient, because the relationship of the behaviour at time t and (t+1) will be linear unless there is some really unexpected therapeutic effect, e.g. that heavy smokers give up smoking more easily than medium smokers.

In the Markov formulation probabilities of the different states are predicted:

$$u_{1i} = u_{01}\, p_{1i} + u_{02}\, p_{2i} + u_{03}\, p_{3i} + \dots \qquad \text{Markov model} \qquad (1)$$

Now that the states are represented by values on a variable, this variable is predicted from values on the same variable at earlier stages and the model is called an autoregressive model.

$$x(t) = a \cdot x(t-1) + e(t) \qquad \text{first-order autoregressive model} \qquad (2)$$

Current behaviour, x(t), is made dependent on earlier behaviour, x(t-1), but not on time itself, as in curve fitting. (The term e(t) is the change component, systematic or random.)

$$x(t) = b \cdot t + e(t) \qquad \text{linear regression in curve fitting} \qquad (3)$$

Table 3. Hypothetical simplex and its inverse

R					R^{-1}				
1.00	.90	.81	.73	.67	5.25	-4.75	0	0	0
.90	1.00	.90	.81	.73	-4.75	9.45	-4.75	0	0
.81	.90	1.00	.90	.81	0	-4.75	9.45	-4.75	0
.73	.81	.90	1.00	.90	0	0	-4.75	9.45	-4.75
.67	.73	.81	.90	1.00	0	0	0	-4.75	5.25

The coefficient a in the autoregressive model (2) is the proportion of behaviour retained from one trial to another and is equal to the correlation coefficient derived from the transition matrix if the variables are standardized+.

It should be mentioned that summarizing the whole transition matrix by a single correlation coefficient must mean losing information. Mean changes, in particular, are eliminated. Leaving aside this important aspect of the therapeutic process for a while, let us look more closely at the correlation structure in a time series.

It can be shown that from an autoregressive model like (2) the correlation between ordered trials (time) takes on a peculiar form. An example is shown in Table 3. If the correlation between adjacent trials is r, then the correlation between trials 1 and 3, or 2 and 4, or 3 and 5 will be r^2 (see Footnote on page 222). Generally trials m steps apart will correlate r^m. This means that the values in the correlation matrix are tapering off from the main diagonal to the north-east and south-west corners.

This kind of correlation structure was called a simplex by GUTTMAN (1954) in the context of mental abilities. The inverse of a simplex or a correlation matrix generated by a first-order autoregressive process is also noteworthy: All elements except those in the main diagonal and just above and below are zero (see MORRISON, 1967, p. 296). The fact that the elements of the inverse are closely related to partial correlations implies here that correlations between trials separated by one and more steps vanish if the variable on the trials between is held constant (partialled out). In a therapeutic time series, this means early behaviour components that show up again at later stages must also be observable at all stages in between; otherwise a first-order Markov or autoregressive model is not adequate to describe the data, and partial correlations between current and earlier behaviour (e.g. of the form $r_{13.2}$) must be different from zero. In this case there are behaviour components that occur at some time, remain latent for a while, and then occur again later.

GABRIEL (1962) devised a statistical test for correlation matrices like these to check whether the partial correlations that bridge a certain number of trials are significantly different from zero. This enables one to test for behaviour components that remain latent for 1, 2, 3, etc. trials before occurring again.

+ The first-order autoregressive model for standardized variables is:

$$z(t) = a \cdot z(t-1) + e(t)$$

The correlation $r_{12} = E(z_1 \cdot z_2)$ is then:

$$E(z_1 \cdot z_2) = E(z_1 \cdot (r \cdot z_1 + e_2)) =$$

$$a \cdot E(z_1{}^2) + E(z_1 \cdot e_2) = a + o$$

(assuming errors e_1, e_2 etc. independent of variables z_1, z_2 etc.)

similarly $r_{13} = E(z_1 \cdot z_3)$ is

$$E(z_1 \cdot (a \cdot z_2 + e_3)) = a\, E(z_1 \cdot z_2) + E(z_1\, e_3) = a^2$$

and so on.

V. Analysis of Therapies for the Modification of Smoking Behaviour

Now some experimental data will be discussed in connection with the model described.

In an experiment reported elsewhere (BRENGELMANN, 1972), eight different therapies were used to reduce cigarette consumption. All were done in group sessions:

1. Faradic shock contingent to smoking behaviour was applied (smoking, reaching for the package etc.). EA
2. Behaviour control was implemented (not smoking before breakfast, buying only small packets etc.). BC
3. Behaviour control (2) and after the sixth week additional faradic shock sessions as in (1). BC + EA
4. Negative practice: Smoking for 30 min to metronome in a closed room. NP
5. Covert sensitization: Aversive images (cancer, vomiting) were induced and associated to smoking. CS
6. A kind of nondirective therapy: people talked freely about smoking and therapeutic measures. ND
7. Control group. Cigarette consumption was simply counted. CO
8. Pharmaco-therapy: Lobeline was given in decreasing doses starting with 2 mg six times daily. LO
9. A placebo was given in the same way as in (8). PL

The therapies were given twice weekly for 6 consecutive weeks and once for the following 2 weeks. The booster sessions were held 5 and 11 weeks after therapy finished. All subjects (Ss) gave weekly reports on daily cigarette consumption for 13 weeks (including intermediate baselines). Weekly averages per S were used for this analysis.

According to what has been said about data-generating models (autoregressive or Markov) for analysing time series, besides mean differences, correlations should be helpful in investigating the time course of therapeutic effects. Roughly four events may be distinguished.

1. No mean change and high correlations (in the range of the reliability of those data) between adjacent trials: this means behaviour generally did not change. No effect. (See e.g. Fig. 4, weeks 8-13.)
2. No mean change and a correlation appreciably lower than the reliability: average behaviour did not change, but some Ss went down as others went up. There are individual differences with respect to direction of change. (See e.g. Fig. 5, weeks 10 and 12.)
3. Mean change and high correlation: all Ss went down or up (depending on the sign of the mean difference) by about the same amount. A general effect is present. (See e.g. Fig. 6, week 3.)
4. Mean change and a correlation appreciably lower than the reliability: most of the Ss changed but at different rates. Effects are more pronounced for some people than for others. Some Ss might even have changed in the opposite direction to the majority. (See e.g. Fig. 6, week 2.)

In cases (2) and (4) utilization of individual differences should enhance therapeutic efficacy. With data like reported number of cigarettes smoked per day, the reliability is close to 1. Actually, correlations between two consecutive weeks were often greater than .95. Major drops in the correlations between adjacent trials can be observed after the therapeutic measures have been applied for the first time with the nondirective (ND), placebo (PL) and Lobeline (LO) groups. These drops were accompanied by large mean changes, compared to the control group. All Ss reacted to therapies in the same direction, but at different rates, rank order of Ss with respect to cigarette consumption changes for these groups. For the Lobeline and placebo groups this continues. In the covert sensitization (CS) group there is a drop in the correlation from weeks 4 to 5 and 5 to 6. This occurred when a new stimulus (cancer) was introduced and given with the old stimulus (vomiting) together (week 5) and then alone (from week 6 on). Time intervals of 1, 3 and 4 weeks occurred after weeks 1, 9 and 11, respectively. In these instances correlations drop slightly, indicating the time spacing (see Figs. 1-9). From this it is apparent that major events in the therapeutic time course, which are not necessarily reflected by the mean curve, can be detected by studying the simple correlations.

The analysis of partial correlations (Table 4) shows that only the cigarette consumption of the control group may be described as a Markov or autoregressive process of order one. No behaviour components that have been latent for a while appear again, mainly because behaviour remained unchanged throughout. In the eight treatment groups, however, partial correlations point back up to 10 weeks (ND). This means that behaviour components (smoking habits) must have submerged and then come up again after the therapy lost its effectiveness. It is not only that smoking in general increases again, but the initial rank order of consumption is gradually reestablished too. This is more obvious when the simple correlations with the first baseline are compared with their hypothetical counterparts under the assumption of zero partial correlations. This is derived as follows: Equation (4) gives the formula for partial correlations:

$$r_{31.2} = (r_{31} - r_{32} \cdot r_{21}) / \sqrt{(1 - r_{32}^2)(1 - r_{21}^2)} \tag{4}$$

If (4) is zero, the correlation between trials 1 and 3 must be in the product of the correlation $r_{12} \cdot r_{23}$. If r_{13} differs appreciably from this product, something is transmitted from week 1 to week 3 which is not observable at week 2, and the expected partial correlation must be nonzero. This argument may be extended to time gaps of more than one week. Correlation with baseline should fade away very much like the cumulative product of correlations between successive weeks, if a first order autoregressive model is valid (see also Footnote on p. 223).

Actual baseline correlations follow the model in the control group (CO) covert sensitization (CS) and negative practice (NP) therapies. In the behaviour control (BC), electric aversion (EA) and nondirective (ND) therapies, the correlations with first baseline are much higher than the first-order model predicts. Despite the obvious success in reducing cigarettes consumption, the underlying smoking habits seem not to be extinguished completely and are reestablished after a while.

Interestingly enough, the baseline correlations and the mean curve take a parallel time course in most groups (see Figs. 1-9). This means that, to the extent that smoking behaviour increases on average, Ss return to their old rank with respect to cigarette consumption. It is the same people who smoke at the beginning and at the end of a therapy, although this is not so in the initial phases of therapeutic success.

Table 4. Significance of partial correlations for nine therapies for the modification of smoking behaviour (last column). Major drops in correlations according to time spacings (columns 2-4) and other reasons (column 5)

		1 W	3 W	4 W	major drops in correlation	no. of weeks partial correlations go back
	n	$r_{1,2}$	$r_{9,10}$	$r_{11,12}$		
Electric aversion (EA)	41	.85	.90	.96	$r_{4,5}$=.83	2
Behaviour control (BC)	45	.78	.81	.69		2 3
Behaviour control + EA	53	.78	.63	.76	$r_{5,6}$=.75	2 3 (5) (6)
Negative practice (NP)	48	.78	.86	.88		2 3
Covert sensitization (CS)	45	.92	.65	.74	$r_{5,6}$=.76 $r_{6,7}$=.74	2
Nondirective (ND)	40	.34	.62	.77		2 3 (4) 9 10
Control group (CO)	30	.91	.94	.85		1
Lobeline therapy (LO)	27	.75	.95	.87	$r_{2,3}$=.56	1 3
Placebo group (PL)	26	.46	.81	.81	$r_{2,3}$=.66	2

VI. Concluding Remarks

Markov models are recommended for the analysis of therapy experiments. They allow for prediction of spontaneous remission and therapeutic efficacy. Their validity may be checked empirically. If therapeutic effects are measured on a discrete or continuous variable, the order of the Markov process may be inferred from the correlation structure of the time series. Other features of the therapeutic effects, which are not reflected in mean changes, might be detected from correlations like time spacing and therapeutic manipulations. High partial correlations with earlier behaviour, as in the examples discussed, indicate superficial extinction of habits. An ideal therapy should show significant mean change without any partial correlations being significant. Then it might be presumed that therapeutic effects will endure and that extinction had been profound.

Fig. caption for Fig. 1-9:

Time course of therapeutic effects over 13 weekly averages.
left ordinate = correlations
right ordinate = no. of cigarettes
o-------o = means
o———o = correlations of adjacent time points
•———• = correlations with baseline (1)
•-------• = Markov model for correlations with baseline (1)
BL = baselines
T = therapeutic sessions
(T) = booster sessions (half time duration)

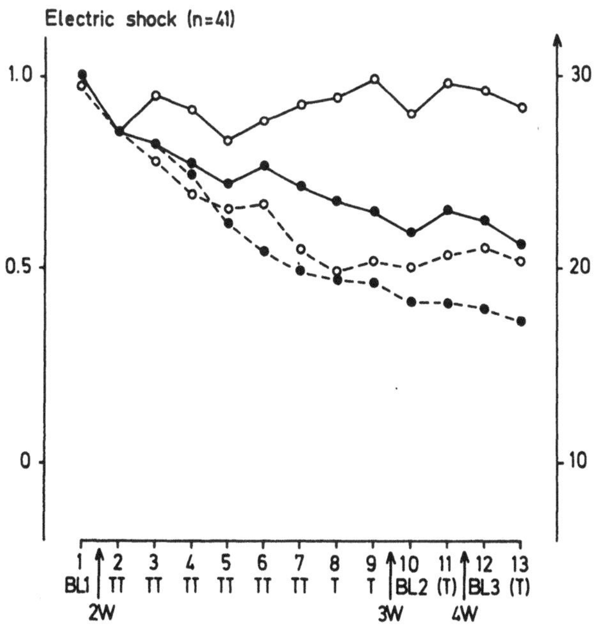

Fig. 1.

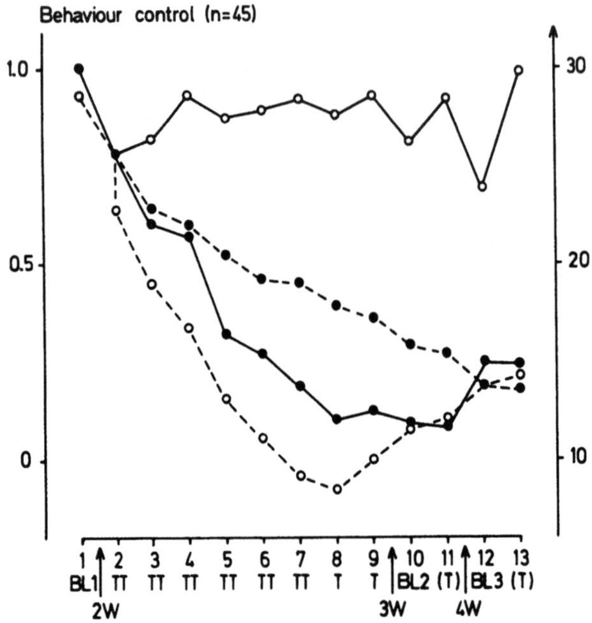

Behaviour control (n=45)
1.0
0.5
0
30
20
10
1 BL1
2 TT
3 TT
4 TT
5 TT
6 TT
7 TT
8 T
9 T
10 BL2
11 (T)
12 BL3
13 (T)
2W
3W
4W

Fig. 2.

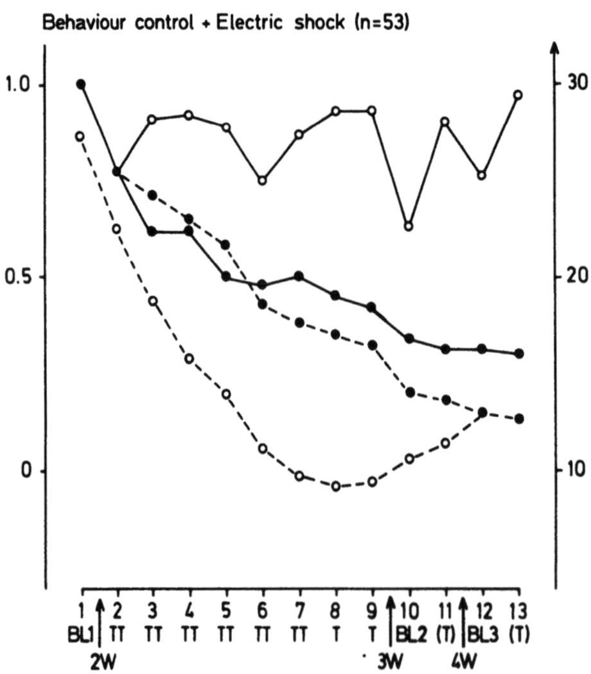

Behaviour control + Electric shock (n=53)
1.0
0.5
0
30
20
10
1 BL1
2 TT
3 TT
4 TT
5 TT
6 TT
7 TT
8 T
9 T
10 BL2
11 (T)
12 BL3
13 (T)
2W
3W
4W

Fig. 3.

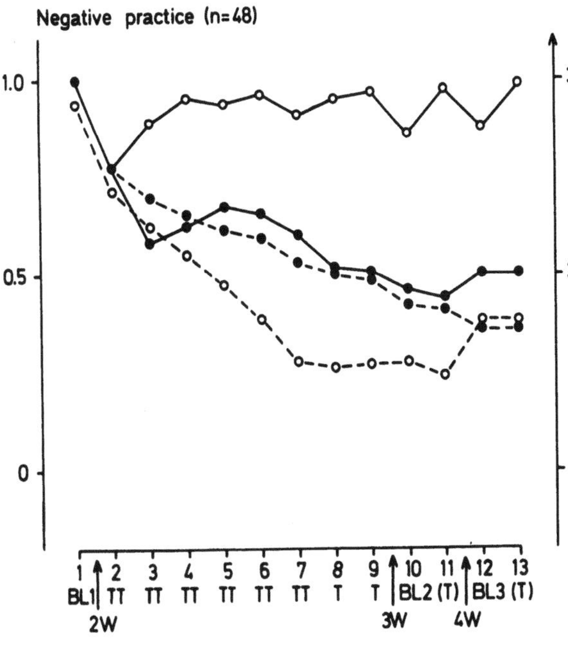
Negative practice (n=48)
1.0
0.5
0
30
20
10
1 BL1
2W
2 TT
3 TT
4 TT
5 TT
6 TT
7 TT
8 T
9 T
3W
10 BL2
11 (T)
4W
12 BL3
13 (T)

Fig. 4.

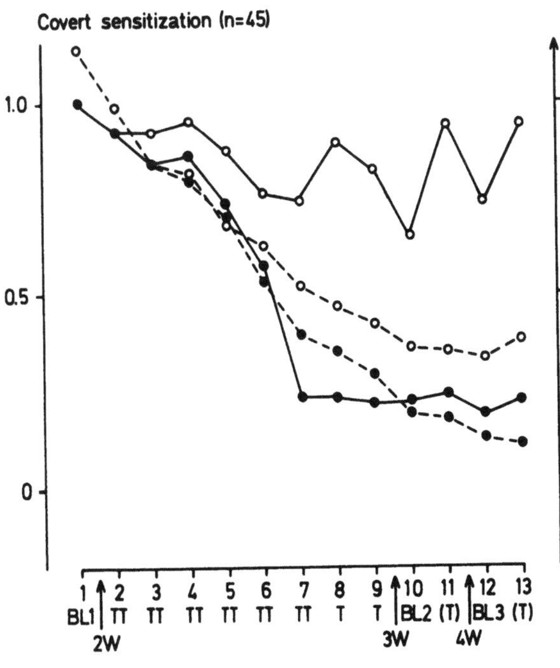
Covert sensitization (n=45)
1.0
0.5
0
30
20
10
1 BL1
2W
2 TT
3 TT
4 TT
5 TT
6 TT
7 TT
8 T
9 T
3W
10 BL2
11 (T)
4W
12 BL3
13 (T)

Fig. 5.

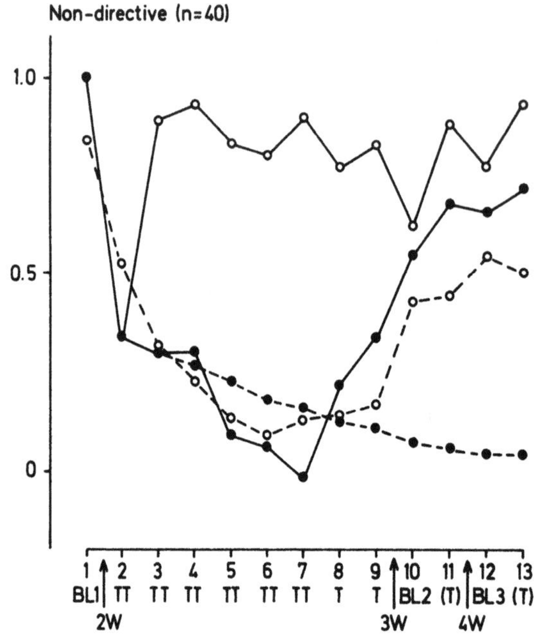
Non-directive (n=40)
1.0
0.5
0
30
20
10
1 BL1
2 TT
3 TT
4 TT
5 TT
6 TT
7 TT
8 T
9 T
10 BL2
11 (T)
12 BL3
13 (T)
2W
3W
4W

Fig. 6.

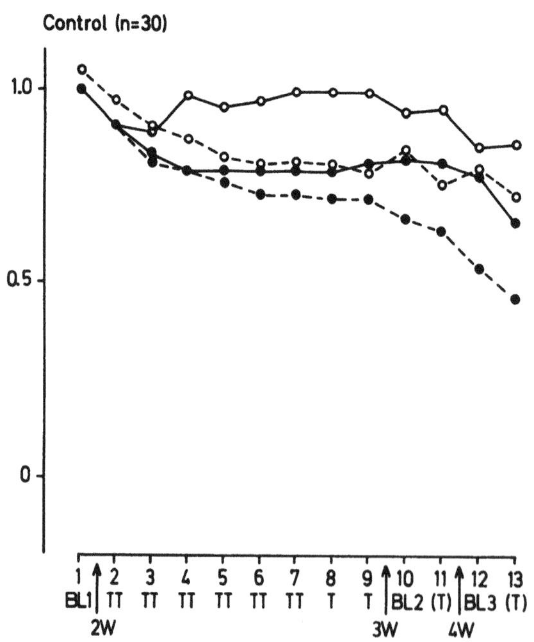
Control (n=30)
1.0
0.5
0
30
20
10
1 BL1
2 TT
3 TT
4 TT
5 TT
6 TT
7 TT
8 T
9 T
10 BL2
11 (T)
12 BL3
13 (T)
2W
3W
4W

Fig. 7.

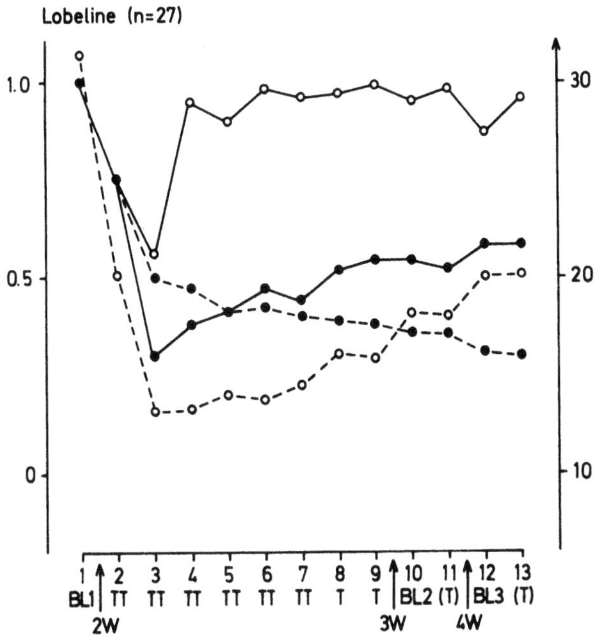
Lobeline (n=27)
1.0
0.5
0
30
20
10
1 BL1
2W
2 TT
3 TT
4 TT
5 TT
6 TT
7 TT
8 T
9 T
3W
10 BL2
11 (T)
4W
12 BL3
13 (T)

Fig. 8.

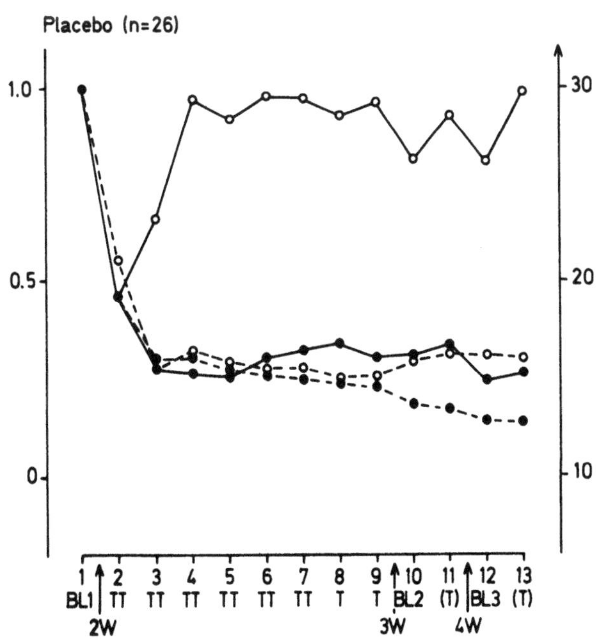
Placebo (n=26)
1.0
0.5
0
30
20
10
1 BL1
2W
2 TT
3 TT
4 TT
5 TT
6 TT
7 TT
8 T
9 T
3W
10 BL2
11 (T)
4W
12 BL3
13 (T)

Fig. 9.

References

ANDERSON, T.W., GOODMAN, L.A.: Statistical inference about Markov chains. Amer. math. Statist. 28, 89-114 (1957).
ATKINSON, R.C., BOWER, G.H., CROTHERS, E.J.: An Introduction to Mathematical Learning Theories. New York: Wiley 1965.
BRENGELMANN, J.C.: The therapy of smoking. Paper presented at the 2nd European Conference on Behaviour Modification, Wexford, Ireland 1972.
BROWNSBERGER, C.N.: Clinical versus statistical assessment of psychotherapy. Behav. Sci. 16, 421-428 (1965).
GABRIEL, K.R.: Ante-dependence analysis of an ordered set of variables Ann. math. Statist. 33, 201-212 (1962).
GOTTMANN, J.M., MacFALL, R.M., BARNETT, J.T.: Design and analysis of research using time series. Psychol. Bull. 72, 299-346 (1969).
GUTTMANN, L.: A new approach to factor analysis: the radex. In: LAZARSFELD, P.E. (Ed.): Mathematical Thinking in the Social Sciences. Free Press: 1954.
HALPERIN, S., LISSITZ, R.W.: Statistical properties of Markov chains: a computer program. Behav. Sci. 16, 244-247 (1971).
HARRIS, C.B.: Problems in Measuring Change 1962.
HERTEL, R.K.: Application of stochastic process analyses to the study of psychotherapeutic processes. Psychol. Bull. 77, 421-430 (1972).
HOEL, P.G.: A test for Markov chains. Biometrica 41, 430-433 (1954).
KEMENY, J.G., SNELL, J.L.: Finite Markov Chains. Princeton, N.J.: van Nostrand 1960.
MORRISON, D.F.: Multivariate Statistical Methods. New York: McGraw Hill 1967.
RODDA, B.E., MILLER, M.C., BRUHN, J.B.: Prediction of anxiety and depression patterns among coronary patients using a Markov process analysis. Behav. Sci. 16, 482-489 (1971).
SUPPERS, P., ATKINSON, R.C.: Markov Learning Models for Multiperson Interactions. Stanford: Stanford University Press 1960.

Mathematical Models for Evaluation of Therapies+

N. MAI

I. Introduction

In applying therapies to psychological disorders, there are many situations in which one has to choose between different courses of action.

For example, a therapist who attempts to reduce the fears of his neurotic patients has to choose between different therapeutic techniques like desensitization, implosion or modelling. Additionally, he may turn to group therapy in order to help more people within the same amount of time. Fortunately, results reported in the literature (RACHMAN, 1971) will make his decicions easier, but they are unlikely to provide a clear answer to his problem. He is forced to evaluate a mass of results for his own purposes, and he may easily find that one or other factor he considers important has not previously been touched upon.

Let us take also the problem of an agency, such as a research institution or a mental health organization, planning a therapeutic programme for drug addicts. Because of limited resources, it is not possible to do all the things that promise the desired effect. The organization has to choose between different combinations of actions or allocations of resources. Compared to the first example, here there are very few data about the relative efficacy of different therapeutic actions. Nevertheless, the organization has to make a decision.

The necessity of choosing between different actions defines a decision situation. Looking for the best alternative, a decision maker (DM)++ has to consider the outcomes or consequences of his action alternatives. In many practical problems the DM will recognize that the actual consequences of his actions depend on the state of certain variables about which he has incomplete information. In such situations he has to decide, in the face of uncertainty, which of the possible outcomes may actually occur. The formal structure of decisions under uncertainty characterizes many practical problems in a wide variety of contexts, for example, military and economic planning. The theory of decisions under uncertainty includes different axiomatic systems (see, for example, PRATT et al.,

---

+ This study is part of a project in the "Sonderforschungsbereich 24, sozial- und wirtschaftspsychologische Entscheidungsforschung der Universität Mannheim". The research was supported by a research grant of the Deutsche Forschungsgemeinschaft.

++ The notion of a "decision maker" is here used in its broadest sense. The DM can be an individual, a group of individuals or an organization.

1964) by means of which it is possible to develop powerful tools for solving decision problems.

The theory has to deal with at least two problems: (1) the judgment of uncertainty and its reduction by new information; (2) evaluation of outcomes or consequences resulting from a given action.

In this paper the discussion is restricted to the evaluation problem.

In a practical evaluation problem one needs at least judgments of the type

$$A > B \quad (1)$$
$$A < B \quad (2)$$
$$A \sim B \quad (3)$$

which means that consequence A is preferred to B (1) or the reverse (2), or that a DM is indifferent between A and B (3). Nevertheless, in complex decision situations, as in the foregoing examples, a DM might find it very hard to state clearly which of the consequences of two action alternatives he prefers. In the example of the therapist who has to choose between different therapeutic techniques, he might prefer therapy A to B in respect to one aspect of the consequences, for example, probability of success. But on the other hand, considering the duration of treatment, he might prefer B to A. Thus, if there are many aspects of consequences, the overall evaluation of therapies A and B in the form of a preference might be difficult. As a result the DM may make inconsistent (intransitive) judgements and in consequence inaccurate decisions. Transitivity here means:

$$\text{If } A \gtrsim B \quad \text{and } B \gtrsim C, \quad \text{then } A \gtrsim C \quad (4)$$

There might be other sources of error in the evaluation task if the consequences vary in many different aspects. People often use simplistic evaluation strategies, considering only some of the relevant aspects. This might result in consistent preference judgment, but if relevant information were neglected, this might also lead to inadequate decisions. Therefore a DM confronted with complex evaluations might look for aids to avoid inconsistent and/or inadequate judgments.

II. Aiding the Decision Maker. Multiattributive Utility Theory (MAUT)

1. General Ideas

The general idea underlying all decision-aiding systems is to break complex judgments down into simpler judgments and then recombine these components to the overall judgment by a formal (mathematical) rule (e.g. RAIFFA, 1968). The problem in constructing such a system is twofold: how should a DM break his problem down into components that are easier to handle, and which formal rule should be applied for recombining the components. The justification of a certain rule for breakdown and recombination is a theoretical problem. Besides this, there are practical scaling problems including the selection of adequate response modes for human judgments.

The evaluation of complex, multidimensional outcomes of consequences is the subject of a relatively new theory, called "Multiattributive Utility Theory" (MAUT) (for an introduction, see V. WINTERFELDT, 1971). As far as practical aids for the DM are concerned, the following sequence of steps is proposed by this theory:

1. List the dimensions (j = 1, 2, ..., m) which are considered important in the evaluation task (e.g. probability of success, duration of therapy, costs, etc.).
2. Assign to each dimension a number (a_j) reflecting its relative importance in the evaluation (e.g. a DM may judge duration of therapy as more important than comfort for patient).
3. Assign to each value (x_i) in each dimension j a number $u(x_{ij})$ reflecting the utility of this value (e.g. values (x_i) in the dimension "probalitity of success" are .85 for therapy A, .70 for B and .78 for C).

These three steps describe a rule for breaking down the complex evaluation. A two-stage rating procedure is proposed; the importance of each dimension and the utility of each variable stage are to be judged. The importance and utility have to be judged only once, since the evaluation of the different action alternatives can be done by computer, using a formal combination rule. The application of the formal combination rule constitutes step (4) of the analysis.

By MAUT, an additive model is proposed for combining the component judgements. The overall utility U_i of consequences of action i (i = 1, 2, ..., n) are given by:

$$U_i = a_1\, u(x_{i1}) + a_2\, u(x_{i2}) + \dots\, a_j\, u(x_{ij}) + \dots + a_m\, u(x_{im}) = \sum_{j=1}^{m} a_j\, u(x_{ij}) \qquad (5)$$

2. Theoretical Approaches

What is the justification for using such a simple formal rule? There are different axiomatic approaches to the multiattribute utility problem. LUCE and TUKEY (1964), KRANTZ (1964) and SAYEKI (1970) developed their systems in the context of conjoint measurement, RAIFFA (1969) and FISHBURN (1965) in a context of expected utility models. Without going into detail on the differences between the axiomatic systems, it might be sufficient to state that all systems prove the existence of the additive model under the condition of mutual independence of demensions. (Besides this, the different systems use certain other conditions of minor importance.) Independence is used here in the utility sense and does not mean causal independence or stochastic (statistical) independence. Duration of therapy and cost of therapy are certainly related in a causal sense, but this fact does not necessarily imply dependence in the utility sense. Independence in the utility sense means that the same utility rating is assigned to the values (x) of a dimension (j) regardless of the values of other dimensions.

A specific value of the dimension "duration of therapy", say 6 weeks, will get the same utility rating whether it occurs in therapy A, B or C. If this is not true, then the dimension "duration" must interact with at least one other dimension. If interaction of this kind does occur, the simple additive model is not valid. Independence is here introduced in a more informal or preliminary way. In the different axiomatic systems formalized definitions of independence and also different tests are available to check the independence condition (FISHBURN, 1965; KRANTZ and TVERSKY, 1971). The axiomatic approaches are not developed explicitly for constructing systems to aid the DM, but they can be used as guidelines for them. If independence can be shown empirically, the additive model is justified. But actual tests of independence are extremely laborious and therefore often impracticable.

There is another approach to the multiattributive utility problem whose main concern is the development of practical decision aids. This approach, advocated by EDWARDS (1970) and HUBER and GUSTAFSON (1971), justifies the additive rule not on an axiomatic but also on an empirical basis. In simulation studies YNTEMA and TORGERSON (1961) have shown that additive models also do a very good job in situations where the independence assumption does not hold. The usefulness of additive models has been demonstrated in a wide variety of problems (for summaries, see SLOVIC and LICHTENSTEIN, 1971; GOLDBERG, 1968). EDWARDS (1970) further justifies this approach by its feasibility for practical applications. The necessary judgments are much simpler than the overall evaluation, and furthermore, the evaluation can be done by different experts for different dimensions, which might be especially important where the DM is an organization. Nevertheless, the merits of the whole approach have to be shown empirically. Validation of MAUT includes some special problems, even if MAUT is implemented on an axiomatic basis. Some of these problems will be discussed below. For the moment let us discuss briefly the problem of our second example concerning programme planning for drug addicts. We concentrate on psychological treatment and therefore assume that all patients are physically cured.

3. Some Extensions

After a preliminary discussion about the application of MAUT to their problem, our organization may recognize that there are great difficulties in estimating the required importance weights. In contrast to the example of selecting therapy for fear reduction, it appears much more difficult to clearly describe the overall goal of treatment in the case of drug addicts. Obviously there are many different subgoals, for example, reduction of psychological drug dependence, compensation for behavioural deficits, establishment of social activities etc.

Confronted with these difficulties, our organization may question the usefulness of the breakdown rule proposed by MAUT. But before the organization decides to forget all about MAUT and to base the necessary choices solely on overall human evaluations, some possible extensions of MAUT should be considered.

Suppose a more specific discussion of the goal problem has led to the following preliminary structure of the problem: Within the overall goal of an effective programme, a set of subgoals is differentiated. It is recognized that these subgoals differ in importance. Furthermore, it seems useful to distinguish between different policy areas (psychological therapy sessions, working, social activities, entertainment etc.), each of which contributes to one or more subgoals. In each area different actions are possible and any combinations of such actions define the programme policies to be evaluated. Fig. 1 demonstrates such an oversimplified structure[+].

If one considers the policy areas as the aspects or dimensions in which programme policies vary, assuming independence of values between areas, the similarity of this approach to the simpler version of MAUT will be apparent. The main difference lies in the assessment of importance weights. The importance weights are broken down into a hierarchic structure. The policy areas contribute to the subgoals, which contribute to the overall goal. If the hierarchy is constructed in a meaningful way,

[+] In an actual analysis one may decide to divide the subgoal "compensation for behavioural deficits" over different areas of deficits. Also it might be useful to refine the policy areas, but for our theoretical arguments this does not matter.

it is much easier to estimate the necessary weights indicated in Fig. 1. If the weights are appropriately scaled, the final weights in the evaluation task can be calculated following the path of connections. For example, consider only one action alternative, say K, under the policy area "social activities". To evaluate the contribution of K to the overall goal, one first assigns a number to K representing the value (utility) of K in the policy area "social activities". This policy area contributes to a certain degree (indicated by a_{31}) to the subgoal "reduction of psychological drug dependence", and this subgoal contributes to the degree a_1 to the overall goal. But the policy area in question contributes also to some degree, namely a_{32}, to the second subgoal, which is connected by a_2 to the overall goal. Formally, the overall evaluation of K is given by:

$$U_K = a_1 \cdot a_{31} \cdot u(K) + a_2 \cdot a_{32} \cdot u(K) \qquad (6)$$

Hopefully, this demonstrates how the difficulty in estimating importance weights can be reduced and, by implementation of MAUT, become meaningful in complex situations. For the special requirements and restrictions of this extension of MAUT the reader is referred to a paper by VESPER and SAYEKI (1971), which discusses this approach in some detail in the context of company investment planning.

III. Some Experimental Problems in Investigating MAUT

Application of MAUT as an aid in complex evaluation is a fairly new undertaking. There are only a few experiments explicitly using MAUT. On the other hand, there is a very extensive literature demonstrating the power of the additive model in human information processing (SLOVIC and LICHTENSTEIN, 1971).

Empirical validation of MAUT seems difficult, at least for situations where its application as an aid to decision-making is proposed. These situations can be characterized by the absence of an accepted outside criterion for evaluation. If such a criterion exists and can be assessed, use of MAUT would be meaningless.

For the axiomatic approaches to MAUT, it is possible to test such assumptions as independence, although this might involve a prohibitively large effort. But in the axiomatic approach, a single violation of one assumption is sufficient to invalidate the whole model. From a pragmatic point of view, however, the model might still be useful.

Furthermore, if the assumptions hold, nothing is said about the quality of the scaling procedures used and the reliability of the judgments made.

To test MAUT, most authors decided to investigate restricted situations where outside criteria are available. HUBER and GUSTAFSON (1971) developed a severity index with MAUT, for burned patients, using mortality as an outside criterion in a validation study. Most experiments of interest here used as outside criterion the overall evaluations or actual choices of the subject and compared MAUT with alternative models, such as the normal regression model or multiplicative models. HUBER et al. (1969), using experienced professional staff as Ss, investigated the evaluation of hypothetical hospital wards varying in 7 factors. HOEPFL and HUBER (1970) had students rate hypothetical teaching professors varying in 6 dimensions. GREEN et al. (1972) studied housewives' preferences for three-dimensional descriptions of retail discount cards, and EINHORN et al. (1972), the evaluation of political candidates. All these studies demonstrate that the additive model does a very good job in predicting overall evaluations. These studies to some extent support the validation of MAUT, but their main contribution concerns such technical details as usefulness of different scaling procedures and response modes.

IV. Concluding Remarks

Some important parts of MAUT have been omitted from the preceding discussion. Among these are practical scaling procedures for utilities and importance weights, and the problem of combining the judgements of different experts.

Considering the state of experimental validation and the fact that in MAUT subjective judgments are combined by a very simple formal rule, one might be sceptical about the usefulness of the whole approach. It should be remembered, however, that MAUT is proposed for situations where no "objective" evaluation criteria (whatever this means) are available. Therefore MAUT should always be compared with the unaided, intuitive human judgment in the same situation.

At its least, MAUT can be seen as a guide to structuring the evaluation task. This may be especially important if the evaluations are done by a group of experts. Very often different people evaluate things differently. By using MAUT, a group of experts may be helped to find the points on which they disagree; they can then concentrate discussion on these aspects.

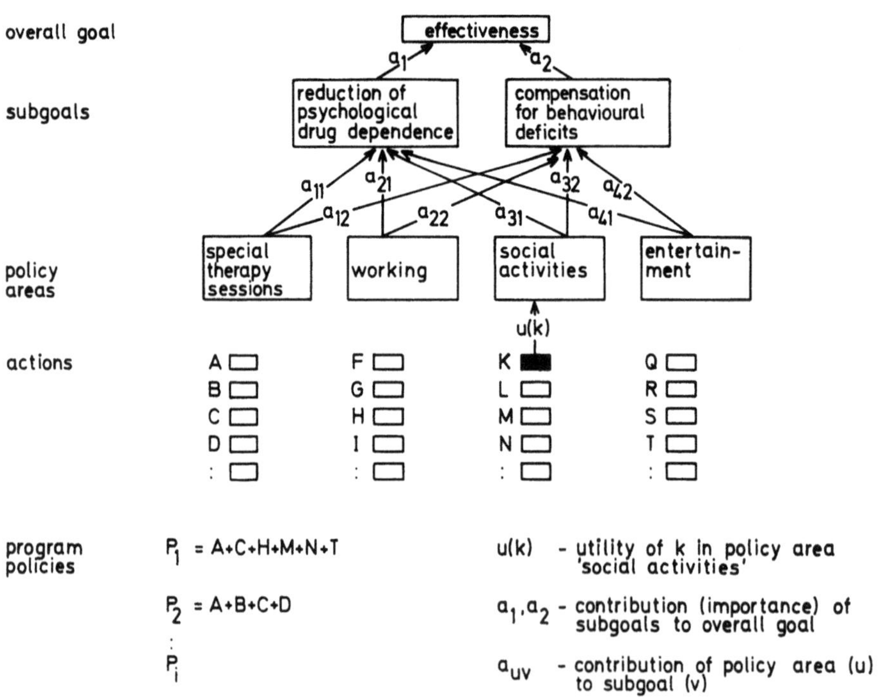

Fig. 1. Example for structuring an evaluation problem

Using the theoretical work on MAUT and on decision analysis in general it is possible to offer a wide variety of consistency checks to make you sure that the final evaluation will be in agreement with the accepted principles of choice behaviour.

References

EDWARDS, W.: Evaluation of unperformed social acts via multi-attribute utilities. Memorandum, Engineering Psychol. Lab. 1970.

EINHORN, H.J., KOMORITA, S.S., ROSEN, B.:Multidimensional models for the evaluation of political candidates. J. exp. soc. Psychol. 8, 58-73 (1972).

FISHBURN, P.C.: Independence in utility theory with whole product sets. Operations Research 13, 28-45 (1965).

FISHBURN, P.C.: Methods of estimating additive utilities. Management Science 13, 435-453 (1967).

GOLDBERG, L.R.: Simple models or simple processes? Amer. Psychol. 23, 483-496 (1968).

GREEN, P.E., CARMONE, F.J., WIND, Y.: Subjective evaluation models and conjoint measurement. Behav. Sci. 17, 288-299 (1972).

HOEPFL, T.R., HUBER, G.P.: A study of self-explicated utility models. Behav. Sci. 15, 408-414 (1970).

HUBER, G.P., GUSTAFSON, D.H.: Some effects to apply behavioural decision theory in the medical care field. In: PHILLIPS, L.D., LOVIE, D., KIDD, J.B. (Eds.): Proceedings of the Third Research Conference on Subjective Probability, Utility and Decision Making. London, Sept. 1971 (in press).

HUBER, G.P., SAHNEY, V.K., FORD, D.L.: A study of subjective evaluation models. Behav. Sci. 14, 483-489 (1969).

KRANTZ, D.H.: Conjoint measurement: The Luce-Tukey-axiomatization and some extension. J. Math. Psychol. 1, 248-277 (1964).

KRANTZ, D.H., TVERSKY, A.: Conjoint-measurement analysis of composition rules in psychology. Psychol. Rev. 78, 151-169 (1971).

LUCE, R.D., TUKEY, J.W.: Simultaneous conjoint measurement: A new type of fundamental measurement. J. Math. Psychol. 1, 1-27 (1964).

PRATT, J.W., RAIFFA, R., SCHLAIFER, R.: The foundations of decisions under uncertainty: An elementary exposition. J. Amer. statist. Ass. 59, 353-375 (1964).

RACHMAN, S.: Effects of Psychotherapy. New York: Pergamon Press 1971.

RAIFFA, H.: Decisions Analysis. Introductory Lectures on Choice under Uncertainty. Reading, Mass.: Addison-Wesley 1968.

RAIFFA, H.: Preferences for multiattribute alternatives. Rand-Memorandum RM-5868, DOT/RC 1969.

SAYEKI, Y.: Allocation of importance: An axiom system. Technical Report. Dept. Psychol., Univ. Washington 1970.

SLOVIK, P., LICHTENSTEIN, S.: Comparison of Bayesian and regression approaches to the study of information processing in judgment. Org. Behav. hum. Perf. 6, 649-744 (1971).

VESPER, K.H., SAYEKI, Y.: A quantitative approach for decision analysis. Technical Report. Dept. Psychol., Univ. Washington 1971.

VON WINTERFELDT, D.: Multiattributive utility theory. Unveröffentl. Diplomarbeit, Hamburg 1971.

YNTEMA, D.B., TORGERSON, W.S.: Man-computer cooperation in decisions requiring common sense. IRE Transactions on human factors in electronics HFG-2, 20-26 (1961).

An Approach to the Experimental Investigation of Some Parameters of Systematic Desensitization of the Individual Patient

J.P.N. PHILLIPS and P.M. KENYON

I. Introduction: Previous Work

Although systematic desensitization is usually spoken of as a single procedure, there are so many parameters which can be varied that it would be more accurately described as a family of procedures. PAUL (1969) refers to four identifiable procedural "packages" (due to WOLPE, to LAZARUS and RACHMAN, to LANG and LAZOVIK, and to PAUL respectively), and gives a table, 3 pages long, of major parameters. Six of these, shown in Table 1, were termed "crucial" by LAZARUS (1964) who made a number of eminently sensible suggestions based on clinical experience, but not explicitly supported by experimental evidence. Other parameters, as well as some of the 6 of LAZARUS, have also been investigated experimentally, as shown in Table 2.

II. Critique

With so many variables which may affect the course and outcome of desensitization, it is clear that more work is needed to determine the most efficient combination of parameters, so as to make the therapy as rapid and as long-lasting as possible, and to make it effective in as many as possible of the cases where it now fails.

Unfortunately, the approach of the majority of the studies cited in Table 2 does not appear to be the most suitable to achieve this aim, for two reasons. Firstly, they deal with the elimination of atypical

Table 1. Six "Crucial Procedural Factors in Desensitization Theory" (from LAZARUS, 1964)

(1) How should repeated signalling of anxiety be handled?

(2) When no signalling occurs, how long should the patient be asked to visualize the individual items on his anxiety hierarchy?

(3) How long should the relaxation interval be between the presentation of scenes?

(4) Is there an optimal number of scenes which should be presented at any given session?

(5) What is the mean or recommended duration of desensitization sessions?

(6) Is there an optimum interval that should elapse between sessions?

Table 2. Some Experimental Studies of Parameters of Systematic Desensitization

Suggestion and Therapeutically Oriented Instructions

VALINS & RAY, 1967; LEITENBERG et al., 1969; MARCIA et al., 1969; McGLYNN et al., 1969; OLIVEAU et al., 1969; McGLYNN & MAPP, 1970; McGLYNN & WILLIAMS, 1970; HOWLETT & NAWAS, 1971; LOMONT & BROCK, 1971; McGLYNN et al., 1971; McGLYNN, 1972; MILLER, 1972; NAWAS, 1972.

Effective Components of Desensitization: Relaxation and Counterconditioning

RACHMAN, 1965; COOKE, 1966a; LARSEN, 1966; LOMONT & EDWARDS, 1967; SCHUBOT, 1967; DAVISON, 1968; KRAPFL & NAWAS, 1969; MILLER & NAWAS, 1970; NAWAS et al., 1970a; NAWAS et al., 1970b; SUE, 1972.

Therapist vs. Automated Desensitization

KRAPFL & NAWAS, 1969; DONNER, 1970.

Individual vs. Group Desensitization

PAUL & SHANNON, 1966; PAUL, 1968.

Standard vs. Individualized Hierarchies

EMERY & KRUMBOLTZ, 1967; McGLYNN et al., 1970; McGLYNN, 1971.

Stimulus Intensity

WOLPE, 1963; WATTS, 1971.

Mode of Stimulus Presentation

COOKE, 1966b; RITTER, 1968; BANDURA et al., 1969; O'NEILL & HOWELL, 1969.

Length of Stimulus Presentation

PROCTOR, 1969; WATTS, 1971.

Verbal Reward

WAGNER & CAUTHEN, 1968; LEITENBERG et al., 1969; OLIVEAU et al., 1969.

Spacing of Sessions

RAMSAY et al., 1966; LANYON et al., 1968.

---

fears in atypical subjects. Usually some experimentally convenient, clear-cut and isolated fear is chosen (most often fear of snakes) rather than the experimentally awkward, vague and diffuse phobias which are more likely to occur in practice. Furthermore, these fears, although intense, are not really phobic symptoms; they are, rather, subclinical, in the sense that the experimental subjects did not spontaneously seek treatment for them, but simply volunteered to act as subjects in an experiment. Indeed, there was often an inducement for them to volunteer, such as being paid, or fulfilling a course requirement[+]. The subjects,

[+] Since this paper was written, a study became available which found clear differences between the symptomatology of psychiatric phobic patients and that of normal volunteers with phobic fears (McALLISTER and OLLEY, 1972).

moreover, are almost always not psychiatric patients, but usually students, most often white American female college students in classes in general psychology (although one study, O'NEILL and HOWELL, 1969, did use male sex offenders incarcerated in a high security hospital). Of all the investigations in Table 2, the only ones which dealt with actual symptoms of psychiatric patients are those by WOLPE (1963) and WATTS (1971): the extent to which the findings of the others are valid for such symptoms and patients is thus an open question.

The second reason why the approach of the majority of these studies appears unsuitable is that they deal with groups of patients rather than with single cases. The disadvantage here is that little account is taken of individual differences. Therefore, even when one mode of desensitization is superior to another for all subjects, the between-subjects variance may well be so large as to swamp any differences due to the therapeutic variable, so that an insignificant treatments effect is obtained. More seriously, different patients can and do respond quite differently to desensitization, so that a (significant or insignificant) treatments effect in a particular experiment may conceal the fact that in reality one level of a parameter is for some patients more effective than another, for some equally effective, and for some less effective. For these and similar reasons, both CHASSAN (1960, 1967) and SHAPIRO (1961, 1963, 1964a, 1966, 1969, 1970) have repeatedly urged the use of single-case rather than group experiments in clinical psychological research. Of all the investigations in Table 2, the only ones to deal with single cases were again those of WOLPE (1963) and WATTS (1971).

III. An Approach: Examples

The purpose of the present paper is to indicate an approach to the investigation of some parameters of systematic desensitization, whose aim is to overcome these disadvantages by carrying out experiments on the desensitization of symptoms of individual patients. The approach will first be illustrated by three specific examples and then discussed in more general terms.

1. Example 1

The first example was an experiment (or, more correctly, two experiments put together) to investigate the effects of extra relaxation after anxiety signals. In the first half, the extra relaxation consisted of maintaining the scene presented until the anxiety signal was withdrawn instead of stopping it immediately (cf. GEER and SILVERMAN, 1967): in the second, the interval before the next presentation of the scene, 2 min, was lengthened by 1 min for each anxiety signal to that scene.

The patient was a 23-year-old married woman under treatment by desensitization for frigidity. The experiment was carried out on the middle 24 items of a 29-item hierarchy of sexual situations, and followed the design shown in Table 3(a)[+]. Half the items (the third, fifth, ninth, tenth, etc.) were presented with normal relaxation after anxiety signals,

[+] Some of those who heard this paper reported difficulty in following the statistical analyses, which presume familiarity with systematic designs and analysis of covariance. The reader who has any doubts on this score should immediately reread the account of analysis of covariance in any standard textbook of statistics (e.g. WINER, 1962, Chap. 11); systematic designs are less frequently treated, but a very clear description is given by MAXWELL (1958) Chap. 10.

Table 3. Mrs. F. Sexual Situations

	Relaxation	
	Normal	Extra
	3	4
	5	6
	9	7
	10	8
	11	12
	13	14
	16	15
	18	17
	19	21
	20	22
	24	23
	26	25
Sum	174	174
Sum of Squares	3098	3098

(a) Experimental Design (for explanation see text)

	Cumulative Presentations to Desensitization			
Item	Normal	Extra	Anxiety Signals	Scale Value
3	79		1	0.5169
4		61	0	0.5277
5	63		0	0.5287
6		91	1	0.5602
7		87	0	0.5905
8		89	0	0.6239
9	93		0	0.6432
10	95		0	0.6935
11	100		1	0.7769
12		102	0	0.7851
13	111		1	0.8007
14		109	0	0.8065
15		113	0	0.8457
16	115		0	0.8617
17		117	0	0.8695
18	124		0	0.9105
19	134		1	1.0669
20	150		1	1.0686
21		142	0	1.1062
22		152	1	1.4876
23		148	0	1.8768
24	154		0	2.2740
25		156	0	2.5350
26	158		0	2.6104
Mean	$114.66\dot{6}$	$113.91\dot{6}$		

(b) Results (for explanation see text)

Table 3. (Continuation)

Source	d.f.	S.S.	V.E.	F	p
	1	18.4127	18.4127	< 1	N.S.
Linear Trend	1	19678.1294	19678.1294	851.809	<.001
Quadratic Trend	1	9.6837	9.6837	< 1	N.S.
Residual	19	438.9300	23.1016		

(c) Analysis of Covariance of Cumulative Presentations to Desensitization with Presence/Absence of Anxiety Signal as Covariate

whilst the remaining half (the fourth, sixth, seventh, eighth, etc.) were presented with extra relaxation, as described above. The results of the experiment are given in columns 2 and 3 of Table 3(b), which shows the cumulative number of presentations to desensitization of each individual item, i.e. the total number of presentations of all items by the last trial on which a given item was presented. Before proceeding to an analysis of these results, it is necessary to mention two other relevant factors.

Trend: In any such experiment in which a sequence of observations is obtained from a single subject, it is possible that there is some sequential trend in the data which might affect the results: certainly here the nature of the dependent variable, namely cumulative presentations to desensitization, makes it virtually certain that the observations will increase in value as the hierarchy is ascended. This was foreseen and provided for in the design, which is a systematic design (COX, 1951) balanced for linear and quadratic trend, as can be seen from the fact that the sums and sums of squares of the two columns of Table 3(a) are the same. This means that any linear and quadratic trends in the data may be assessed independently of the experimental treatment.

A Failure of Control: A problem which cannot be overcome experimentally is that, if the patient never signals anxiety to certain items, then the independent variable, here namely normal/extra relaxation after anxiety signals, will be rendered inoperable. As may be seen from col. 4 of Table 3(b), where a one indicates that there was at least one anxiety signal and a zero that there was none, this happened extensively in the present experiment. The problem can be partly overcome by treating this column of ones and zeros as an extra variable on which the items could not be matched, and whose effects must therefore be controlled statistically by parcelling it out in an analysis of covariance. However, a rather extensive attenuation of the power of the experiment cannot be avoided.

The results of the analysis of covariance+ shown in Table 3(c) are essentially negative. The effect of extra relaxation is not significant, possibly because this variable was rendered largely inoperative, or possibly not. There is a highly significant linear trend in the data, which is further discussed below (Preliminary Results. Stimulus Intensity): there is no significant quadratic trend.

+ The fact that in this and both of the two following examples an analysis of covariance happens to be necessary might give rise to the impression that this is always the case; however, in most experiments of this kind an analysis of variance is sufficient.

2. Example 2

The second example is an experiment designed to investigate separately the two variables put together in Example 1: (1) the time before withdrawal of items after an anxiety signal, and (2) the interval between presentations of the items. The patient was a 30-year-old married man under treatment by desensitization of anxieties in a rather diffuse set of situations. The experiment was carried out on a 24-item hierarchy of items concerned with "being alone in public", and followed the design shown in Table 4(a), where the items are classified by columns according to variable (1), in seconds, and by rows according to variable (2), in minutes⁺. The design, which is a magic rectangle (essentially similar in principle to a systematic design: PHILLIPS 1964, 1968a, b) is balanced for linear (but not for quadratic) trend, as can be seen from the fact that all the columns have the same sum, and so do all the rows.

The results of the experiment are shown in Table 4(b), both sequentially, in a layout analogous to Table 3(b), and in a rectangle, so as to exhibit the means due to the two variables.

The results of the analysis of covariance are shown in Table 4(c), and are very similar to those of Example 1, the only significant effect being a very highly significant linear trend in the data.

3. Example 3

In the third example the same two variables were investigated as in the second, as well as the effects of special relaxation instructions after an anxiety signal. The patient was a 49-year-old married man under treatment for desensitization of feelings of physical tension in a number of situations involving driving, walking, standing or waiting. The experiment was carried out on the last 32 items of the 37-item "standing" hierarchy, and followed the design shown in Table 5(a). For all the items in the block marked "Ordinary", an item was withdrawn after an anxiety signal with the words: "Stop visualizing that, relax completely again, not thinking of anything in particular". For the block marked "Special" the instructions were: "Stop visualizing that, relax completely again, not thinking of anything in particular. Relax away all the tension that occurred just then, until it's absolutely gone. Keep on relaxing until you're still more deeply relaxed than before you visualized that scene. And even then don't stop, keep on relaxing more and more, deeper and deeper all the time", or some similar paraphrase. The design, which is again a magic figure design, is balanced for linear (but not quadratic) trend, as may be seen from the fact that all columns and all rows have the same sum, and so do all corresponding pairs of cells in the two blocks.

The results of the experiment are shown in Table 5(b), both sequentially, and also in subtables exhibiting the means due to the main effects of the three variables and their first-order interactions.

The results of the analysis of covariance, shown in Table 5(c), are very similar to those of the first two examples, the only significant effect being a highly significant linear trend in the data.

⁺ Note that this variable is unavoidably inoperative for the first presentation of a session; the slight bias resulting therefrom has been ignored.

Table 4. Mr. Y. Being Alone in Public

Time before Withdrawal

		0"	2"	4"	6"	8"	10"	Sum
Interval before Presentation	1'	12	13	4	20	21	5	75
	2'	1	24	9	17	16	8	75
	3'	18	7	15	2	10	23	75
	4'	19	6	22	11	3	14	75
	Sum	50	50	50	50	50	50	

(a) Experimental Design (for explanation see text)

Time before Withdrawal

		0"	2"	4"	6"	8"	10"	Mean
Interval before Presentation	1'	56	58	18	88	146	20	64.33
	2'	7	112	36	100	81	32	61.33
	3'	79	30	64	5	41	123	57.00
	4'	86	34	107	62	16	60	60.83
	Mean	57.00	58.50	56.25	63.75	71.00	58.75	

Item	Cumulative Presentations to Desensitization	Anxiety Signal	Scale Value
1	7	1	0.3436
2	5	0	0.3680
3	16	1	0.4054
4	18	1	0.4473
5	20	0	0.4476
6	34	1	0.4756
7	30	0	0.5032
8	32	0	0.5123
9	36	0	0.5132
10	41	1	0.5944
11	62	1	1.0437
12	56	1	1.1413
13	58	0	1.1560
14	60	0	1.1643
15	64	0	1.2121
16	81	1	1.2251
17	100	1	1.6182
18	79	0	1.6947
19	86	0	1.7959
20	88	0	2.4586
21	146	1	2.5641
22	107	1	3.0144
23	123	1	3.0681
24	112	0	3.8105

(b) Results (for explanation see text)

Table 4. (Continuation)

Source	d.f.	S.S.	V.E.	F	p
Time before Withdrawal	5	236.5719	47.3144	< 1	N.S.
Interval before Presentation	3	119.5168	39.8389	< 1	N.S.
Linear Trend	1	32105.5127	32105.5127	287.817	<.001
Residual	13	1450.1306	111.5485		

(c) Analysis of Covariance of Cumulative Presentations to Desensitization, with Presence/Absence of Anxiety Signal as Covariate

IV. Discussion of the Approach

It can be seen from these examples that the approach to the investigation of parameters of desensitization advocated here consists simply of an application, to the items of a hierarchy of an individual patient, of ordinary experimental method. This method consists of observing the effects on a dependent variable of systematically manipulating certain independent variables of interest, whilst holding others constant or, if they cannot be held constant, controlling for them either by the design of the experiment or, if this is not possible, statistically, by parcelling out their effects. Since this experimental method is familiar, it is only necessary to consider those special problems which arise specifically here, firstly because we are dealing with sequences of observations from a single subject, and secondly, even more specifically, because we are dealing with systematic desensitization.

1. Problems Arising with Single-Subject Repeated-Measures Experiments

There are two difficulties peculiar to single-subject repeated-measures experiments: (1) the possibility of a sequential trend in the data, and (2) the possibility of a lack of the independence assumed by analysis of variance (and most other statistical techniques as well).

The former difficulty can readily be overcome by the use of an appropriate experimental design which permits assessment of trend independently of other effects, as has already been illustrated in the foregoing examples. Systematic designs (COX, 1951) are appropriate for a fairly complicated (i.e. linear, quadratic, cubic, or even higher order) trend with a relatively simple design, usually a one-way design with just two different levels of the independent variable, whilst magic figure designs (PHILLIPS, 1964, 1968a, b) are suitable for a simple (usually only linear) trend with relatively complicated designs, e.g. two- or three-way factorial, or Latin or Graeco-Latin square designs.

The difficulty of possible lack of independence is more serious, since violations of the independence-of-errors assumption can markedly affect the distribution of the F ratio, and hence the validity of the conclusions derived from analyses of variance, whilst not much appears to be known about how to compensate for such violations (SCHEFFÊ, 1959). However, it is important to understand this difficulty properly so as not to exaggerate its importance. The mathematical model underlying analysis of variance is that every observation is the sum of various components,

Table 5. Mr. J. Standing

		Ordinary: Time before Withdrawal 0"	3"	6"	9"	Sum		Special: Time before Withdrawal 0"	3"	6"	9"	Sum
Interval	3/4'	15	30	12	29	86	3/4'	28	13	31	14	86
before	1 1/2'	8	25	19	34	86	1 1/1'	35	18	24	9	86
Presen-	2 1/4'	26	11	33	16	86	2 1/4'	17	32	10	27	86
tation	3'	37	20	22	7	86	3'	6	23	21	36	86
	Sum	86	86	86	86		Sum	86	86	86	86	

(a) Experimental Design (for explanation see text)

Ordinary		Time before Withdrawal 0"	3"	6"	9"	Mean
Interval	3/4'	103	189	90	178	140.00
before	1 1/2'	63	151	111	230	138.75
Presen-	2 1/4'	164	67	216	113	140.00
tation	3'	240	127	142	50	139.75
	Mean	142.50	133.50	139.75	142.75	139.6250

Special		Time before Withdrawal 0"	3"	6"	9"	Mean
Interval	3/4'	169	81	201	92	135.75
before	1 1/2'	221	125	155	55	139.00
Presen-	2 1/4'	101	203	65	187	139.00
tation	3'	38	153	140	223	138.50
	Mean	132.25	140.50	140.25	139.25	138.0625

Mean of Ordinary and Special		Time before Withdrawal 0"	3"	6"	9"	Mean
Interval	3/4'	136.0	135.0	145.5	135.0	137.875
before	1 1/2'	142.0	138.0	133.0	142.5	138.875
Presen-	2 1/4'	132.5	135.0	140.5	150.0	139.500
tation	3'	139.0	140.0	141.0	136.5	139.125
	Mean	137.375	137.000	140.000	141.000	

Item	Cumulative Presentation to Desensitization	Anxiety Signal	Scale Value
6	38	1	0.6229
7	50	1	0.6745
8	63	1	0.6758
9	55	1	0.7046
10	65	1	0.7534
11	67	1	0.7552
12	90	1	0.8237
13	81	1	0.8675
14	92	1	0.8748
15	103	1	0.8924
16	113	1	0.9652
17	101	0	0.9816

Table 5. (Continuation)

Item	Cumulative Presentation to Desensitization	Anxiety Signal	Scale Value
18	125	1	0.9829
19	111	0	0.9850
20	127	1	0.9857
21	140	1	1.0159
22	142	1	1.0360
23	153	1	1.0976
24	155	1	1.1306
25	151	0	1.1810
26	164	1	1.1908
27	187	1	1.2067
28	169	0	1.2304
29	178	1	1.3304
30	189	1	1.3373
31	201	1	1.3727
32	203	1	1.3749
33	216	1	1.5871
34	230	1	1.6314
35	221	1	1.6790
36	223	0	1.8558
37	240	1	2.8674

(b) Results (for explanation see text)

Source	d.f.	S.S.	V.E.	F	p
Relaxation Instruction	1	1.3399	1.3399	< 1	N.S.
Time before Withdrawal	3	69.9039	23.3013	< 1	N.S.
Interval before Presentation	3	40.1352	13.3784	< 1	N.S.
R x T	3	48.1541	16.0514	< 1	N.S.
R x I	3	97.9214	32.6405	< 1	N.S.
T x I	9	404.9671	44.9963	1.272	N.S.
Linear Trend	1	95283.6168	95283.6168	2692.571	<.001
Residual	7	247.7132	35.3876		

(c) Analysis of Covariance of Cumulative Presentations to Desensitization, with Presence/absence of Anxiety Signal as Covariate

each due to a specific level or combination of levels of one (or more) of the independent variables being manipulated, plus an error term, and it is only if these error terms are correlated that we have lack of independence. In psychological terms, errors are correlated only if the extent to which the subject happens by chance on one occasion to respond at a level above or below what may be expected purely on the basis of the independent variables affects his chance deviation from expectation on another occasion. Thus, violations of the independence-of-errors assumption are not a certainty with repeated-measures designs, but only a risk. Unfortunately, in the present state of our knowledge they seem to be a risk which will have to be run until statistical tools are developed for dealing with them; the only alternative would be to abandon any attempt at such experimentation.

2. Problems Arising with Systematic Desensitization

The problems which arise specifically because we are dealing with systematic desensitization may conveniently be classified into those connected with the independent variables and those connected with the dependent variable(s).

Independent Variables: There is one main limitation on the independent variables which can be investigated by the approach we suggest: they must be capable of variation from item to item of a hierarchy. Thus, the effects of parameters which can only be manipulated globally, such as the last two of LAZARUS's 6, the optimum number of scenes per session and the interval between sessions, and also therapeutically oriented instructions, relaxation training and standard versus individualized hierarchies, would be either very difficult or impossible to determine by this method.

Dependent Variables: The dependent variable we have used, namely cumulative number of presentations to desensitization, is for two reasons far from satisfactory, although we have not been able to define a better one.

Firstly, the aims of the investigations are to improve our theoretical understanding of what makes systematic desensitization effective, and to determine that combination of parameters which will in practice produce the fastest and most lasting real-life cure of the patient's phobia, so that an index of his behaviour in the treatment session is not the most appropriate measure.

For example, the criterion for desensitization for each item initially used for earlier hierarchies with the patient of Example 2 was two consecutive presentations without an anxiety signal. However, he reported that situations which had been successfully desensitized were starting to cause him anxiety again (cf. WOLPE, 1961; AGRAS, 1965; RACHMAN, 1966), and it was hypothesized that this would be overcome with overlearning relaxation responses to the items by using a stricter criterion for their desensitization, in other words, the first two presentations of the given item in a session should be without anxiety signals. The expedient appeared to be successful, but this was only manifest in the cessation of reports of such relapses, not in the desensitization sessions themselves.

Unfortunately a real-life criterion of desensitization of each individual hierarchy item is usually impracticable with patients, since their exposure to the different situations is subject to uncontrollable day-to-day contingencies. For example, the higher items in the hierarchy of this patient concerned having to be in various towns for his company.

A second reason why cumulative number of presentations to desensitization is not satisfactory is that it is only one of a number of possible indices of the desensitization procedure which could be used, as may be seen from Table 6(a), which contains the raw data for Table 4. Another index, which has been used by WATTS (1971), is the non-cumulative number of presentations of each individual item, as shown in Table 6(b). This is sometimes correlated with cumulative presentations, as in Example 2, where $r = 0.44$, $p < 0.5$, and sometimes not, as in Examples 1 and 3, where $r = -0.03$ and $r = 0.08$, respectively. We have analysed

Table 6.

14/5	4/6	11/6	17/6	25/6	2/7	6/8	3/9	10/9	17/9	1/10	8/10	15/10	29/10	3/12	21/1	25/2
1 √	1 X	3 X	6 X	6 X	10 X	11 X	11 X	16 X	16 X	17 √	17 X	21 X	21 √	21 √	21 √	21 X
X	X	X	√	X	X	√	X	√	X	X	X	√	√	X	X	X
X	3 X	4 X	X	9 X	11 √	√	15 X	X	17 √	X	21 √	X	X	X	X	24 X
2 X	√	X	X	X	X	X	X	X	X	21 √	√	X	X	24 √	24 X	X
X	X	5 X	7 X	10 √	√	X	16 √	17 X	X	√	√	24* √	24 √	√	√	
	X	X	X	X	X	12 X	√	√	19 X	X	X	X	X	X	X	
	4 √	6 √	8 X	X	X	X	√	X	X	X	X	√	X	X	X	
	X	√	X		12 √	13 X	X	X	20 X	22 √	22 X	√				
	X	X			X	X	X	18 X	X	X	X	√				
		X			X	14 X		X		X	23 √	23 X				
						X					X	X				
											X					
											24 X					
											X					

(a) Protocols of the desensitization sessions for Mr. Y

Key √ Anxiety Signal

X No Anxiety Signal

* Note that item 24 was presented on 15/10 in error for 23, and found not to be desensitized.

Table 6. (Continuation)

Item	Cumulative	Non-Cumulative
1	7	5
2	5	2
3	16	6
4	18	5
5	20	2
6	34	10
7	30	2
8	32	2
9	36	2
10	41	5
11	62	12
12	56	5
13	58	2
14	60	2
15	64	2
16	81	11
17	100	12
18	79	2
19	86	2
20	88	2
21	146	25
22	107	5
23	123	5
24	112	2

(b) Cumulative and Non-Cumulative Presentations to Desensitization

our data using this index also: the only essential difference in the results was that the linear trend in the data became insignificant. The reader should have no difficulty in deriving further indices, say taking into account the number of anxiety signals or the number of sessions. The situation would, of course, be even more complicated if two or more hierarchies were being desensitized in parallel.

V. Preliminary Results

In discussing our (very) preliminary results, it is convenient to deal separately with stimulus intensity, which plays a rather special role, and then with all other variables.

1. Stimulus Intensity

WOLPE (1963) found that with hierarchies which were objectively quantifiable, such as distance from a fearful object or situation, distance from a safe point, or number of phobic objects, the graph of cumulative presentations to desensitization plotted against this objective quantification was describable by a power function, as illustrated in Fig. 1. He related this to STEVENS' (1957, 1962) psychophysical power law:

$$\psi = k\,\phi^n$$

where ψ is psychological magnitude, ϕ is physical magnitude and k and n are constants (the graph will be positively accelerated if $n > 1$, a straight line if $n = 1$ and negatively accelerated if $n < 1$). Whilst none

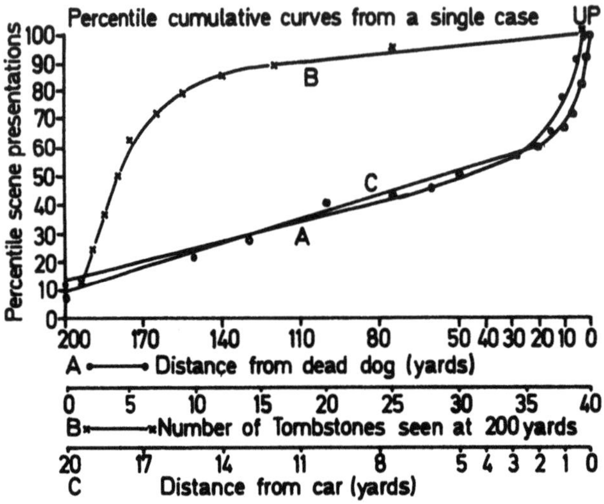

Fig. 1 (From WOLPE, 1963)

of the three hierarchies in the present examples was objectively quantifiable, psychological scale values of the items were obtained by asking the patient to make pair-comparison-ratio judgments of their intensities (PHILLIPS, 1971); these are shown in the final columns of Table 3(b), 4(b) and 5(b). It may be deduced from WOLPE's interpretation that the graph of cumulative presentations to desensitization, plotted

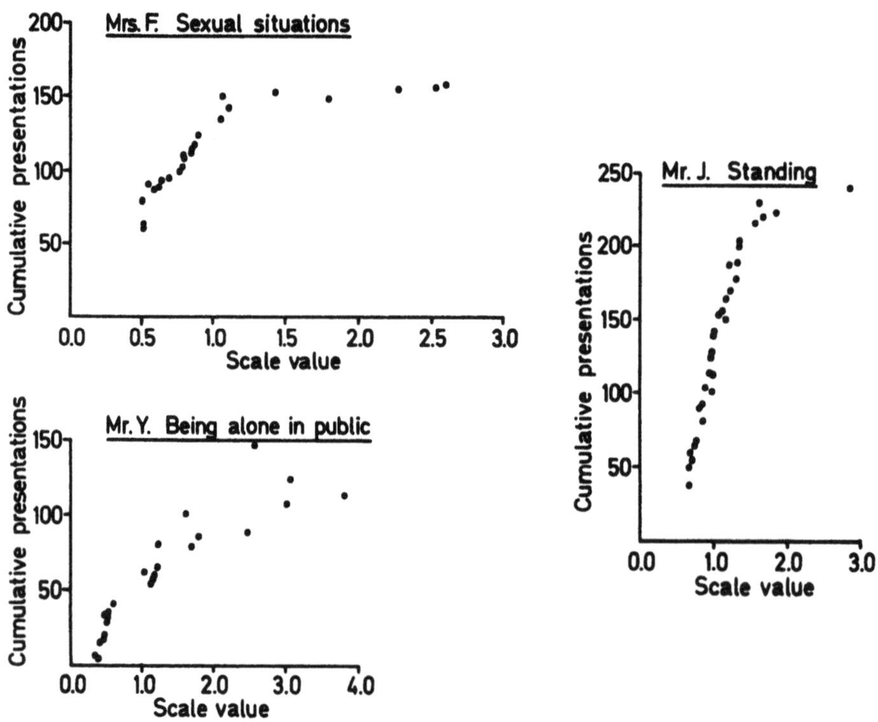

Fig. 2.

against the psychological intensities of the stimuli, should be a straight line. We have not found this to be the case, as illustrated by Fig. 2, which shows these graphs for the data of Tables 3, 4 and 5. Instead, in our data, cumulative presentations to desensitization are linearly related simply to item number, as illustrated in Fig. 3+, and this relationship does not appear to be an artefact of the correlation between item number and scale value, for the latter is a positively accelerated and sometimes saltatory function of the former, as illustrated in Fig. 4.

It should be noted that here item intensity is a variable which, although inevitably present, we have not manipulated. However, WATTS (1971) investigated it as an independent variable, both by itself and in combination with length of presentation.

2. Other Variables

In the small number of experiments we have so far carried out, the effects of parameters other than stimulus intensity have been uniformly insignificant. It would, of course, be entirely premature, and contrary to the findings of, say, WATTS (1971) to conclude that all these para-

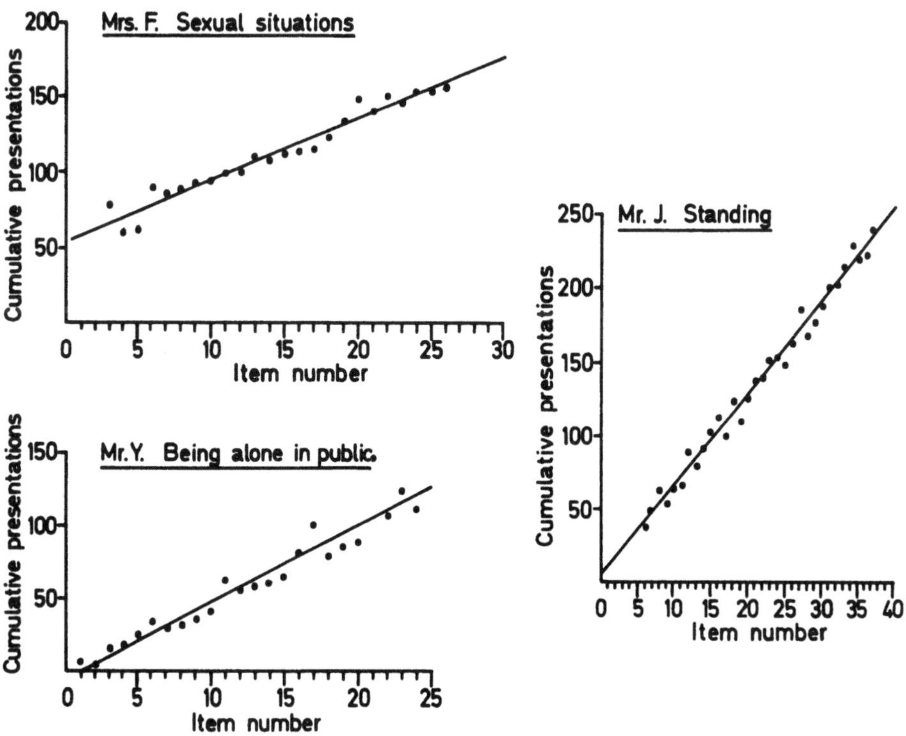

Fig. 3.

+ The fact that the straight line for Example 1 clearly does not pass through the origin, as it does for Examples 2 and 3, is probably attributable to the fact that prior to item 3 (the first item in Table 3) of this example, some items from another hierarchy had been inextricably included in the desensitization.

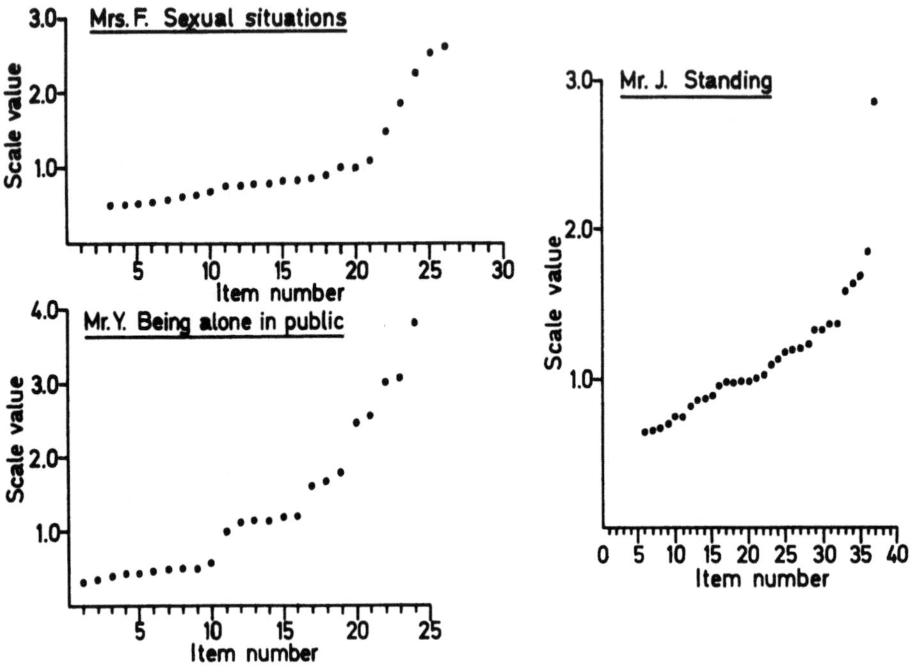

Fig. 4.

managed to find levels of them which are operative. The approach we advocate is, indeed, fraught with difficulties and full of unsolved problems, as may be seen from the preceding examples. It does, however, offer the possibility of making the therapeutic desensitization of every reasonably large hierarchy at the same time an experiment which may be of both therapeutic and scientific value.

References

AGRAS, W.S.: An investigation of the decrement of anxiety responses during systematic desensitization therapy. Behav. Res. Ther. 2, 267-270 (1965).

BANDURA, A., BLANCHARD, E.B., RITTER, B.: Relative efficacy of desensitization and modeling approaches for inducing behavioral, affective and attitudinal changes. J. Pers. Soc. Psychol. 13, 173-199 (1969).

CHASSAN, J.B.: Statistical inference and the single case in clinical design. Psychiatry 23, 173-184 (1960).

CHASSAN, J.B.: Research Design in Clinical Psychology and Psychiatry. New York: Appleton-Century-Crofts 1967.

COOKE, G.: Identification of the efficacious components of reciprocal inhibition therapy. Diss. Abstr. 27, 1618-B (1966a).

COOKE, G.: The efficacy of two desensitization procedures: an analogue study. Behav. Res. Ther. 4, 17-24 (1966b).

COX, D.R.: Some systematic experimental designs. Biometrika 38, 312-323 (1951).

DAVISON, G.C.: Systematic desensitization as a counterconditioning process. J. abnorm. soc. Psychol. 73, 91-99 (1968).

DONNER, L.: Automated group desensitization - a follow-up report. Behav. Res. Ther. 8, 241-247 (1970).

EMERY, J.R., KRUMBOLTZ, J.D.: Standard versus individualized hierarchies in desensitization to reduce test anxiety. J. cons. Psychol. 14, 204-209 (1967).
GEER, J.H., SILVERMAN, I.: Treatment of a recurrent nightmare by behavior-modification procedures: a case study. J. abnorm. soc. Psychol. 72, 188-190 (1967).
HOWLETT, S.C., NAWAS, M.M.: The effects of subject expectancy on the outcome of desensitization. In: RUBIN, R.D., FENSTERHEIM, H., LAZARUS, A.A., FRANKS, C.M. (Eds.): Advances in Behavior Therapy - 1970. New York: Academic Press 1971.
KRAPFL, J.E., NAWAS, M.M.: Client-therapist relationship factor in systematic desensitization. J. consult. clin. Psychol. 33, 435-439 (1969).
LANYON, R.I., MANOSEVITZ, M., IMBER, R.R.: Systematic desensitization: distribution of practice and symptom substitution. Behav. Res. Ther. 6, 323-329 (1968).
LARSEN, S.E.: Strategies for reducing phobic behavior. Diss. Abstr. 26, 6850 (1966).
LAZARUS, A.A.: Crucial procedural factors in desensitization therapy. Behav. Res. Ther. 2, 65-70 (1964).
LEITENBERG, H., AGRAS, W.S., BARLOW, D.H., OLIVEAU, D.C.: Contribution of selective positive reinforcement and therapeutic instructions to systematic desensitization therapy. J. abnorm. soc. Psychol. 74, 113-118 (1969).
LOMONT, J.F., BROCKS, L.: Cognitive factors in desensitization. Behav. Res. Ther. 9, 187-195 (1971).
LOMONT, J.F., EDWARDS, J.E.: The role of relaxation in systematic desensitization. Behav. Res. Ther. 5, 11-25 (1967).
MARCIA, J.E., RUBIN, B.M., EFRAN, J.S.: Systematic desensitization: expectancy change or counterconditioning? J. abnorm. soc. Psychol. 74, 382-387 (1969).
MAXWELL, A.E.: Experimental Design in Psychology and the Medical Sciences. London: Methuen 1958.
McALLISTER, H., OLLEY, M.: Are phobics ill? Paper presented to the second European conference on Behaviour Modification, Wexford, Ireland.
McGLYNN, F.D.: Individual versus standardized hierarchies in the systematic desensitization of snake-avoidance. Behav. Res. Ther. 9, 1-5 (1971).
McGLYNN, F.D.: Systematic desensitization under two conditions of induced expectancy. Behav. Res. Ther. 10, 229-234 (1972).
McGLYNN, F.D., MAPP, R.H.: Systematic desensitization of snake-avoidance following three types of suggestion. Behav. Res. Ther. 8, 197-201 (1970).
McGLYNN, F.D., MEALIEA, W.L., NAWAS, M.M.: Systematic desensitization of snake-avoidance under two conditions of suggestion. Psychol. Rep. 25, 220-222 (1969).
McGLYNN, F.D., REYNOLDS, E.J., LINDER, L.H.: Experimental desensitization following therapeutically oriented and physically oriented instructions. J. Behav. Ther. Exp. Psychiat. 2, 13-18 (1971).
McGLYNN, F.D., WILLIAMS, C.W.: Systematic desensitization of snake-avoidance under three conditions of suggestion. J. Behav. Ther. Exp. Psychiat. 1, 97-101 (1970).
McGLYNN, F.D., WILSON, A.L., LINDER, L.H.: Systematic desensitization of snake-avoidance with individualized and non-individualized hierarchies. J. Behav. Ther. Exp. Psychiat. 1, 201-204 (1970).
MILLER, H.R., NAWAS, M.M.: Control of aversive stimulus termination in systematic desensitization. Behav. Res. Ther. 8, 57-61 (1970).
MILLER, S.B.: The contribution of therapeutic instructions to systematic desensitization. Behav. Res. Ther. 10, 159-169 (1972).

NAWAS, M.M: The effects of subject expectancy on the outcome of desensitization. In RUBIN, R.D., FENSTERHEIM, H., LAZARUS, A.A., FRANKS, C.M.: Advances in Behavior Therapy - 1970. New York: Academic Press 1972.

NAWAS, M.M., FISHMAN, S.T., PUCEL, J.C.: A standard desensitization program applied to group and individual treatments. Behav. Res. Ther. 8, 49-56 (1970a).

NAWAS, M.M., WELSH, W.V., FISHMAN, S.T.: The comparative effectiveness of pairing aversive imagery with relaxation, neutral tasks and muscular tension in reducing snake phobia. Behav. Res. Ther. 8, 63-68 (1970b).

OLIVEAU, D.C., AGRAS, W.S., LEITENBERG, H., MOORE, R.C., WRIGHT, D.E.: Systematic desensitization, therapeutically oriented instructions and selective positive reinforcement. Behav. Res. Ther. 7, 27-33 (1969).

O'NEILL, D.G., HOWELL, R.J.: Three modes of hierarchy presentation in systematic desensitization therapy. Behav. Res. Ther. 7, 289-294 (1969).

PAUL, G.L.: Two year follow-up of systematic desensitization therapy in groups. J. abnorm. soc. Psychol. 73, 119-130 (1968).

PAUL, G.L.: Outcome of systematic desensitization II: controlled investigations of individual treatment, technique variations, and current status. In: FRANKS, C.M. (Ed.): Behav. Therapy. Appraisal and Status. New York: McGraw Hill 1969.

PAUL, G.L., SHANNON, D.T.: Treatment of anxiety through systematic desensitization in groups. J. abnorm. soc. Psychol. 71, 124-135 (1966).

PHILLIPS, J.P.N.: The use of magic squares for balancing and assessing order effects in some analysis of variance designs. Applied Statistics 13, 67-73 (1964).

PHILLIPS, J.P.N.: A simple method of constructing certain magic rectangles of even order. Math. Gazette 52, 9-12 (1968a).

PHILLIPS, J.P.N.: Methods of constructing one-way and factorial designs balanced for trend. Applied Statistics 17, 162-170 (1968b).

PHILLIPS, J.P.N.: A simple method of obtaining a ratio scaling of a hierarchy. Proceedings of the Third B.E.A. Conference on Behavioural Modification 1971.

PROCTOR, S.: Duration of exposure to items and pretreatment training factors in systematic desensitization. In: RUBIN, R.D., FRANKS, C.M. (Eds.): Advances in Behavior Therapy - 1968. New York: Academic Press 1969.

RACHMAN, S.: Studies in desensitization - I: The separate effects of relaxation and desensitization. Behav. Res. Ther. 3, 245-251 (1965).

RACHMAN, S.: Studies in desensitization - III: Speed of generalization. Behav. Res. Ther. 4, 7-15 (1966).

RAMSAY, R.W., BARENDS, J., BREUKER, J., KRUSEMAN, A.: Massed vs. spaced desensitization of fear. Behav. Res. Ther. 4, 205-207 (1966).

RITTER, B.: The group treatment of children's snake phobias using vicarious and contact desensitization prodecures. Behav. Res. Ther. 6, 1-6 (1968).

SCHUBOT, D.E.: The influence of hypnotic and muscular relaxation in systematic desensitization of phobias. Diss. Abstr. 27, 3681-B - 3682-B (1966).

SHAPIRO, M.B.: The single case in fundamental clinical research. Brit. J. med. Psychol. 34, 255-262 (1961).

SHAPIRO, M.B.: A clinical approach to fundamental research with special reference to the study of the single patient. In: SAINSBURY, P., KREITMAN, N. (Eds.): Methods of Psychiatric Research. Oxford: Oxford University Press (1963).

SHAPIRO, M.B.: The measurement of clinically relevant variables. J. psychosom. Res. 8, 245-254 (1964a).

SHAPIRO, M.B.: The single case in psychological research: a reply. J. psychosom. Res. 8, 283-291 (1964b).
SHAPIRO, M.B.: The single case in clinical-psychological research. J. genet. Psychol. 74, 3-23 (1966).
SHAPIRO, M.B.: A clinically oriented strategy in individual-centred research. Brit. J. soc. clin. Psychol. 8, 290-291 (1969).
SHAPIRO, M.B.: Intensive assessment of the single-case. The inductive-deductive approach. In: MITTLER, P. (Ed.): Psychological Assessment. London: Methuen 1970.
SCHEFFÉ, H.: The Analysis of Variance. New York: Wiley (1959).
STEVENS, S.S.: On the psychophysical law. Psychol. Rev. 64, 153-181 (1957).
STEVENS, S.S.: The surprising simplicity of sensory metrics. Amer. Psychologist 17, 29-39 (1962).
SUE, D.: The role of relaxation in systematic desensitization. Behav. Res. Ther. 10, 153-158 (1972).
VALINS, S., RAY, A.A.: Effects of cognitive desensitization on avoidance behavior. J. Pers. soc. Psychol. 7, 345-350 (1967).
WAGNER, M.K., CAUTHEN, N.R.: A comparison of reciprocal inhibition and operant conditioning in the systematic desensitization of a fear of snakes. Behav. Res. Ther. 6, 225-227 (1968).
WATTS, F.: Desensitization as an habituation phenomenon: I. Stimulus intensity as determinant of the effects of stimulus lenghts. Behav. Res. Ther. 9, 209-217 (1971).
WINER, B.J.: Statistical Principles in Experimental Design. New York: McGraw Hill 1962.
WOLPE, J.: The systematic desensitization treatment of neuroses. J. nerv. ment. Dis. 132, 189-203 (1961).
WOLPE, J.: Quantitative relationships in the systematic desensitization of phobias. Amer. J. Psychiat. 119, 1062-1068 (1963).

Discriminant Function Analysis of the SOM+

J.T. QUINN, P.J. GRAHAM, J.J.M. HARBISON and H. McALLISTER

The Sexual Orientation Method (SOM) was introduced in 1966 by FELDMAN and his associates as a questionnaire measure intended to assess the relative levels of homo- and heteroerotic orientation of patients. It is based on a combination of the semantic differential technique of OSGOOD (1957) and the personal questionnaire technique of SHAPIRO (1961). As FELDMAN et al. say: "We have followed the basic approach of the former, but have changed the method of presentation so as to gain the advantage of detecting departures from internal consistency afforded by the latter, as well as basing our scoring system on Shapiro's."

The questionnaire will not be described in detail here. It originally consisted of 120 paired comparisons, 60 of which dealt with the concept "Men are sexually to me" and 60 with the concept "Women are sexually to me". In the scoring of the SOM, FELDMAN et al. list 8 consistent patterns of response and treat all the remaining possible response patterns as being inconsistent. Scores of 1 to 8 are assigned to each response pattern and thus scores varying from 6 (min.) to 48 (max.) are possible for each of the sexual orientations. PHILLIPS (1968), however, has suggested that the scoring system originally described by FELDMAN et al. is based on unjustified scaling assumptions and that this scoring system may treat as inconsistent patterns that are, in fact, consistent. He suggests modifications to the SOM, which remove a need for these assumptions but give the same number of consistent response patterns. This system has a further advantage of decreasing the number of judgments required of the subject from 120 to 84, although it loses some information on internal consistency. In an earlier paper (WOODWARD et al., 1973), we demonstrated the comparability of the two scoring systems with groups of normal and homosexual subjects.

The present paper is a discussion of the efficiency of SOM in discriminating between various known diagnostic groups in terms of their sexual orientation scores. The statistical technique used in this paper is discriminant analysis; this can be used when one has a set of measures or scores on individuals who are known to belong on the basis of other evidence to more than one group. The aim of this analysis is to establish whether, and to what extent, individuals can be allocated to the original groups on the basis of their scores on SOM. The first part investigates the efficiency of SOM in discriminating between groups of normals and homosexuals; in the second part a five-way discrimination is carried out between groups of normal subjects, homosexuals,

+ This research was carried out as part of an M.R.C.-supported project M.R.C. G970/340/C) under the general direction of Professor J.G. Gibson. Four of us (J.J.M.H., P.J.G., J.T.Q., H.McA.) constitute a research team. No seniority of authorship is implied by the order of names on this paper.

psychiatric controls, impotent males and the husbands of frigid women. The third part of the paper investigates whether this five-way discrimination can be made more efficient by adding personality measures (Cattell 16PF Scale). There is some suggestion in the literature (FELDMAN and MacCULLOCH, 1971) that the personality of homosexual patients may help in any discrimination process.

In the first part of the study two groups of male subjects participated. The first comprised 43 individuals referred to the Department of Mental Health with sexual orientation problems, the second, a group of 43 unselected non-psychiatric controls matched in terms of age and intelligence with the homosexual groups.

Each subject completed the SOM in its normal 120-item form, which was then computer-scored to produce both PHILLIPS and FELDMAN homosexual, heterosexual and inconsistency scores.

These two sets of scores were then used in two separate discriminant function analyses, using the Queen's University of Belfast's I.C.L. 1907 computer.

Table 1 contains the results of the discriminant analysis, which utilized all 4 variables derived from the SOM (heterosexual score, homosexual score, heterosexual inconsistencies and homosexual inconsistencies).

Each subject can then be allocated to his most appropriate group in terms of the 4 variables from the discriminant scores obtained. Table 1 indicates that both scoring systems of SOM produce remarkably accurate discrimination and are equally efficient with regard to the present group of subjects. Both discriminant analyses correctly classify 84 out of 86 subjects (a misclassification rate of under 3 %) from the two groups. One subject is misclassified from both the normal and the homosexual groups in each analysis, the same subjects being misclassified each time.

Five groups of male subjects were involved in the second study. The groups comprised: 25 unselected normal men (N); 25 homosexual patients who had been referred for treatment (A); 25 male psychiatric controls, who did not have a sexual problem as the main presenting complaint (C); 25 men who presented with potency problems (I); 25 husbands of women who were referred with problems of frigidity (S).

Each subject completed SOM in the 120-item form, and both FELDMAN and PHILLIPS scores were obtained for homosexual orientation, heterosexual orientation, homosexual inconsistencies and heterosexual inconsistencies. These scores were then employed in a five-way discriminant analysis.

Table 2 shows the 4 scores obtained from each of the 5 diagnostic groups. The means and standard deviations are in terms of the PHILLIPS scoring system. The results of the two discriminant analyses are shown in Table 3. It can be seen that there is little difference in the efficiency of either the PHILLIPS or the FELDMAN scoring system, and that both succeed very well in discriminating between homosexual subjects and all others. Table 3 indicates that over 80 % of the homosexual group were correctly classified as homosexual by both scoring systems, and that under 3 % of the remaining 100 subjects were classified as homosexual by either of the methods of scoring. It can be seen that the analysis does not succeed in discriminating particularly well between the 4 non-homosexual groups, and to try and increase the overall efficiency of the system, the next study looked at the advantages of adding a further number of variables in the discrimination process.

Table 1. 'Hits and Misses' table derived from discriminant analyses using two criterion groups and (a) FELDMAN's, (b) PHILLIP's scoring systems

a Predicted Group				b Predicted Group		
	Homosexual	Heterosexual			Homosexual	Heterosexual
Homosexual	42	1	Actual Group	Homosexual	42	1
Heterosexual	1	42		Heterosexual	1	42

Table 2. Means, standard deviations and inconsistency scores for the five groups on the SOM

	Heterosexual Scores		Homosexual Scores	
	M	SD	M	SD
F[a]	42.5	8.1	10.0	7.3
A	25.6	9.5	39.8	11.3
N	44.6	5.2	9.4	4.0
I	42.2	5.7	10.1	6.8
C	43.2	5.9	8.8	4.2
Inconsistency Scores: Means and Standard Deviations				
F[a]	1.4	1.8	2.0	1.6
A	1.6	1.9	1.2	1.6
N	0.8	1.0	1.3	1.3
I	1.1	2.1	2.2	1.9
C	1.5	1.9	2.5	1.7

[a] F (husbands of frigid women)
A (homosexual)
N (normal)
I (impotent)
C (psychiatric control)

The same 5 groups also completed the Cattel 16PF, which measures 16 personality traits. Table 4 presents the results of a discriminant analysis, and this time we find that the 16PF is less successful than SOM in discriminating between the homosexual and the other four diagnostic groups. Sixteen out of 25 homosexuals are correctly classified, while 11 out of the 99 non-homosexual subjects are classified as homosexual. The table also shows, in contrast, that the 16PF is more successful than SOM in correctly classifying subjects within the non-homosexual groups (57 out of 99 correct). One subject out of the impotent group had not completed the 16PF.

The final stage of this set of analyses is to combine both tests in a further discriminant analysis. Table 5 shows the results of this analysis. With the combined measures there is a further slight improvement, with 23 of the homosexual group correctly allocated, and only 2 of the remaining 99 subjects misclassified as homosexuals. The combined measures are also the most successful in correctly classifying the non-homosexual groups, with 69 of the 99 subjects being correctly allocated to their respective groups.

Table 3. Discriminant analysis of SOM scores from five groups of males

	Actual Group					
		F[a]	A	N	I	C
Forecast Group (PHILLIPS)	F[a]	3	3	3	2	4
	A	1	21	0	1	0
	N	11	1	17	9	11
	I	0	0	2	3	0
	C	10	0	3	10	10
Forecast Group (FELDMAN)	F[a]	1	2	2	0	1
	A	1	22	0	2	0
	N	10	1	18	9	10
	I	1	0	3	5	3
	C	12	0	2	9	11

[a] F (husbands of frigid women)
A (homosexuals)
N (normal)
I (impotent)
C (psychiatric controls)

Table 4. Discriminant analysis of 16PF scores from five groups of males

	'Hits and Misses' Table					
	Actual Group					
		F[a]	A	N	I	C
Forecast Group	F[a]	16	1	4	1	4
	A	2	16	3	3	3
	N	3	2	13	2	4
	I	1	0	1	14	0
	C	3	6	4	4	14

[a] F (husbands of frigid women)
A (homosexual patients)
N (normal)
I (impotent)
C (psychiatric controls)

Table 5. Discriminant analysis of SOM and 16PF scores from five groups of males

	'Hits and Misses' Table					
	Actual Group					
		F[a]	A	N	I	C
Forecast Group	F[a]	17	0	2	2	3
	A	1	23	0	1	0
	N	2	1	19	2	5
	I	1	0	3	16	0
	C	4	1	1	3	17

[a] F (husbands of frigid women)
A (homosexual patients)
N (normal)
I (impotent)
C (psychiatric controls)

Discussion

The present paper confirms our earlier work, which indicated that the shorter PHILLIPS SOM is as efficient as the original 120-item scale in discriminating between various diagnostic groups of subjects, and it would appear that future work should concentrate on the shorter scale. Recently SAMBROOKS and MacCULLOCH (1972) reached a similar conclusion.

Obviously further work is needed to cross-validate the results of the present discrimination analyses. New subjects are needed within each of the various known diagnostic groups; these subjects could then be given eigenvalues derived from the present analysis, and allocated to their respective predicted groups in terms of these eigenvalues. It would then be possible to cross-validate the efficiency of the discrimination in terms of these new subjects.

The results of the five-way discrimination confirm the usefulness of SOM and its remarkable efficiency in discriminating between homosexual subjects and other diagnostic groups. It is interesting that the impotent group of patients was clearly distinct from the homosexual group, as there have been suggestions that latent homosexuality is one aspect of impotence. The addition of personality factors to the discrimination yields some interesting information. It can be seen that the overall discrimination between the homosexual and other groups is not improved, but that within the other 4 diagnostic categories the personality variables greatly improve the efficiency of the statistical technique. Obviously much more could be done within this area, and we are currently adding more variables to the various groups to see how far we can improve the effectiveness of the present system.

Finally, our work indicates the power of a combination of modern methods of psychological assessment and complex statistical techniques in helping the diagnostic process. We indicated earlier (HARBISON et al., 1973) how we feel that psychometrics can be used within behaviour modification; the present paper is an extension of this approach.

References

FELDMAN, M.P., MacCULLOCH, M.J.: Homosexual Behaviour, Therapy and Assessment. Oxford: Pergamon Press 1971.

FELDMAN, M.P., MacCULLOCH, M.J., MELLOR, VALERIE, PINSCHOF, J.M.: The application of anticipatory avoidance learning to the treatment of homosexuality: 3 The sexual orientation method. Behav. Res. Ther. 4, 289-299 (1966).

HARBISON, J.J.M., McALLISTER, H., QUINN, J.T., GRAHAM, P. JOAN: Psychological assessment of sexual dysfunction. In: BRENGLEMANN, J., TUNNER, W. (Eds.): Behavioural Therapy. München:

OSGOOD, C.E., SUCCI, G.J., TANNENBAUM, P.: The Measurement of Meaning. Illinois: University of Illinois Press 1957.

PHILLIPS, J.P.N.: A rate on the scoring of the sexual orientation method. Behav. Res. Ther. 6, 121-123 (1968).

SAMBROOKS, JEAN, MacCULLOCH, M.J.: A modification of the sexual orientation method. Brit. J. soc. clin. Psychol. (in press).

SHAPIRO, M.B.: Manual of the Personal Questionnaire. London: Institute of Psychiatry 1961.

WOODWARD, R., McALLISTER, H., QUINN, J.T., GRAHAM, P. JOAN, HARBISON, J.J.M.: A comparison of two scoring systems for the S.O.M. Brit. J. soc. clin. Psychol. (in press).

[illegible]

[illegible]

[illegible] ...sociation of ... [illegible]

[illegible]

[illegible]

[illegible]

VIII. Methodological Problems in Behaviour Modification

Behaviour is Behaviour is Behaviour

D.F. PECK

I. Introduction

Behaviour modification has a short but factious history and, as with any innovation that challenges established ideas, it has encountered its quota of scepticism. Three important questions have emerged. Firstly, from a theoretical viewpoint: "Can behaviour modification work?" This question arose on the part of those who regarded problematic behaviour as the public manifestation of internal conflicts and pathologies, and who thought that "symptom substitution" would inevitably occur if only the "symptom"was removed. This and related problems have been adequately answered elsewhere (e.g. BANDURA, 1969), and it is safe to conclude: "Yes, behaviour modification can work."

The second question is: "Does behaviour modification work?" It is unfortunate but true that there have, to date, been too few well-controlled studies to enable us to answer this question definitively; nevertheless it is possible to state a tentative: "Yes, behaviour modification does work."

This paper is concerned with the third question, i.e. "What are the limits of the behaviour modification approach?" In other words: "What kinds of behaviour are amenable to an environmental approach and what kinds are not?"

Early work in the general area of behaviour therapy (at least in the UK) was virtually restricted to "neurotic" and "charactor" disorders, which was reflected in the textbooks of the period (e.g. EYSENCK and RACHMAN, 1965). Little or nothing was done in other areas. More recently, WHITE (1972) has stated "Those suffering from structural defects and others from physiological disorders are generally beyond the immediate scope of anything but medicine. Even people suffering from milder disorders than brain lesions or psychosis, such as generalised anxiety, are beyond purely psychological." By summarizing work that has been done on "testing the limits" of the behavioural model, we intend to show that this pessimism and narrow outlook is unwarranted and represents a premature restriction of the ambit of behaviour modification.

II. Brain Damage

LINDSLEY (1964) pointed out the fallacies in the doctrine of "Similia similibus curantur" or "like cures like", that is, if disordered behaviour is consequent upon a particular pathological process, the most efficacious approach to the amelioration of the problem would be by methods directly related to the pathological agent. On the contrary, he argues that although a deficit may have its roots in, for example, a neurological disorder, this does not at all imply that the best or the only way to alleviate the deficit is by neurological methods. No one would doubt that brain damage has marked effects on behaviour; however, to say that the behaviour we observe after brain injury is a direct consequence of, or is caused by brain injury is, according to LINDSLEY, a very naive way of conceptualizing brain - behaviour relationships. There are now a large number of studies which indicate that a behaviour modification approach to brain-damaged individuals can be very fruitful. Despite this, numerous reports appear in the literature in which brain-damaged individuals are specifically excluded from the study, with little or no justification being given.

CONNOLLY (1968) has applied operant techniques to the shaping of motor skills in cerebral palsied (or spastic) children. He described a device which consisted of a clown's face with a very large nose; the nose acted as a target which could be increased or decreased in size. Initially the children are required to hit the large target with a hand within a given time limit after the onset of a light. Success (i.e. hitting the target) is reinforced by flickering a light in the clown's eye, and playing a pre-recorded message such as "do that again, Johnnie", or laughter.

Once the basic response is established, the size of the target is gradually reduced by small amounts until the child can reliably hit a small target; the time limit is simultaneously reduced. Cerebral palsied children can be trained to develop a remarkable degree of control over their arm movements, even though their motor difficulties have a definite neurological basis. Furthermore, the beneficial effects of this training apparently generalize a broad range of motor tasks, and tend to be stable. (CONNOLLY, 1970, p. 356). KOLDERIE (1971) has outlined how behaviour modification techniques can be applied to a wide variety of problems associated with cerebral palsy, and RICE et al. (1968) give details of the application of behavioural modification techniques to a severly spastic retarded child.

Behavioural techniques have also been successfully applied to aphasic patients. TAYLOR and SANDS (1966) reported considerable improvement in 21 out of 25 of a group of severly impaired aphasic patients, using programmed instruction. All of the patients derived some benefit from the programme, even if it was only how to write their own name. None of the patients had shown any improvement with traditional forms of therapy. Similar work has been reported by GOODKIN (1969) and GRAY and FYGETAKIS (1968), amongst others.

Hyperactivity is generally considered, at least in certain cases, to be due to brain damage (e.g. BARKER, 1971). Nevertheless, several reports have indicated that hyperactive behaviour can be environmentally controlled, despite its putative organic basis. (PATTERSON, 1965; PIHL, 1967). PIHL and SHORE(1971) investigated this question experimentally; previous reports had indicated that increased motor activity in experimental animals often resulted after bilateral lesions in the septal area, and PIHL and SHORE set out to examine the "relationship between neurologically altered activity levels and the effect of contingencies for movement and non-movement". Eight hooded rats were subjected to bilateral lesions in the septal area, and their activity level was then monitored under 4 conditions: (1) postoperative free movement, (2) aversive sound contingent upon movement, (3) aversive sound contingent on non-movement, (4) a second period of aversive sound contingent on movement. They found that the septal lesions doubled the pre-operative or baseline activity scores (as expected), that aversive sound for movement reduced activity to below the pre-operative level, and that aversive sound for non-movement greatly increased the amount of activity. Their conclusions were as follows: "There is an interactive effect between neurological functioning and environmental contingencies on activity level. In terms of theories of septal functioning, whether one assumes that the effect of lesioning is to produce an over-reactivity to stimuli or that an inhibitory control center has been removed, the resultant activity changes remain susceptible to environmental manipulation," and that "It could well be that, like the effect of neurological damage in this study, environmental contingencies can abet and limit neurologically generated hyperactivity in individuals showing the hyperactive child syndrome."

It would appear therefore that the presence of brain pathology should in no way preclude a direct behaviour modification approach to the consequent problem behaviour, a conclusion reinforced in a study by HALBERSTAM and ZARETSKY (1969), who maintained that "both the aged and the brain-damaged patients appear to have learning potential that does not differ from that of younger rehabilitation patients, although special conditions may be needed in order to make maximal use of this potential." However, a study by SALZINGER et al. (1970) has shown that these "special conditions" need not be very complex. They trained the parents of brain-injured children in behaviour modification techniques and reported that "All parents who carried out the modification programmes reported success in changing their children's behaviour." Other neurological problems that seem to be amenable to an environmental approach are epilepsy (e.g. FORSTER, 1966) and Huntington's chorea (MacPHERSON, 1967).

It has been unequivocally established that neuronal regeneration does not occur to any significant degree in the vertebrate brain and spinal chord. However, neurophysiologists have recently found evidence, not for regeneration itself but for reorganization or the formation of new neuronal connections after lesions (RAISMAN, 1969; WALL and EGGER, 1971). This "neuronal plasticity" supports the possibility, at the neurophysiological level, that relearning may occur even after severe lesions. It has been suggested by OAKLEY (1971) that it is possible to operantly train rabbits whose cortex has been completely removed. Thus, a number of studies on both humans and lower animals indicate complex relearning can take place even after gross cortical lesions.

III. Physical Rehabilitation

Behaviour modification is not, of course, restricted to the types of problem behaviour that could bring one to a psychiatric clinic. Indeed, there are now a number of studies showing that these techniques can have a considerable part to play in general medical problems, problems that again would not seem at first sight to be amenable to the operant approach. WRIGHT et al. (1969) describe the application of operant techniques to long-standing difficulties in decannulation after tracheostomy in 2 infants; using a social reinforcement technique they were able to reinstate normal breathing within 3 weeks, despite numerous unsuccessful previous attempts by a variety of methods. They were particularly impressed by these successes, since they claim that cannula "addition" appears to be an 'involuntary or autonomically' mediated response." TROTTER and INMAN (1968) conducted a controlled study into the efficacy of positive reinforcement in the treatment of 12 quadriplegic and 12 paraplegic patients, and found that "the use of a planned programme of positive reinforcement appeared to promote greater increases in upper-extremity muscular strength than did the usual physical therapy program." Similarly, TROMBLY (1966) applied operant techniques to the orthotic training of quadriplegic patients.

IV. Severe Subnormality

The diagnosis of severe subnormality used to, and occasionally still does engender an air of therapeutic defeatism. LINDSLEY (1964) argued, however, that the current performance of severely retarded patients, in particular that of children, can give little or no guide to learning potential. He argues that a special prosthetic environment is required, and abnormal children reared in average environments have therefore had little or no opportunity to acquire complex behavioural repertoires; to quote "Retardation is not the property of the child but of an inadequate child environment relationship. It is our ability to design suitable environments for exceptional children, that is retarded. Classrooms should be tailored to children - not children adjusted to classrooms. Retarded behaviour is penalised and sub-skills ignored in environments designed for agerage children. In prosthetic environments tailored to their skills, exceptional children will behave adjustively, efficiently, and with full human dignity."

There is now an enormous amount of empirical evidence to support this view. BERKOWITZ et al. (1971), for example, trained 14 boys, whose ages ranged from 9 to 17, and whose Vineland Social Ages ranged from 1.3 to 1.7 years, to feed themselves: they concluded that regardless of IQ level, any child physically capable of holding a spoon and raising it from plate to mouth is also capable of learning to feed himself. Similarly, LOYND and BARCLAY (1970) trained an 8-year-old microcephalic girl to walk; her IQ was estimated to be below 25. THOMPSON et al. (1970) trained an entire ward of 67 patients, whose mean IQ was 23 (or was unmeasurable by any standard test) in self-care, self-feeding, speech, toileting and reduction in assaultive behaviour, with considerable success. Finally TATE and BAROFF (1967) indicate that subnormal children are capable of being trained to produce highly complex electrical products.

It would appear therefore that the IQ concept has no important part to play in behaviour modifcation. Irrespective of intellectual level as measured by standard psychometric tests, severly subnormal children and adults can be trained to perform a variety of complex behaviours. Why are IQ tests inappropriate? THRONE (1970) maintained that "radical behaviourists ordinarily forego the use of transmuted standardised intelligence test scores, constituting as they do extrapolations twice removed from in situ behavioural events. They are second-order theoretical values derived from first-order theoretical values (raw performance scores on tests), they do not reflect actual performance even under average circumstances. To use such scores as hypothetical treatment indices requires a dangerous and unnecessary interpretative exercise totally at variance with basic radical behaviourist strategy. Why risk interpretative error with hypothetical indices when actual indices may be obtained in the course of treatment? Moreover standardized intelligence test scores are uninterpretable unless obtained under the average circumstances prevailing for the standardisation sample prior to and during testing." In other words, we are using incompletely reliable techniques to measure indirectly and partially erroneously a hypothetical abstraction, based upon the scores of children obtained in normal circumstances. However, it is obvious that subnormal children do not and never have operated in normal circumstances, so the test is being applied to a different population from that on which it was standardized. Clearly, to use IQ scores as predictive indices of how to deal with problem behaviour associated with severe subnormality is fraught with danger. Why risk an interpretative error using hypothetical indices of behaviour, when we can study the actual behaviour in the first place? If we really wish to make a direct contribution to the welfare of severely subnormal patients, should we not sell our Binets and WAIS's, and spend the proceeds on event recorders and "Smarties".

V. Schizophrenia

Schizophrenia is generally regarded as a serious form of mental illness, in which genetic and biochemical factors are considered to be very important; however, the evidence for this, particularly biochemical factors, is by no means unequivocal (WYATT et al., 1971). Nevertheless there are now many studies which indicate that behaviour labelled as psychotic or schizophrenic is subject to environmental manipulation. This work has been extensively discussed elsewhere (e.g. ULLMANN and KRASNER, 1969), and it would be unnecessary duplication to repeat it here. It is perhaps worthwhile to point out that the three main "symtoms" of schizophrenia have all been shown several times to be at least partially under the control of their consequences. BUCHER and FABRICATORE (1970) report a case in which a schizophrenic patient was provided with a portable shock device, and instructed to shock himself at the onset on the "voices". Reported hallucinations were completely eliminated while the patient was in hospital, but reappeared some time after his discharge. SLADE (1972) found a marked relationship between self-rated tension and the experience of auditory hallucinations in an acute schizophrenic; a programme of systematic desensitization led to a marked reduction in the frequency of hallucinations. Similar work has been reported by RUTNER and BUGLE (1969) and ALUMBAUGH (1971). However, WEINGAERTNER (1971) has cast doubt upon the learning mechanisms responsible for the changes reported in these studies. It should be noted also that on the whole these studies were on single patients and any conclusions drawn should be regarded as being very tentative.

More adequately controlled studies have been conducted on the modification of delusional speech. WINCZE et al. (1970) used a token reinforcement technique to reduce the frequency of delusional speech in 10 paranoid schizophrenics using a classical counterbalanced ABA design, and AYLLON and HAUGHTON (1964) and KENNEDY (1964) employed an extinction procedure that substantially reduced the proportion of delusional speech.

Thought disorder has also proved to be modifiable by operant techniques. GORHAM et al. (1970) found marked improvement in "disorganised thinking" and "unusual thought content" after the introduction of a token economy scheme. MEICHENBAUM (1969), in a large-scale controlled study, demonstrated that token reinforcement is effective in increasing the level of abstraction to proverbs, and decreasing the amount of "sick talk"; evidence for response and stimulus generalization was also obtained. Similar results have been reported by WAGNER (1968).

As with schizophrenia, depression is considered to have a biochemical origin. Again, however, there is much evidence to show that depressive behaviour can be modified by an operant approach; this has recently been briefly reviewed by SEITZ (1971), who refers to 8 different behavioural approaches to depression.

To summarize to this point, there is now much evidence from studies of clinical problems to indicate that, irrespective of any putative aetiological factor, many types of problem behaviour remain amenable to an environmental, particularly an operant, approach. This conclusion is further supported by a number of recent non-clinical studies, now to be discussed, whose implications seem to lead us in the same direction.

VI. Autonomic Learning

From a theoretical and practical viewpoint, one of the most interesting and important developments in psychology during the 1960's was the demonstration that autonomic functions can be brought under operant control. Previously it had been categorically stated that functions such as blood pressure, skin potential, intestinal contraction etc. were involuntary and that unelicited autonomic responses were not therefore amenable to modification by reinforcement (e.g. KIMBLE, 1961). Despite some methodological shortcomings in the early work (KATKIN and MURRAY, 1968), it is now firmly established that autonomic learning can take place in both humans and in the lower animals, and that such factors as skeletal operants (TROWILL, 1967), other autonomic functions (ENGEL and CHISM, 1967) and "cognitive" factors (CRIDER et al., 1969) cannot be regarded as mediators of the change in automonic functions during operant training. A recent review by DI CARA (1970) stated that "we have produced, through instrumental training, increases and decreases in heart rate, blood pressure, intestinal contractions, control of blood-vessel diameter, and rate of formation of urine;" further, this list is by no means exhaustive. If, then, autonomic functions can be, as seems to be the case, modified by operant techniques, it would follow that the same techniques could be used in the treatment of some cardiovascular disorders: BENSON et al. (1971) used operant techniques to lower systolic blood pressure in 7 patients with essential hypertension, and achieved significant decreases in 5 of them; however, no attempt was made to follow up the patients outside the laboratory situation. Similarly, WEISS and ENGEL (1971) used operant techniques to control the inotropic action of patients with premature ventricular contractions. There is now some evidence to show that the beneficial changes obtained in the laboratory do generalize to other situations and are persistent (ENGEL, 1972).

Equally important is the related work on the operant control of cortical activity. DEWAN (1966) demonstrated that subjects could achieve sufficient control over their electroencephalographic traces to activate a typewriter, and a series of papers by FETZ and his co-workers (e.g. FETZ, 1969; FETZ and FINOCCHIO, 1971) have shown that the rate of firing of single neurones can be increased by the differential reinforcement of high rates of neuronal discharge. Furthermore, there is evidence that evoked potentials can be brought under operant control in both cats (FOX and RUDDELL, 1968) and humans (ROSENFELD et al., 1969).

VII. Personality

Discussing the problem of whether human behaviour is determined by broad dispositional personality traits or is specific to the situation in which it occurs, EYSENCK (1953) stated "the problem ceases to be a theoretical one, and becomes instead quantitative and empirical".

MISCHEL (1969) examined the relevant empirical evidence and concluded: "The initial assumptions of trait-state theory were logical, inherently plausible, and also consistent with common sense and intuitive impressions about personality. Their real limitation turned out to be empirical - they simply have not been supported adequately, and highly generalised behavioural consistencies have not been demonstrated and the concept of personality as broad response dispositions is thus untenable." A review of socio-behavioural studies led him to further conclude that behaviour is situationally determined, and not the result of enduring predispositions; that is, it is under stimulus control, and not internal control. Similar conclusions have been drawn by reviewers of allied fields; WICKER (1969), after an extensive review of the literature, suggested that it might be best to "abandon the attitude concept in favour of directly studying overt behaviour." BERSOFF (1971), with special reference to intelligence, also argues against the "assumption of trans-situational consistency of behaviour," and makes a plea for "psychosituational assessment," or the direct assessment of behaviour "as it is elicited through interaction with specific stimulus situations." These comments clearly have marked implications for clinical psychologists; it is a futile activity to use assessment procedures to discover patterns of behaviour that are consistent in a wide variety of different stimulus situations, when there is insufficient evidence (despite an enormous amount of research) to demonstrate their existence. The observation of actual behaviour in specific stimulus situations (i.e. behavioural assessment) appears to lead to much greater accuracy in predicting, and makes fewer assumptions (GOLDFRIED and KENT, 1972). It is therefore of greater utility for behaviour modifiers in practical, clinical situations.

VIII. Summary and Conclusions

It is hoped that the impression has not been given that contingency management is omnipotent; clearly, behaviour modification is not a cure-all. Failures are common, and in many areas the results of behaviour modification approaches, despite very intensive and long-term work, remain disappointing; for example, RITVO et al. (1971) have reported on the somewhat limited results with autistic children after a 5-year follow-up, and LICHTENSTEIN (1971) points to the repeated failures of a behaviour modification approach to smoking. The intention of this paper is not to restate the Watsonian excessive claims of the omnipotency of the behavioural approach, but simply to make a plea that the therapeutic possibilities of a behavioural approach should not be discounted, but should at least be examined over a broad range of problems.

This review has marshalled evidence from a large number of studies in widely disparate fields; the common theme throughout is the suggestion that a behavioural approach is feasible in many more areas than had previously been thought. It does not appear to matter whether abnormal patterns of behaviour are associated with brain damage, physical disability, severe retardation, psychoticism or biochemical abnormalities; nor whether behaviour is alleged to the result of personality predispositions, attitudes or measured intelligence; nor whether the behaviour involves skeletal movements of the whole organism, responses of the autonomic nervous system, or even of a single neurone. If behaviour is emitted, it is at least potentially amenable to environmental manipulation. In short, behaviour is behaviour is behaviour.

The implications for the practice of clinical psychology are clear: What an organism <u>has</u> does not appear to be as relevant a consideration as to what an organism does, and behaviour modifiers should focus their attention accordingly. We need to reconsider the value of the concepts of personality, intelligence, brain damage etc. The use of these concepts tends to put constraints on our approach to problem behaviour by generating an unwarranted feeling of hopelessness and futility in therapeutic endeavour. Instead of attempting to assess the behavioural predispositions that obtain across many stimulus situations, we should be looking at behaviour as it actually occurs in specific situations, and devising modification schemes from this viewpoint. Furthermore, assessment must be related to treatment or it is a waste of time. Our ability to tackle problem behaviour of various sorts, and to help people to achieve a dignified, independent and fully human existence, will be a function of how quickly clinical psychology can rid itself of the notion of the primacy and immutability of the internal control of behaviour.

References

ALUMBAUGH, R.V.: Use of behaviour modification techniques towards the reduction of hallucinatory behavior: a case study. Psychol. Rec. 21, 415-417 (1971).

AYLLON, T., HAUGHTON, E.: Modification of symptomatic verbal behavior of mental patients. Behav. Res. Ther. 2, 87-97 (1964).

BANDURA, A.: Principles of Behaviour Modification. London: Holt Rinehart & Winston 1969.

BARKER, P.: Basic Child Psychiatry. London: Staples Press 1971.

BENSON, H., SHAPIRO, D., TURSKY, B., SCHWARTZ, G.E.: Decreased systolic blood pressure through operant conditioning techniques in patients with essential hypertension. Science 173, 740-742 (1971).

BERKOWITZ, S., SHERRY, P.J., DAVIS, B.A.: Teaching self-feeding skills to profound retardates using reinforcement and fading procedures. Behav. Ther. 2, 62-67 (1971).

BERSOFF, D.: "Current functioning" myth: an overlooked fallacy in psychological assessment. J. consult. clin. Psychology 37, 391-393 (1971).

BUCHER, B., FABRICATORE, J.: Use of patient-administered shock to suppress hallucinations. Behav. Ther. 1, 382-385 (1970).

CONNOLLY, K.: Applications of operant conditioning to the measurement and development of motor skill in children. Develop. Med. Child Neurol. 10, 6, 697-705 (1968).

CONNOLLY, K.: Mechanisms of Motor Skill Development. London: Academic Press 1970.

CRIDER, A., SCHWARTZ, G.E., SHNIDMAN, S.: On the criteria for instrumental autonomic conditioning: a reply to Katkin and Murray. Psychol. Bull. 71, 455-461 (1969).

DEWAN, E.M.: Communication by voluntary control of the electroencephalogram. Proceedings of the Symposium of Biomedical Engineering 1, 349-351 (1966).

DI CARA, L.V.: Learning in the autonomic nervous system. Scientific American 222, 1, 30-39 (1970).

ENGEL, B.T.: Operant conditioning of cardiac function: a status report. Psychophysiology 9, 161-177 (1972).

ENGEL, B.T., CHISM, R.A.: Cardiovascular effects of respiration. Psychophysiology 4, 83-89 (1967).

EYSENCK, H.J.: The Structure of Human Personality. London: Methuen 1953.

EYSENCK, H.J., RACHMAN, S.: The Causes & Cures of Neurosis. London: Routledge & Kegan Paul 1965.

FETZ, E.E.: Operant conditioning of cortical unit activity. Science 163, 955-958 (1969).

FETZ, E.E., FINOCCHIO, D.V.: Operant conditioning of specific patterns of neural and muscular activity. Science 174, 431-435 (1971).

FORSTER, F.M.: Conditioning in sensory evoked seizures. Condit. Reflex 1, 224-234 (1966).
FOX, S.S., RUDELL, A.P.: Operant controlled neural event: formal and systematic approach to electrical coding of behavior in brain. Science 162, 1299-1302 (1968).
GOLDFRIED, M.R., KENT, R.N.: Traditional versus behavioral personality assessment: a comparison of methodological and theoretical assumptions. Psychol. Bull. 77, 6, 409-420 (1972).
GOODKIN, R.: Changes in work production, sentence production and relevance in an aphasic through verbal conditioning. Behav. Res. Ther. 7, 93-99 (1969).
GORHAM, D.R., GREEN, L.W., CALDWELL, L.R., BARTLETT, E.R.: Effect of operant conditioning techniques on chronic schizophrenics. Psychol. Rep. 27, 223-234 (1970).
GRAY, B.B., FYGETAKIS, L.: Mediated language acquisition for dysphasic children. Behav. Res. Ther. 6, 263-280 (1968).
HALBERSTAM, J.L., ZARETSKY, H.H.: Learning capacities of the elderly and brain-damaged. Arch. phys. Med. 50, 133-139 (1969).
KASSORIA, I.C.: A new approach to mental illness. Science Journal 5, 68-74 (1969).
KATKIN, E.S., MURRAY, E.N.: Instrumental conditioning of autonomically mediated behavior. Theoretical and methodological issues. Psychol. Bull. 70, 52-68 (1968).
KENNEDY, T.: Treatment of chronic schizophrenia by behavior therapy: case reports. Behav. Res. Ther. 2, 1-6 (1964).
KIMBLE, G.A.: Hilgard & Marquis' Conditioning and Learning. New York: Appleton-Century-Crofts 1961.
KOLDERIE, M.L.: Behavior modification in the treatment of children with cerebral palsy. Phys. Ther. 51, 10, 1083-1091 (1971).
LICHTENSTEIN, E.: Modification of smoking behavior: Good designs - ineffective treatments. J. cons. clin. Psychol. 36, 163-166 (1971).
LINDSLEY, O.R.: Direct measurement and prosthetics of retarded behavior. Journal of Education, 147, 1, 62-81 (1964).
LOYND, B., BARCLAY, A.: A case study in developing ambulation in a profoundly retarded child. Behav. Ther. 8, 207 (1970).
MacPHERSON, E.L.R.: Control of involuntary movement. Behav. Res. Ther. 5, 143-145 (1967).
MEICHENBAUM, D.H.: The effects of instructions and reinforcement on thinking and language behavior of schizophrenics. Behav. Res. Ther. 7, 101-114 (1969).
MISCHEL, W.: Personality and Assessment. New York: Wiley & Sons 1960.
OAKLEY, D.A.: Instrumental learning in neodecorticate rabbits. Nature 233, 185-186 (1971).
PATTERSON, G.R.: An application of conditioning techniques to the control of a hyperactive child. In: ULLMANN, L.P., KRASNER, L. (Eds.): Case Studies in Behavior Modification. New York: Holt, Rinehart & Winston 1965.
PIHL, R.O: Conditioning procedures with a hyperactive child. Neurology (Minneap.) 17, 421-423 (1967).
PIHL, R.O., SHORE, H.: The aversive control of lesion-altered locomotor activity in the rat. Psychol. Rec. 21, 507-512 (1971).
RAISMAN, G.: Neuronal plasticity in the septal nuclei of the adult rat. Brain Res. 14, 25-48 (1969).
RICE, H.K., McDANIEL, M.W., DENNEY, S.L.: Operant conditioning techniques for use in the physical rehabilitation of the multiply handicapped retarded patient. Phys. Ther. 48, 4, 342-346 (1968).
RITVO, E.R., LEVITT, M., LEVITT, B., WINGARD, J.: Operant conditioning therapy of autism: a 5 year clinical follow-up study. Journal of Autism and Childhood Schizophrenia 1, 3 (1971).
ROSENFELD, J.P., RUDELL, A.P., FOX, S.S.: Operant control of neural events in humans. Science 165, 821-823 (1969).
RUTNER, I.T., BUGLE, C.: An experimental procedure for the modification of psychotic behavior. J. consult. clin. Psychol. 33, 651-653 (1969).

SALZINGER, K., FELDMAN, R.S., PORTNOY, S.: Training parents of brain-injured children in the use of operant conditioning techniques. Behav. Ther. 1, 4-32 (1970).
SEITZ, F.C.: Behavior modification techniques for treating depression. Psychotherapy: Theory, Research and Practice 8, 181-183 (1971).
SLADE, P.D.: The effects of systematic desensitization on auditory hallucinations. Behav. Res. Ther. 10, 85-91 (1972).
TATE, B., BAROFF, G.: Training the mentally retarded in the production of a complex product: a demonstration of work potential. Expectional Children 3, 405-408 (1967).
TAYLOR, M.L., SANDS, E.: Application of programmed instruction to the language training of severely impaired aphasic subjects. National Society for Programmed Instruction Journal 5, 5, 10-11 (1966).
THOMPSON, T., GRABOWSKI, E., ERRICKSON, E., JOHNSON, R.: Operant conditioning program for chronically institutionalised profoundly retarded adult males. Proceedings, 78th Annual Convention of the American Psychological Association, 783-784.
THRONE, J.M.: A radical behaviorist approach to diagnosis in mental retardation. Mental Retardation Abstracts 8, 2-5 (1970).
TROMBLY, C.A.: Principles of operant conditioning: related to orthotic training of quadriplegic patients. Amer. J. occup. Ther. 20, 5, 217-220 (1966).
TROTTER, A.B., IMMAN, D.A.: The use of positive reinforcement in physical therapy. Phys. Ther. 48, 4, 347-352 (1968).
TROWILL, J.A.: Instrumental conditioning of the heart rate in the curarised rat. J. comp. physiol. Psychol. 63, 7-11 (1967).
ULLMANN, L.P., KRASNER, L.: A psychological Approach to Abnormal Behavior. New Jersey: Prentice-Hall 1969.
WAGNER, B.W.: The training of attending and abstracting responses in chronic schizophrenics. J. exp. Res. Person. 3, 77-88 (1968).
WALL, P.D., EGGER, M.D.: Formation of new connexions in adult rat brains after partial deafferentation. Nature 232, 542-545 (1971).
WEINGAERTNER, A.H.: Self-administered aversive stimulation with hallucinating hospitalised schizophrenics. J. consult. clin. Psychol. 36, 422-429 (1971).
WEISS, T., ENGEL, B.T.: Operant conditioning of heart rate in patients with premature ventricular contractions. Psychosom. Med. 33, 301-321 (1971).
WHITE, J. GRAHAM: What is wrong with clinical psychology? Bull. Brit. Psychol. Soc. 25, 101-106 (1972).
WICKER, A.W.: Attitude versus actions: the relationship of verbal and overt behavioral responses to attitude objects. J. soc. Issues 25, 41-78 (1969).
WINCZE, J.P., LEITENBERG, H., AGRAS, W.S.: A sequential analysis of the effects of token reinforcement and instructions on the delusional behavior of chronic paranoid schizophrenics. Proceedings of the Annual Convention of the American Psychological Association, 5 (part 2), 737-738 (1970).
WRIGHT, L., NUNNERY, A., EICHEL, B., SCOTT, R.: Behavioral tactics for reinstating natural breathing in infants with tracheostomy. Pediat. Res. 3, 275-278 (1969).
WYATT, J., TERMINI, B.A., DAVIS, J.: Biochemical and sleep studies of schizophrenia: a review of the literature - 1960-70. Part 1: Biochemical studies. Schizophrenia Bulletin. No. 4, 10-44 (1971).

Therapist Variables in the Desensitization of Clinically Phobic Patients

P.D. EVANS and A.M.P. KELLAM

Research into desensitization usually draws a distinction between what are termed specific factors and what are termed nonspecific factors. Specific factors are those which form part of the definition of the procedure: graded presentation of stimuli, relaxation, active visualization, and so on. Nonspecific factors make up the somewhat ill-defined class of elements where the common property of each is simply its exclusion from the class of specific factors. Of all nonspecific factors, those involving relationship with a therapist have been thought to be the most important of those in need of investigation. The argument that desensitization success derives from the therapist - patient relationship has, however, been steadily and systematically eroded. Early controlled studies, albeit with nonclinical volunteer phobics, have shown that factors accruing from continuous relationship with a therapist are not <u>sufficient</u> conditions of success in desensitization. LANG and LAZOVIK (1963), LANG et al. (1965) and PAUL (1966) all utilized some variety of placebo control. The argument base on relationship in its strongest form has been dismissed as a result of these studies. Instead, the debate centres on whether relationship is a necessary condition of success; or, if not <u>necessary</u>, the extent to which it may be facilitatory.

To test whether relationship variables play a necessary role in the efficacy of desensitization suggests the simple comparison of treatment with a therapist and without. This, in turn, implies automation of the procedure. Much of the work on automated desensitization has been reported by LANG and his colleagues (LANG, 1968, 1969a; LANG et al., 1970). With reference to automation, LANG (1969a) writes: "The fact that a programmed device can 'sit in' for the experimenter during a fundamental part of the therapy process is the strongest kind of evidence that it is the specific program of instruction, and not the therapist or relationship variables, that is the viable aspect of desensitization therapy." This statement clearly points to the theoretical value of trials of automated therapy. Similar statements have been made by MIGLER and WOLPE (1967). It would be wrong, however, to think that all nonspecific factors of importance are eliminated by automation. Automation of desensitization usually means the automation of the mechanical part of the procedure, leaving minimal therapist contact in the devising of hierarchies and the assessment of the patient's condition and progress. Variables such as expectation of success can still operate and be manipulated under conditions of minimal therapist contact (see WILKINS, 1971). But, even if automated trials cannot eliminate all therapist- and relationship-derived factors, they do reduce the field to short-term ones. Controlled trials of automated desensitization have been reported by KRAPFL (1968), DONNER and GUERNEY (1969), and LANG et al. (1970). Results tended on the whole to show little if any significant difference between automated and non-automated treatment groups. However, all these studies were accomplished using nonclinical volunteer subjects, and it is open to further question whether clinical patients would respond similarly to automated desensitization. As DONNER and GUERNEY (1969) point out, there is a need for controlled clinical trials in this area. For this reason, as well as for reasons concerning the obvious practical implications of automation in the clinic (economy, opportunity to treat patients on a large scale, and so on), it was decided to undertake a controlled trial of automated desensitization with clinically phobic patients.

I. Method

Patients were referred for inclusion in the trial over a period of 21 months. Twenty-four patients took part in the trial. When they had been referred, patients were classified into three groups on the basis of the type of phobia they were suffering from. These "diagnostic" groups were simple phobics, social phobics, and agoraphobics. Referrals were made from Whitchurch Hospital, Cardiff, by the second author. Only patients whose main problem was phobic anxiety and who showed no signs of being psychotic were referred for inclusion. Otherwise depressed or neurotic patients who had phobias as subsidiary symptoms were not included.

The design of the experiment demanded two treatment groups. Patients in the one group received desensitization in the usual way: the procedure was administered personally by a therapist. Patients in the other group received a semi-automated form of treatment, in which instructions during therapy were delivered by pre-recorded tapes. Control groups were not possible for ethical reasons.

Once a patient had been referred, he was automatically assigned to the treatment group contrary to that of the preceding patient of the same diagnostic group. In other words, if an agoraphobic patient were assigned to the Therapist-Absent group, the next agoraphobic would be assigned to the Therapist-Present group. Thus it was possible to limit the agoraphobics to half of each treatment group (without this limitation, agoraphobics would probably have swamped the sample). No such controls were put on simple or social phobics[+]; the final balance between these patients in the two treatment groups reflects the true referral pattern. Finally, a period of 16 treatment sessions was set as the maximum duration of treatment. This was felt to be sufficient time to guarantee clinically significant improvement.

II. Patients

All were outpatients. All were treated at the Psychology Department, University College, Cardiff: 12 patients were in the Therapist-Present group, 12 in the Therapist-Absent group. The patients turned out to be adequately matched between groups on variables which might have influenced outcome (Table 1), although the rating of the main phobia was more severe on average in the Therapist-Absent group.

The Therapist-Present group comprised 6 patients with agoraphobia, 3 with social phobias, and 3 with simple phobias (claustrophobia, blood

---

[+] For this purpose only, social phobics and simple phobics were put together to form an 'other phobic' group of comparable size to the agoraphobic group.

Table 1. Treatment groups before therapy

	Therapist-Present	Therapist-Absent
Duration of Illness (yrs)	5.2	4.5
Mean Age	38.0	34.2
Males	4	3
Females	8	9
Agoraphobics	6	6
Social Phobics	3	2
Simple Phobics	3	4
Neuroticism	16.8	18.4
Extraversion	12.0	12.3
Initial Severity on Self-Ratings	8.5	9.8
Initial Severity on Psychiatrist's Ratings	8.4	9.1

and contamination). The social phobics all shared a common attribute: they were afraid of doing certain things in public, such as eating, using public conveniences, and so on. The Therapist-Absent group comprised 6 agoraphobics, 2 social phobics, and 4 simple phobics (claustrophobia and fear of dogs, spiders and becoming pregnant). All agoraphobias were of moderate severity. Typically these patients could not leave the house unaccompanied. They could, however, attend for treatment as long as initially at least, they were accompanied. They were not usually crippled by depression or chronic anxiety.

III. Treatment

1. The Therapist-Absent Treatment

Patients in this group received their therapy in a soundproof room, entirely on their own. They were shown into the room by the therapist, told to make themselves as relaxed as possible on an adjustable couch, and given a button-press which they were told controlled the administration of the therapy. It was stressed that the therapist would not need to be present, but could be summoned in an emergency by repeatedly pressing the button on and off. They were also told that the treatment was completely automated and controlled by computers and logic circuits (which incidentally were present in the adjoining room, though they were not in fact part of this experiment). In reality, the treatment was only semi-automated, and when the patient was shut in the therapy room, the therapist stayed unseen in the adjoining room and controlled a tape recorder in accordance with the signals given by the patients' button-presses. The button-press in fact controlled only a light.

The whole procedure began with an interview and a practice session in relaxation. The patient was shut in the therapy room and a prepared relaxation tape was played to him.

On ascertaining that the patient could experience a reasonable level of relaxation (in terms of verbal report and observation over a closed circuit TV monitor) and visualization, the first interview was concluded. In future sessions, after being relaxed, the patient was instructed to imagine anxiogenic items from pre-recorded hierarchies, which had been drawn up before therapy in the usual way. Each patient was seen personally by the therapist for 10 min a week at another time. This minimal therapist contact was necessary for assessment purposes and/or the discussion and modification of hierarchies, if necessary.

In dealing with the delivery of hierarchies the automated method was quite systematic. If anxiety was signalled, the tape was immediately released and instructions to stop imagining and relax were given. The scene would then be re-presented. If anxiety was signalled again, the same procedure would be initiated. If anxiety was signalled on 3 consecutive occasions, the tape would be taken back to the penultimate and successfully concluded item. Progression forward along the hierarchy, after the scene had originally provoked anxiety, was accomplished only after 3 consecutive presentations of the scene without any elicited anxiety.

Sessions lasted for between 25 and 30 min. No sessions were concluded with an unresolved item. Sessions always began with a presentation of the last successfully concluded item. Sessions were on a weekly basis It has been mentioned that patients in this group did receive minimal therapist contact, thus relationship factors of some kind might have been operative. It was not, however, the purpose of this trial to investigate all such variables. It is quite possible that nonspecific factors such as "expectation of success", which could be manipulated under conditions of minimal therapist contact, might prove to be important (LEITENBERG et al., 1969). If this is so, a different kind of clinical trial would be needed to show it.

2. The Therapist-Present Treatment

In practically every respect this treatment paralleled the Therapist-Absent treatment except that the procedure was carried out by the therapist in person. The relaxation induction procedure was the same. Rules governing forward progression and backtracking in the hierarchy were identical. Patients in this group were likewise seen personally once a week for about 10 min in addition of the treatment sessions. The reasons for this were the same.

Patients in both groups were given prior to therapy a short theoretical explanation of the treatment rationale, designed to encourage an expectation of success. All patients, regardless of treatment group, were given exercises to do as homework. This always involved their reality-testing items they had already dealt with in imagination. It might be argued that this blurs the distinction between desensitization and other methods, although desensitization in practice is not as isolated as is sometimes thought. Moreover, the 2 treatment groups were equally exposed to these additional methods, and the experiment therefore is only contaminated if one has reason to believe that desensitization is less influential in a patients's recovery than the additional aids used. There is no reason to believe that this is true.

Patients taking drugs were confined to the agoraphobic and social phobic groups. The drugs were mainly diazepam or chlordiazepoxide. Since the proportions of patients with different kinds of phobias in the two treatment groups were almost equal, differences in medication could hardly account for any differences that might be found between treatments.

IV. The Therapist

Since the therapist was also the experimenter+, accusations of unintentional bias might be made. The only retort to this is that this was a trial of two methods of delivering a therapy, not of two methods of therapy. Perhaps this issue is less loaded with bias, although that, it must be admitted, is only opinion. Also it might be argued that this sort of criticism is at its strongest when applied to less systematic and clearly definded methods, e.g. interpretive group methods.

V. Assessment

1. Self Ratings of Phobic Behaviour - Rationale, Construction and Administration

There are three systems through which fear is expressed (LANG, 1968; MATHEWS, 1971): physiological, cognitive and behavioural. Measurement of change in all three systems would have been ideal in a study of this kind, but time did not allow this. It was decided that the behavioural (or overt-motor) system was the one that seemed to be the most important. A consideration of the way we ascribe the word 'fear' makes it clear that we tend to give behavioural evidence precedence over evidence from the other two systems. If a person shows signs of autonomic activity in a situation but does not consistently avoid that situation, we might conclude that he is apprehensive (existed?) but we should probably deny him the use of the word 'fear'. On the other hand, if a person constantly avoids a situation yet denies he is afraid, but cannot otherwise explain his avoidance, we should probably question his (cognitive) judgment. When discharging a patient from treatment one would like to say, using any criteria, that fear has been diminished or eliminated. In the absence of being able to make such a strong statement, one should like to say at least that the person avoids his phobic situations less often. One might even surmise that, since the patient is no longer avoiding situations, he will be in an excellent position to extinguish any residual fear responses.

For these reasons, the self-ratings in this study were based solely on verbal report of behaviour. The rating of overt behaviour is recognized to be more reliable than the rating of mood or feeling (KNOWLES, 1963). Ratings were based on the analysis of a form of Personal Questionnaire, using, for each patient, 3 statements about behaviour which were felt to be indicative of low, middling and high degrees of phobic disturbance. It was assumed that the low statement of one patient was comparable with the low statement of another, and likewise for the middling and high statements. The validity of this assumption lay ultimately in the agreement of self-ratings with other means of assessment. From each of the 3 statements, 3 further statements were derived. The latter were presented in paired-comparison form to assess the applicability on a 4 point scale of each of the 3 primary statements. The procedure is best elucidated by looking at the typical agoraphobic questionnaire. The following 3 statements were first derived:

1) I cannot go out alone even into the street outside (H)

2) I cannot go shopping alone at the local village shops (M)

3) I cannot go shopping alone in the town centre. (L)

+ The first author

The endorsement of statement (1) would indicate a severe degree of agoraphobia, whilst statement (3) would have to be endorsed to some extent by anyone with claims to be agoraphobic.

It will be appreciated that the use of statements of this sort is well paralleled in the case of outside raters who use the information contained in statements of this kind as a guide to the subject's position on a subjective scale. The difference is that here an attempt is made to structure more exactly the mapping of information about behaviour to the final rating. Each of the statements was used as a basic for three further statements which, through paired-comparison presentation, roughly indicated whether a statement was true, half-true, half-untrue, or untrue. Thus, the original statement "I cannot do X" would give rise to the following three statements:

On the whole, I cannot do X

I sometimes can do X

On the whole, I can do X.

Thus one finished up with 3 sets of 3 statements. Paired-comparison presentation meant that assessment of each primary statement was by means of 3 cards which might look like this:

A) On the whole, I cannot do X B) I sometimes can do X	Card 1
A) I sometimes can doe X B) On the whole I can do X	Card 2
A) On the whole I cannot do X B) On the whole I can do X	Card 3

Two other sets of 3 cards dealt with the other two primary statements.

Patients were asked to consider whether the A or B statement best represented their current behaviour, and to show their choice by moving the card to the left (A - appropriate) or to the right (B -appropriate). The sum of the 3 primary statements scores (each ranging from 1 to 4) could give rise to 10 different meaningful totals. These totals constituted the final 10-point rating scale.

Self-ratings were made prior to therapy, at 4 weeks and 8 weeks and every other week during therapy. The final rating was a follow-up, on the average 14 months after discharge.

2. Psychiatrist's Ratings

A more global assessment of each patient's condition was made by the referring psychiatrist+, who was of course blind with regard to treatment group of the patient. The psychiatrist's ratings were meant to counterbalance the deliberate behavioural bias of the self-ratings and to give equal attention to the 'felt anxiety' of the patient. The scale ranged from 10 (very severe) to 2 (cured). The rating of the main phobia was supplemented by ratings of subsidiary symptoms, if present. The first psychiatrist rating was made from tape recordings of the first interview with the therapist. The interview format was structured. Each symptom category was introduced with a particular question, and each question was put in the same order. The psychiatrist had seen each patient previously at the referral interview and so was in some position

+ The second author

to know him adequately. It would have been preferable for the rating to have been done on the basis of a further interview with the psychiatrist in person, but other duties prevented this. Assessment at the referral interview would have been unsatisfactory. Not all patients seen were suitable for referral. The time between referral and being taken into the trial was not constant. Psychiatrist's ratings were also made at discharge and follow-up. These were based on personal interviews between the psychiatrist and the patient.

3. Other Means of Assessment

In addition to ratings, a battery of tests was administered before treatment, these included the E.P.I. (Form B), the 'Faces' test (LIGGETT, 1957), and a prognosis questionnaire for desensitization (GELDER et al., 1967). The first two tests were also given at discharge and follow-up.

VI. Results

1. Drop outs

In all, 7 patients dropped out of the trial. Two moved away from the district after a week of treatment; one was hospitalized with a slipped disc. The remaining patients made the excuse that they had made sufficient progress to manage without further treatment. Although this was to some extent true, they did not reach the criterion of 'cure' on the self-ratings.

Of these 7, 4 had been assigned to the Therapist-Absent group, and 3 to the Therapist-Present group. There was thus no evidence of a differential rate of dropping out between the two groups. Data from all these subjects were excluded from the final analysis. Patients who dropped out were replaced by adopting the procedure of assigning the next patient (agoraphobic or other phobic, accordingly) to the treatment group in which the drop-out patient had been placed.

2. Treatment Effects on the Self-Rating Measure

Ratings (not counting follow-up) were taken on up to 7 occasions. For purposes of analysis, if a patient was discharged on the criterion of having achieved a rating of 1 on the scale, he was assumed to maintain that score for all occasions of measurement thereafter, e.g. if he achieved a score of 1 on occasion 6 and was discharged, his score for occasion 7 was assumed to be 1.

Before the treatment began the mean intensity of the main phobia in the treatment groups turned out to be somewhat different. (A 't' test applied to the scores of both groups on occasion 1 was significant in its result.) The actual means for the groups on all of the seven occasions are shown in Table 2.

Differences between the 2 treatment methods were investigated by means of analysis of variance, with appropriate adjustments for repeated measures (WINER, 1962). Parametric statistics were used for two reasons. Although rating scales seldom give one the right to assume one's data conform to all the requirements of parametric tests, the F test in particular is generally recognized to be quite robust even with respect to large violations of its assumptions. More importantly, non-parametric tests with the sophistication to deal with multifactorial repeated-measures designs have not, as far as the author knows, been developed.

Table 2. Self-rating means for treatment groups on the seven occasions

Group	Occasions						
	1	2	3	4	5	6	7
Therapist-Present	8.5	5.3	3.6	2.9	2.5	2.1	2.0
Therapist-Absent	9.8	6.2	4.1	3.4	2.8	2.7	2.7

The analysis of variance for treatment effects (treatments; treatments x diagnostic groups; treatments x diagnostic groups x occasions; treatment x occasions) was insignificant on all counts. In particular, the treatment x occasions F ratio was somewhat less than unity. The progress of the two groups across time is shown in Fig. 1.

The patients in the Therapist-Absent group were slightly more severe at the start of treatment and the difference was in the same direction afterwards, though it was no longer significant and completely accounted for by two patients.

3. Treatment Effects on Psychiatrist's Rating

Psychiatrist's ratings were taken before and after treatment and at follow-up. Follow-ups for all measures are reported later. At the start of treatment the mean main phobia intensities of the two groups were slightly different in the same direction as on the self-ratings. Ratings for both groups before and after treatment are shown in Table 3.

Once again, results were subjected to analysis of variance. No treatment factors or interactions were significant. The psychiatrist's ratings then confirm the impression of the self-ratings, that there exist no meaningful differences in outcome that are in any way dependent on the method of desensitization used. The correlation of psy-

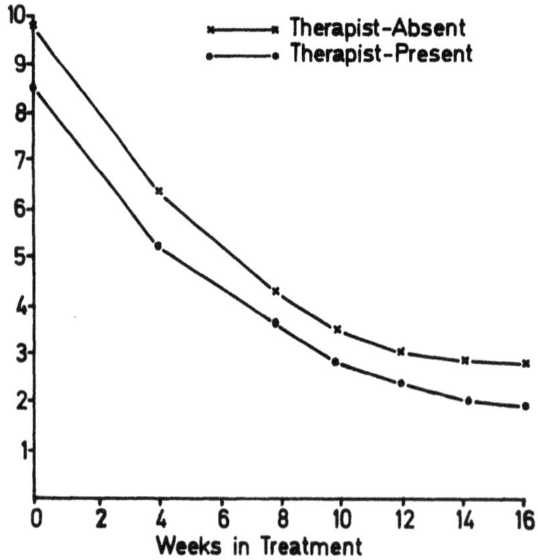

Fig. 1. Progress of treatment groups over time as measured by self-ratings

Table 3. Mean psychiatrist's rating for treatment groups before and after treatment

Group	Before	After
Therapist-Present	8.4	3.5
Therapist-Absent	9.2	4.3

chiatrist's ratings and self-ratings was .53 (before treatment) and .88 (after treatment). It will be remembered that the psychiatrist's rating was meant to give a global assessment of the patient, and this might have been reflected in the different degree of correlation before and after treatment. It could be that, when the patient is ill, the intensity of his suffering in terms of felt anxiety etc. does not perfectly correspond with the intensity of his phobic behaviour. It might then happen that a patient's general improvement is commensurate with the amount of successful behaviour modification. In other words, there is more variability in the way patients feel about the presence of their behavioural symptoms, than in the way they feel about the relative absence of those symptoms.

4. Follow-ups

Follow-ups were done after the main trial had finished. Thus the time elapsing between the end of treatment and follow-up was variable. The reason for adopting this procedure was that the period of follow-up, on average, should be as long as circumstances allowed. Possible disadvantages were a differential relapse rate, and difficulties in establishing contact with patients discharged a long time previously. Neither of these difficulties was in fact realized. The range of the follow-up period was 14 months, with a lower limit of 6 months. In all, 18 out of the original 24 patients were followed up; 4 could not be contacted, and 2 had received further therapy meanwhile.

Before treatment, after treatment, and follow-up scores for patients on both ratings were subjected to analysis of variance. No treatment effects of any kind were significant. There was a slight tendency for some relapse to occur between discharge and follow-up, but differences between before-therapy scores and follow-up were still highly significant. There was some evidence, on the self-ratings at least, to suggest that 'recovered' patients tended to stay the same, whereas patients who had made some improvement but had not been rated as fully recovered tended to relapse just a little. This is summarized in the following contingency table (Table 4).

Table 4.

At End of Treatment	At Follow-Up	
	No Relapse	Relapse
Completely Symptom-Free	9	5
Not Completely Symptom-Free	0	4
Fisher-Yates Test of Significance: *p* .05		

5. Other Results

The type of phobia (diagnostic group) did affect outcome to some extent, but in no way interacted with treatment method. Social phobics were significantly worse than simple phobics in terms of trend analysis on the self-ratings. They also differed marginally in terms of gross differences between before and after scores. Agoraphobics and simple phobics differed in the pattern of progress across time (trend analysis), with agoraphobics taking longer to improve, but did not differ in the absolute amount of progress. These results are fully reported elsewhere.

'Neuroticism' and 'extraversion' changes were apparent in treatment. The former decreased significantly; the latter increased. These changes were still apparent at follow-up. There was no evidence that the two treatments differentially affected change on either dimension, nor were treatment effects noticeable with regard to 'Faces Test' records.

Few patients were rated by the psychiatrist for clinically significant subsidiary symptoms. Such ratings as were available were too few for statistical analysis, but in no way did they seem to be affected by treatment differences. In fact, all subsidiary symptoms seemed to show a pattern of improvement related to improvement in the main phobia even though the therapy was in no way addressed to them. This has been a common finding in desensitization research.

VII. Discussion

The negative result obtained has important implications. First, it echoes the results of previous researchers in this area, that the removal of the therapist from the administration of desensitization does not appear to affect the outcome in any way. Secondly, it confirms that this is equally true for phobic patients in the clinic, despite expectations that perhaps relationship with an understanding therapist would be more important for this class of subject. It seems then that long-term therapist or relationship variables do not play any clinically significant role in accounting for the success of desensitization; transference phenomena are the obvious variables which can be ruled out, at the very least for the kind of patient treated in this trial.

Does a study of this kind lend support to WOLPE's explanation of desensitization in terms of counterconditioning? Not necessarily. First, it is likely that much of the success of desensitization derives from a variety of nonspecific factors - perceived encouragement and support, sufficient expectation of success and so on - which are still demonstrably present even under conditions of minimal therapist contact. It is probable that this is true of most therapies. Secondly, the significant contribution of the specific method of desensitization, though not in doubt, does not necessarily entail any particular interpretation of its mode of action. Thus the enthusiasm of some early researchers for automation as a means of demonstrating the clear connexion between the desensitization method and certain conditioning principles needs now to be tempered in the light of studies which have (a) shown up the ubiquity of nonspecific factors even when automation is used, and (b) cast doubt on the necessity of many of the specific elements of the desensitization method. This whole area of problems has been ably reviewed by WILKINS (1971). Nevertheless, successful automation does narrow down future research to less complex nonspecific factors, which do not involve lengthy therapist - patient interaction. It will, hopefully, not be too long before it is possible to give a comprehensive explanation of just how desensitization works.

References

DONNER, L., GUERNEY, B.G.: Automated group desensitization for test anxiety. Behav. Res. Ther. 7, 1-13 (1969).

GELDER, M.G., MARKS, I.M., WOLFF, H.E., CLARK, M.: Desensitization and psychotherapy in the treatment of phobic states: a controlled clinical inquiry. Brit. J. Psychiat. 113, 53-73 (1967).

KNOWLES, J.B.: Rating methods and measurement of behaviour. In: SAINSBURY, P.H., KREITMAN, N. (Eds.): Methods of Psychiatric Research. Oxford: Oxford University Press 1963.

KRAPFL, J.E.: Differential ordering of stimulus presentation and semi-automated versus live treatment in the systematic desensitization of snake phobia. Diss. Abstr. 28B 3878 (1968).

LANG, P.J.: Fear reduction and fear behaviour: Problems in treating a construct. Res. Psychotherapy 3, 90-102 (1968).

LANG, P.J.: The on-line computer in behaviour research. Amer. Psychol. 24, 236-239 (1969a).

LANG, P.J.: The mechanics of desensitization and the laboratory study of human fear. In: FRANKS, C. (Ed.): Behaviour Therapy: Appraisal and Status. New York: McGraw Hill 1969b.

LANG, P.J., LAZOVIK, A.D.: The experimental desensitization of a phobia. J. abnorm. soc. Psychol. 66, 519-525 (1963).

LANG, P.J., LAZOVIK, A.D., REYNOLDS, D.J.: Desensitization, suggestibility and pseudotherapy. J. abnorm. soc. Psychol. 70, 395-402 (1965).

LANG, P.J., MELAMED, B.G., HART, J.: A psychophysiological analysis of fear modification using an automated desensitization procedure. J. abnorm. soc. Psychol. 76, 220-234 (1970).

LEITENBERG, H., AGRAS, W.S., B , D.H., OLWEAN, D.C.: Contribution of selective positive reinforcement and therapeutic instructions to systematic desensitization therapy. J. abnorm. soc. Psychol. 74, 113-118 (1969).

LIGGETT, : The Faces Test (Self Valuation Test Forms M & F). Newcastle-upon-Tyne: Bealle 1957.

MATHEWS, A.: Psychophysiological approaches to the investigation of desensitization and related procedures. Psychol. Bull. 76, 73-91 (1971).

MIGLER, B., WOLPE, J.: Automated self-desensitization: a case report. Behav. Res. Ther. 7, 27-33 (1967).

PAUL, G.L.: Insight versus Desensitization in Psychotherapy: An Experiment in Anxiety Reduction. Stanford, California: Stanford University Press 1966.

WILKENS, W.: Desensitization: Social and cognitive factors underlying the effectiveness of Wolpe's procedure. Psychol. Bull 76, 311-317 (1971).

WINER, B.J.: Statistical Principles and Experimental Design. New York: McGraw Hill 1962.

An Evaluation of the Factors that Influence Prognosis in Behaviour Therapy

D.K.B. NIAS

I. Psychotherapy Research

This paper outlines some of the problems involved in trying to review the literature on prognosis. LUBORSKY, et al. (1971) have already attempted such a review, but for psychotherapy only. They reviewed 161 quantitative studies and arrived at 3 main conclusions: (1) Patient variables provide the best predictors; patients who do well tend to be in better psychological health, to have higher motivation and to enjoy better educational and social assets, etc. (2) A few therapist variables also affect outcome; therapists who do well tend to have more experience, more empathy and to charge higher fees. As regards patient - therapist interaction, prognosis is improved if they are of similar social class or have similar interests. (3) The type of psychotherapy does not seem to make any difference, e.g. client-centred therapy gives much the same outcome as Adlerian analysis. Only the number of sessions or duration of treatment is clearly related to getting better.

LUBORSKY et al. stated that their review was aimed at improving prognosis by obtaining a better understanding of psychotherapy, a better selection of patients and a better matching of patients and therapists. Unfortunately, they seem instead to have just highlighted the problems involved in a review of this kind.

For a start they were, of course, restricted to published studies, and it is known that significant results tend to get published more often than non-significant results; of their 161 studies only a quarter reported non-significant results. Apart from this limitation, they noted that most of the available studies involved seriously ambiguous designs. For example, results on the importance of empathy may alternatively be interpreted as evidence that improving patients elicit more empathy from their therapist, simply because he is responding to his apparent success. There are many other examples where alternative explanations of this sort are possible. But most striking is their last conclusion that "the more psychotherapy the better"; this result can much more easily be explained in terms of spontaneous remission (EYSENCK, 1972). To quote a more specific example, they suggest that "patients with high anxiety at the initial evaluation or at the beginning of treatment are the ones likely to benefit from psychotherapy". Since it is already known that spontaneous remission is particularly high among anxiety neurotics (not phobics), it becomes apparent that the causal connection with psychotherapy is meaningless, based as it is on studies that have failed to use a control group of "no treatment".

In general, research on psychotherapy has given us very few pointers that are of any practical or theoretical value. How then would an evaluation of behaviour therapy studies make out? The aim of this paper is to outline some of the main problems in this area, and to compare the likely conclusions with those put forward for psychotherapy.

II. Behaviour Therapy Research

Consider first the severity of the disorder. There have been several studies on the effects of this variable on prognosis. For example, MORGENSTERN et al. (1965) found that conditioning treatment of transvestites was less successful for those showing more complex and generalized symptoms. In particular, high scores on Neuroticism and on Slater's Femininity scale indicated a poor outcome. The general rule emerges that the worse patients are to begin with, the poorer the prognosis. This accords well with conclusions based on psychotherapy.

A second category to consider is the more general characteristics of the patient. In contrast to psychotherapy, patient variables have been neglected in behaviour therapy research. However, factors such as motivation would seem relatively unimportant if we take Dr. Marks' suggestion that they act mainly by increasing cooperation in the details of treatment. But if this is the case, then we would need to explain why such variables are found to be very important in psychotherapy, where treatment details appear to be unimportant. Similarly, in physical medicine it is generally believed that psychological factors play a large part in determining why certain patients recover more quickly than others. We heard, for example, that Stirling Moss showed exceptional motivation to recover his racing accident, prompted no doubt by a desire to compete again later in the year when he still had a chance of winning the World Championship series. Although he did not manage this, the fact that he recovered at all was described as "miraculous". Another example was Abebe Bikila who underwent an appendicectomy shortly before the 1964 Olympic Marathon. After the operation he was strapped to a board to prevent the characteristic stoop of patients after stomach surgery. Even so he was not expected to recover in time, but he did and won in world record time.

Clearly it would be interesting to ascertain whether variables such as motivation do help in behaviour therapy, over and above their effect on cooperation; the results from the psychotherapy studies suggest an affirmative answer. Similarly, it would be useful to establish the degree to which therapist variables are important over and above the need to design an effective treatment programme.

A third category to consider is treatment variables. In contrast to the conclusion from psychotherapy that the type of treatment is unimportant, the research on behaviour therapy points to a number of variables that are of predictable importance.

III. Theory and Practice

In behaviour therapy there is a reasonably close association between three aspects of research, namely theory, animal experiments and clinical trials. There are many examples where knowledge has increased through an interaction of these three areas.

For example, EYSENCK's theory of arousal postulates that rate of conditioning should be enhanced by increasing arousal in the CNS. TURNER and YOUNG (1966) indeed found that conditioning treatment for enuresis works faster when a stimulant drug is administered. They also found that this advantage from the drug was, unfortunately, offset by a higher relapse rate. Moreover, there are animal experiments that illustrate this effect for various conditioning procedures; conditioning is facilitated by a stimulant drug but extinction occurs sooner (see TAPP, 1969). This finding has led to the theory of "dissociation" or "stimulus change", which postulates that conditioned responses (CRs) are very dependent on the actual conditions (including the state of the CNS) at the time of acquisition. It follows that, if conditions are maintained, then CRs should be more resistant to extinction. This prediction has been confirmed with animals in that rapid extinction is less apparent when the stimulant drug is continued throughout the experiment, i.e. during both acquisition and extinction trials. It will be interesting to see if this result is replicated with humans.

There are many other examples of the simultaneous development of theory, animal experiments and clinical trials. Thus EYSENCK's (1968) theory of incubation can be used to explain the finding that repetition of a conditioned stimulus (CS) alone does not always lead to extinction, but can instead increase a learned fear. Napalkov first demonstrated this effect in dogs; a single pairing of a CS with an aversive stimulus (UCS) was followed by an increased rise in blood pressure each time the CS was subsequently presented. Incubation theory suggests that the unpleasant nature of the CR itself may be sufficient to act (in place of the UCS) as reinforcement for the CS-CR link. An application for this work may be found in the design of both desensitization and "flooding" treatment, by way of maximizing the conditions under which extinction can occur. WATTS (1971) has provided some direct information on this point by comparing the effects of short and long stimulus presentations for items at high and low levels in desensitization hierarchies.

IV. Role of Attitudes

It may be useful at this stage to draw attention to the role of attitudes in determining treatment. CAINE and SMAIL (1969) have argued that therapists seem to be influenced in their choice of treatment more by their own attitudes than by objective criteria of what works best. Sadly, advances in treatment made possible by research of the type noted above will be of limited use if personal attitudes prevent the wide-scale implementation of such techniques. LILLIE (1973) has reviewed recent evidence for the interaction of social attitudes and treatment preferences in psychiatry.

CAINE and LEIGH (1972) administered the Attitudes to Treatment Questionnaire together with the Wilson-Patterson Conservatism Scale to nurses. Those nurses who believed in a traditional medical approach to treatment (as measured by items relating to discipline, hygiene and formality) tended to score higher on conservatism; this result was obtained three times (Table 1). It was also found that the more liberal nurses believed in a therapeutic community approach, while those who believed in a general psychiatric approach were intermediate on the conservative-liberal dimension. PANAYOTOPOULOS and STOFFELMAYR (1972) conducted a similar study on psychiatrists and found that those who had chosen training in psychotherapy were more liberal and tender-minded. Table 2 gives a comparison of the scores obtained by (i) psychotherapists, and (ii) psychiatrists with a more general training.

Table 1. Conservatism related to formal treatment attitudes in nurses (CAINE and LEIGH, 1972)

	Correlation
75 nurses attending course	.50
94 nurses attending course	.22
72 nurses attending psychiatric course	.44

Table 2. Treatment and social attitudes in psychiatrists (PANAYOTOPOULOS and STOFFELMAYR, 1972)

	20 Psychotherapists	20 Psychiatrists
Physical treatments (ATQ)	35.9	44.4
Group therapy	43.6	41.9
Individual psychotherapy	37.5	37.1
Conservatism (C-Scale)	28.4	37.7
Radicalism (SAI)	9.7	7.7
Tender-mindedness	17.2	13.7

Patients also have their preferences. CAINE and LEIGH found that patients who endorsed attitudes consistent with a behaviour therapy approach were more conservative than those who endorsed group therapy attitudes ($r = .37$, $n = 85$). Moreover, such attitudes may influence the type of therapy that is actually prescribed. CAINE and LEIGH analyzed their data in terms of responses to the item "Socialism" on the Conservatism scale. Patients who anwered "no" to this item tended to be assigned to behaviour therapy (rather than group psychotherapy) more frequently than those who answered "yes" (32 % compared with 15 %). They interpreted this result in terms of the way in which patients present their problems to the doctor. Thus the more conservative patients may put greater emphasis on symptoms (which invites behaviour therapy) rather than on interpersonal difficulties.

Behaviour therapy has tended to be regarded as a radical form of treatment, favoured by younger, more scientifically-minded psychiatrists. However, in the light of the foregoing results it would seem to fit more appropriately into a "conservative" category. Behaviour therapy is certainly a specialist treatment aimed at specific symptoms, which is more in keeping with the traditional medical approach. In contrast, psychotherapy may be regarded as an informal or vague procedure aimed at interpersonal difficulties or symptoms of a mysterious and personal nature. A conservative patient who admits to such problems might be expected to feel responsible for his condition, or at least to feel a loss to his pride and self-esteem, which would make the treatment less acceptable to him.

The type of treatment prescribed may subsequently affect prognosis in a number of peripheral ways because of attitudes instilled by the therapist. CAINE and SMAIL give the example of discharged patients having to report regularly to their GPs to obtain prescriptions. Patients who have received psychotherapy seem less likely to do this because they have been taught a different way of handling their problems; in contrast, physically treated patients may have been taught to look upon their disorder as a constitutionally or genetically determined illness needing drugs. If follow-up prescriptions are a necessary part of treatment, then it is the latter patients who seem likely to have a better prognosis.

In practice, it can thus be said that prognosis will partly depend on the treatment prescribed, which in turn will depend on the patient's attitudes, the attitudes of the doctor he sees, and no doubt also on the type of hospital he visits. If these variables were partialled out, the exact nature of his disorder may be of very minor consequence. A similar point was made by BANNISTER et al. (1964) who analyzed 1000 cases and concluded that, although psychiatrists spend a great deal of time and effort in diagnosis, the type of treatment prescribed usually bears little relationship to the diagnosis made.

V. Methodological Problems

As with psychotherapy, behaviour therapy studies are likewise open to criticisms of methodology and interpretation. In particular, although the behaviour therapy studies may have been carried out by more scientifically-minded researchers, the problem arises that different interpretations are rarely mutually exclusive. Research results may be attenuated or inflated because various other influences are acting in addition to the variables being investigated. This need not be too discouraging, since with increasing knowledge of the way the different variables act we should become better able to arrive at informed judgments of the most likely conclusion.

To illustrate the point about different interpretations not being mutually exclusive, a study has been selected at random. Table 3 presents results obtained from an investigation of individual differences in the readiness with which children learn to swim (HARDY and NIAS, 1971). Difficulties in learning to swim may be seen as analogous to psychiatric problems, since there is a certain element of danger and discomfort to the beginner. Anyway, we selected children who could not swim and proceeded to give them a 10-week course of instruction; from behaviour therapy we adopted the method of graduated progression as the most appropriate form of training. The pupils were finally placed in rank order in terms of how soon they had learned to swim, and were assessed for a total of 13 variables including intelligence, lung capacity and physique. For both boys and girls, Extraversion was the variable most closely related to learning to swim.

As it stands, this study may serve to show how prognostic variables can be useful for swimming teachers in identifying those children most likely to experience difficulty in learning to swim. It may also serve to illustrate the relevance of psychological variables to a physical task, and how the principles of behaviour therapy can be applied to teaching situations. As regards interpretation, however, the correlation with extraversion can be explained in at least three ways: (i) extraverted children may be less afraid of the water because they have not developed conditioned fears to such an extent as introverts; (ii) extraverts may be better at learning motor (as opposed to cognitive) tasks; or (iii) extraverts may simply be more interested in the novelty and challenge of learning to swim. It is difficult to choose between these interpretations, and indeed all three may have played a part. Nevertheless, there are two apparent reasons why the first explanation may not have been relevant in this particular study. First, the children had little or no previous experience of trying to swim, and so would have

Table 3. Correlations with 'learning to swim' (HARDY and NIAS, 1971)

15 boys		14 girls	
Extraversion	.72	Extraversion	.50
Sitting height	.57	Mesomorphy	.49
Height	.45	Intelligence	.38
Lung capacity	.44	Height	-.20
Weight	.39	Physical maturity	-.13
Body surface area	.38	Lung capacity	.12
Intelligence	.37	Body surface area	-.11
Physical maturity	.37	Neuroticism	-.10
Mesomorphy	.33	Endomorphy	-.09
Neuroticism	-.32	Weight	-.05
Ponderal index	-.22	Ponderal index	-.05
Endomorphy	-.17	Ectomorphy	.04
Ectomorphy	-.01	Sitting height	-.02

had little opportunity for 'learning to be afraid'. Second, if there was a fear element, then Neuroticism might have been expected to interact with introversion in retarding learning, but from the correlations obtained this did not appear to be the case. In contrast, another study assessed older children, most of whom had failed to learn in spite of repeated opportunities; these persistent non-swimmers were indeed high on Neuroticism as well as introversion (WHITING and STEMBRIDGE, 1965).

Finally, interpretation may be difficult if the quality in question is not being assessed properly. The work attempting to demonstrate correlations between different types of conditioning may fall into this category. EYSENCK's theory of the link between personality and arousal requires the existence of a general factor of conditionability. But evidence on this point has been largely negative. It would thus be easy to conclude that there is no general factor of conditionability, and that EYSENCK's theory is wrong. However, recent work indicates that if proper attention is paid to parameter values, then this general factor is likely to emerge. The necessity of this requirement is demonstrated by EYSENCK and LEVEY's (1972) finding that, with certain parameter values, extraverts condition better than introverts, i.e. the opposite of the usual result. They did this by increasing the strength of the air puff, increasing the length of time that the buzzer sounded, and using continuous rather than partial reinforcement. Under the opposite conditions, the usual superiority of introverts was obtained. Thus it can be predicted that parameter values need to be roughly equivalent for the purposes of correlating rates of conditioning obtained from different procedures. Without this equivalence a general factor would not be expected.

In conclusion, a review of the factors influencing prognosis in behaviour therapy needs to take many problems into account, but even so seems to provide a number of important conclusions that, relative to the psychotherapy conclusions, are linked to theory in a fairly predictable fashion.

References

BANNISTER, D., SALMON, P., LEIBERMAN, D.M.: Diagnosis-treatment relationships in psychiatry: a statistical analysis. Brit. J. Psychiat. 110, 726-732 (1964).

CAINE, T.M., LEIGH, R.: Conservatism in relation to psychiatric treatment. Brit. J. soc. clin. Psychol. 11, 52-56 (1972).

CAINE, T.M., SMAIL, D.J.: The Treatment of Mental Illness: Science, Faith and the Therapeutic Personality. London: University of London Press 1969.

EYSENCK, H.J.: A theory of the incubation of anxiety/fear responses. Behav. Res. Ther. 6, 309-321 (1968).

EYSENCK, H.J.: A note on 'factors influencing the outcome of psychotherapy'. Psychol. Bull. in press (1972).

EYSENCK, H.J., LEVEY, A.: Conditioning, introversion-extraversion and the strength of the nervous system. In: Biological Bases of Individual Behaviour. New York: Academic Press 1972.

HARDY, C.A., NIAS, D.K.B.: An investigation of physical and personality factors involved in learning to swim. Personality 2, 1-7 (1971).

LILLIE, F.J.: Conservatism, psychiatry and mental distress. In: Psychology of Conservatism (Eds. G.D. WILSON et al.). London: Academic Press 1973.

LUBORSKY, L., CHANDLER, M., AUERBACH, A.H., COHEN, J., BACHRACH, H.M.: Factors influencing the outcome of psychotherapy: a review of quantitative research. Psychol. Bull. 75, 145-185 (1971).

MORGENSTERN, F.S., PEARCE, J.F., LINFORD REES, W.: Predicting the outcome of behaviour therapy by psychological tests. Behav. Res. Ther. 2, 191-200 (1965).

PANAYOTOPOULOS, D.J., STOFFELMAYR, B.E.: Training preferences, social attitudes and treatment orientation among psychiatrists. J. clin. Psychol. 28, 216-217 (1972).

TAPP, J.T. (Ed.) : Reinforcement and Behaviour. New York: Academic Press 1969.

TURNER, R.K., YOUNG, G.G.: CNS stimulant drugs and conditioning treatment of nocturnal enuresis: a long term follow-up study. Behav. Res. Ther. 4, 225-228 (1966).

WATTS, F.: Desensitization as an habituation phenomenon: I. Stimulus intensity as determinant of the effects of stimulus lengths. Behav. Res. Ther. 9, 209-217 (1971).

WHITING, H.T.A., STEMBRIDGE, D.E.: Personality and the persistent non-swimmer. Res. Quart. Amer. Ass. Hlth. phys. Educ. 36, 348-356 (1965)

Prognosis in Behavioural Psychotherapy

I. MARKS

Prognosis refers to the likely future outcome of a disorder in the light of present and past evidence. To be meaningful one needs to specify in some detail what one is prognosticating about. The prognosis for a mongol child may be hopeless with regard to his chromosomal and anatomical aberrations, but fair for the prospects of training him to lead a semi-independent social existence. In compulsive rituals with frequent depression one might be able to eliminate most of the rituals without affecting the tendency to recurrent depression. Prognosis can thus be good for some aspects of a problem but poor for others.

Questions of prognosis commonly involve the probable outcome with and without treatment intervention. The "natural history" of a disorder usually describes the hypothetical outcome without treatment, though so-called "spontaneous remissions" may be due as much to environmental as to endogenous processes. Unfortunately, there are grave difficulties in ascertaining the course of untreated psychiatric problems, and the obvious baseline of the natural history is not usually available to compare with treated samples.

Prognostic factors can be conveniently divided into those which transcend particular problems or techniques (sometimes some of these are called nonspecific variables), and those which are more clearly related to the disorder or treatment technique in question (Table 1).

Table 1. Prognostic factors in behavioural psychotherapy

Variables TRANSCENDING diagnosis or technique
<u>In patient and in therapist:</u>
empathy and warmth
motivation
expectancy
<u>In patient only:</u>
chronicity
discreteness of problem
Variables SPECIFIC to diagnosis or technique:
e.g. free-floating anxiety in phobics, with desensitization (not flooding)
transsexualism in transvestism, with aversion
anxiety during flooding of phobics (irrelevant fear cues only)
etc.

Transcending variables which affect the outcome of behavioural treatment include such intangibles as motivation of the patient and his relatives, expectancy of the patient and the therapist, empathy and warmth of the therapist, and the degree to which the problem is bound up with the patient's life style. Hard data on most of these factors are hard to collect, so that inevitably comments have to be based largely on impressions, not statistical evidence.

Even where transcending variables are shown to correlate significantly with future course in a variety of conditions, the question is whether statistical significance has clinical meaning. The relative size of the contribution of a variable to outcome is important. Empathy and warmth may be pervasive prognostic variables, but how much of the outcome variance is in fact due to them? Is it 10 % or 90 %? A pervasive factor may make but a small contribution, which is necessary but not sufficient by itself for improvement to occur. In a grief reaction confession may cleanse the soul, and empathy and warmth could be of overriding importance in this instance. In compulsive rituals, however, empathy and warmth may simply be the vehicle by which the patient is persuaded to expose himself to the noxious situation so that extinction can occur.

In volunteers, tape-recorded desensitization of phobias had had some success, which is evidence that desensitization can work with minimal empathy and warmth. However, taped flooding has been less successful in phobic volunteers and patients (MARKS, 1972). This may argue equally for the value of attentional variables - patients may listen more carefully to a live therapist than to a taped voice. Therapist empathy and warmth can improve prognosis by ensuring better communication between patient and therapist, allowing better definition of the problem to be treated. This will also increase patient motivation to work harder toward his recovery; a phobic will expose himself to the phobic situation more readily, a compulsive is more likely to desist from his rituals, a sex deviant is more likely to shock his own deviant fantasies, there is a greater chance that a motivated patient with social deficits will seek social situations in which to develop social skills, etc. Therapist empathy and warmth can thus improve prognosis by increasing patient motivation or "gutsiness". Patient warmth may also play a part. A warm patient can make the therapist more inclined to exert his energies in treatment.

Motivation on the part of the patient ensures that he will carry out treatment procedures appropriately, increase the number of practice trials, and so enhance his probability of improving with potent techniques. Motivation is of little value if it makes the patient an ineffective technique diligently all day long. If a compulsive patient is motivated simply to relax well and regularly, his hard work is unlikely to be rewarded by much reduction of his rituals (HODGSON et al., 1972). However, prognosis becomes brighter if the patient is motivated to refrain from carrying out his rituals for long periods so that he learns to tolerate the discomfort engendered by such abstention from rituals. Spouces in contract marital therapy are not likely to fulfil their contracts unless they are motivated strongly to do something about changing their behaviour towards one another. A patient with compulsive gambling has to be able to assiduously shock every urge to gamble, or to deal with such urges by other forms of self-regulation. As most behavioural methods require active participation by the patient in his own treatment, patient motivation is a key prognostic variable which transcends diagnosis and technique. We must be clear, however, that motivation is not a mystic factor which acts merely by being present. In fact, it acts by firing the patient to carry out those activities necessary for his recovery.

We should not forget that therapist motivation acts just like patient motivation. It helps the therapist attend to the often tiresome detail of complex treatment and to support the patient through difficult periods. A therapist trying to complete a treatment series for his M.D. or Ph.D. dissertation is well motivated to do all he can for his patients. His enthusiasm may wane after the degree has been granted, though the patient's treatment needs remain unaltered.

When a patient is poorly motivated for treatment it is usually a waste of time trying to apply behavioural psychotherapy, since failure to cooperate and a high dropout rate are likely to frustrate all therapeutic endeavours. At a time of long waiting lists and few therapists, it is more economic to devote one's time to those patients who are willing to work towards their salvation along with the therapist. With flooding procedures in particular, it is worth placing some obstacles in the path of treatment, stressing the difficulties, to make sure that participating patients will perform the required treatment procedures properly.

It is, of course, an admission of defeat to exclude poorly motivated patients, and we need to develop ways of motivating them towards treatment. In San Francisco, FISHER (1971) found that foster parents would not cooperate in the rehabilitation of their delinquent children until the patients were rewarded with trading stamps for attendance at group meetings to discuss treatment approaches. How motivation is best stimulated depends a great deal upon the problem to be treated, the method selected, and the context of therapy.

Another pervasive variable which is often thought to be of prognostic import is expectancy. Expectancy involves the patient and the therapist. It can be a vague idea that improvement will take place, or that specific manoeuvres will help. Obviously, high expectancy will increase a patient's motivation to cooperate, and may also reduce his subjective feelings of distress. Though expectancy can help treatment along, its importance can be exaggerated. Measures of initial patient expectancy in the flooding of phobic patients have failed to correlate significantly with outcome (STERN and MARKS, 1973a; MATHEWS, 1971).

In brief, transcending variables such as empathy and warmth, motivation and expectancy, both in patient and therapist, all seem to have prognostic import. It is probable that these variables usually act, not of and in themselves, but by the way they increase attention to treatment detail and cooperation in completion of therapeutic manoeuvres by patient and therapist. It is worth remembering that these issues play a similar role in traditional psychotherapy. In that area good prognosis is said to be associated with the YAVIS set of variables - young, attractive, verbal, insightful and successful.

Another prognostic variable which might be thought important, regardless of diagnosis and treatment, is chronicity. Though evidence is not available, it is often held that disturbances of brief duration are easier to treat. In phobias and compulsions this may well be true, and it is possible that treatment time is shorter in such patients. However, once these problems have been present for a year or more, duration need not be important. Specific phobias and compulsions of 20 years' standing can improve dramatically with the same few hours of treatment as those which have only been present for a year (WATSON et al., 1971; MARKS et al., 1971a). The same can apply to other conditions. After years of marital strife couples have been known to readjust dramatically after a few sessions of contract therapy (STUART, 1969; STERN and MARKS, 1973b).

Chronicity is often bound up with another general prognostic factor - the discreteness of the disability in question. The longer a problem has been present, the more time it has had to affect the patient's life style in a myriad of ways, although even problems of several decades' standing can remain very focal. In general, more focal problems are easier to treat. The greater the ramifications of a disorder in the life of a patient and his family, the harder they are to unravel and change. There are several possible reasons for this. The extinction of one fear hierarchy will be faster than that of 5 separate hierarchies. However, we do not know whether a coping set develops which makes 5 hierarchies in one patient easier to extinguish than one hierarchy in 5 patients, or whether on the other hand additional hierarchies compound the time required. Probably this will vary according to the nature of the problem and the patient.

When a problem involves the patient's family, then relatives can affect the prognosis if they need to be drawn into treatment for improvement to occur and be maintained. Chronic compulsive rituals are a case in point, as the following case history illustrates:

The patient was a 30-year-old married woman with a 12-year history of compulsive checking, worsening especially in the 3 years since her marriage. She and her husband slept in separate bedrooms, and they both spent several hours a night carrying out checking rituals at her behest, e.g. whether the lights were off, whether the switches pointed up or down, what side their baby was lying on next door, etc. By day she spent further hours carrying out other rituals alone. The couple ceased buying food tins, milk bottles or newspapers lest the numbers in or on these objects trigger more checking.

At the 1 1/2-hour assessment interview the husband himself suggested that his own actions might be reinforcing his wife's rituals. I explained to the couple the principles of flooding with response prevention, and stressed the difficulty of treatment, that it might involve the husband locking up the wife alone in her bedroom at night and not checking for or reassuring her, and that they would have to resume buying food tins, milk bottles and newspapers. Because of the unpleasantness of the treatment, I told them to ponder the question for 1 week and then to let me know their decision. At this interview both spouses had been warm, attentive and easy to talk to. When they returned 4 weeks later, to my surprise the wife said "I'm 70 % better. We did what you asked. My husband stopped checking for or reassuring me, and I'm now stopping each ritual one by one. We've fitted my bedroom door with a lock and if you wish, my husband and I are prepared for me to be locked in at night." The latter was done, and she was asked to resume buying newspapers, food tins and milk in bottles. By her 3rd appointment a week later nearly all desires to check had disappeared. Her pre-existing frigidity and hostility to her husband continued as before. She developed obvious transference feelings for me, which were not dealt with, and utilized the flooding principle spontaneously to extinguish the few residual rituals we had not discussed. Early in the treatment the husband several times slipped into his reassuring ways and required some role rehearsal with his wife and with me to avoid checking for and reassuring of her which had previously reinforced his wife's rituals. The patient remained well at 6 months follow-up and had ceased asking her husband to check, though her contempt for him remained.

This couple shows how motivation and warmth allow patients and their relatives to carry out the procedures necessary for recovery to occur, and how intimately relatives sometimes have to be involved in the day-to-day transactions of treatment. The prognosis is abetted by an intelligent problem-solving set, as was present in both spouses here.

In this cooperative couple the prognosis was greatly improved by the possibility of carrying out home treatment by proxy through the couple themselves. Often, however, domiciliary visits are essential, and if the staff is not available for this the prognosis worsens considerably. Treatment of problem families right in their home is often important (PATTERSON, 1971) for at least two reasons: (1) cues that trigger abnormal behaviour are often not apparent except in the natural setting; (2) adaptive behaviour can be taught on the spot as soon as it is required, without a gap occuring in the transfer of learning from hospital to home.

Another example where ramification of the symptom in the patient's like makes the prognosis worse is in exhibitionism. When the life style of persistent exposers centres round their deviations, and they have a history of multiple convictions or a high exposure rate, the prognosis is significantly worse for the outcome of exhibitionism after aversion and self-regulation (ROOTH and MARKS, 1973).

The Biblical adage that "to them that hath it shall be given even more...." unfortunately applies to the prognosis in behavioural as in other treatments. Patients with existing problem-solving skills and a reasonable social repertoire seem to cooperate more successfully in complex treatment than those with multiple personality deficits. Patients from very deprived backgrounds can need Herculean efforts to push them to a higher level of social function in an operant program, without ever reaching "take-off point" (MARKS et al., 1971b). The adage is emphasized by LOVAAS' 1967) finding that it is much harder to teach speech to totally mute autistic children than to those with at least a few words at their command. Similarly, in sexual deviants FELDMAN and MacCULLOCH (1971), MARKS et al. (1970) and BANCROFT (1970) found a better heterosexual outcome where deviants had prior heterosexual interest or experience, and fewer neurotic personality traits and higher self-esteem. In keeping with this, ROOTH and MARKS (1973) found that married exhibitionists had a better prognosis. The acquisition of complex social skills takes time, and the therapeutic investment required increases greatly the lower the patient's starting level.

Finally, we come to prognostic variables which are tied to certain problems or techniques rather than to others. One example comes from desensitization and flooding. Desensitization improves patients with more focal phobias without much free-floating anxiety, and whose GSR habituates readily to repeated stimuli (GELDER et al., 1967; LADER et al., 1967; MARKS et al., 1969). These limitations were not found with flooding, which is associated with good results even in patients with free-floating anxiety and other neurotic symptoms (MARKS et al., 1971a; WATSON et al., 1971; STERN and MARKS, 1973a). Table 2 illustrates this contrast in prognoses between two different techniques in the same condition.

Yet another distinction is found in the prognosis with flooding in fantasy using relevant vs. irrelevant fear cues. WATSON and MARKS (1971, Table 3) found that these two methods had different prognostic correlates. Whereas relevant flooding worked better in patients with greater initial anxiety or arousal and did not correlate with anxiety during treatment sessions, outcome to irrelevant flooding did not correlate significantly with arousal before treatment, but correlated positively with anxiety during treatment sessions. These differential prognostic correlates gave a clue that the two procedures might be operating at least in part through separate mechanisms.

To complicate matters further, in obsessive-compulsives, HODGSON et al. (1972) found no significant correlates between initial anxiety level and outcome with flooding and response prevention.

Table 2. Prognostic factors in flooding and desensitization (from MARKS et al., 1971a)

Correlation with variables at start of treatment	Improvement criteria: 1 Main phobia FLO	1 Main phobia DES	2 Heart rate FLO	2 Heart rate DES	3 GSR flucs FLO	3 GSR flucs DES	4 GSR deflec FLO	4 GSR deflec DES
Agoraphobia					-.23	(-.74xx)		
panic attacks - doctors' rating	.32	(-.54x)						
total phobia - doctors' rating	.30	(-.51x)						
anxiety - doctors' rating	.30	(-.54x)						
depression - doctors' rating					.63^{+}	(.12)		
work impairment	.64xx	(-.62xx)			.25	(-.55x)	-.06	(.54x)
leisure impairment					.50	(-.55x)		
sexual impairment	.51x	(-.38)						
social phobia checklist	.55x	(-.32)						
phobia checklist	.52x	(-.50)			.56x	(-.22)		
introversion (EPI)	.62^{+}	(-.36)			.16	(-.57x)		
GSR fluctuations during:								
neutral fantasy			-.09	(-.83xxx)				
neutral talk			-.23	(-.73xx)				
minor phobic fantasy			-.06	(-.73xx)				
GSR maximum deflection during:								
main phobic fantasy					.60^{+}	(.24)	.40	(-.51)x
minor phobic fantasy					.71^{+}	(-.04	.68^{+}	(-.45)
neutral fantasy					.53x	(-.14)	.62^{+}	(-.38)
phobic talk (ips)					.87xxx	(.04)	.71xx	(-.21)
Heart rate increment during:								
minor phobic fantasy	.76xx	(-.78xx)						
phobic talk							.19	(-.53x)
Subjective anxiety during:								
neutral fantasy						(-.78x)		

x = $p < .05$ from correlation of o.   xx = $p < .01$ ips = ipsative measure   FLO = flooding
\+ = $p < .02$ xxx = $p < .001$ DES = desensitization
1 = decrease on 1-5 scale, patient's and doctors' ratings combined
2 = decrease in heart rate, increment during main phobic fantasy (ips)
3 = decrease in spontaneous fluctiations increment during 3rd minute of phobic talk (ips)
4 = decrease in maximum deflection of GSR during 3rd minute of phobic talk (ips).

Table 3. Prognostic factors in flooding with relevant and irrelevant fear cues (from WATSON and MARKS, 1971)

Correlation with variables at start of treatment	Outcome criteria: Phobic talk – Heart rate	Phobic talk – SK.-emd. fluct.	Main phobia Pt. + drs. anxiety + avoidance	Total phobias – Doctors – Anxiety	Total phobias – Doctors – avoidance	Total phobias – Patient – Anxiety	Total phobias – Patient – avoidance	Phobia attitude (evaluative)
Heart rate								
Neutral fantasy	[$-.51^{x}$]							
Neutral talk	$-.54^{x}$	[$-.59^{*}$]					$-.49^{x}$	
Normal fear fantasy			$.59^{*}$					
Phobic fantasy						xx		
Phobic talk				$.54^{x}$			$.50^{x}$	
Skin-conductance fluctuations								
Neutral fantasy			$.74^{xxx}$	$.50^{x}$				
Neutral talk		$.52^{x}$						
Normal fear fantasy				$.50^{x}$				
Phobic fantasy		$.59^{*}$						
Phobic talk		$.63^{xx}$			$.53^{x}$			
Subjective anxiety								
Neutral fantasy						[$-.61^{*}$]		
Neutral talk						[$-.54^{x}$]		
Normal fear fantasy	[$-.68^{xx}$]							
Phobic fantasy		[$-.50^{x}$]						
Sessional anxiety								
During flooding			[$.60^{*}$]		[$.54^{x}$]		[$.56^{x}$]	[$.59^{*}$]
During irrelevant fear			$.51^{x}$					
Mean of both			[$.70^{xx}$]		[$.54^{x}$]		[$.54^{x}$]	[$.66^{xx}$]

(Boxed values are shown in square brackets.)

[a] Correlations with outcome to irrelevant fear are boxed, with outcome to flooding unboxed.
x = $p < .05$ xx = $p < .01$ * = $p < .02$
xxx = $p < .001$. Blank cells denote insignificant correlations

A final example of a diagnostic variable affecting prognosis comes from aversion in transvestites (Fig. 1). There the additional presence of transsexualism - the desire for a bodily sex change as well as the clothes of the opposite sex - augured a uniformly poor outcome with aversion (MARKS et al., 1970).

In summary, transcending variables such as motivation, empathy and warmth, and expectancy, probably act through increasing patient and therapist cooperation in executing the details of treatment operations. Other specific variables apply to certain diagnoses and techniques rather than to others, examples of which have been given.

Abstract: As with any psychological treatment, prognosis in behavioural psychotherapy can be divided into those variables which transcend given diagnoses or techniques, and those which are specific to the condition or treatment method being employed. Transcending (nonspecific) variables include motivation, expectancy, empathy and warmth of patient and of therapist, chronicity of the disorder, and the extent to which it involves the patient's life style and family. Mechanisms of action of these variables are discussed. Specific variables are those such as amount of free-floating anxiety and habituation rate in phobics treated by desensitization or by flooding, presence of transsexualism in transvestites treated by aversion, and ability to speak in autistic children treated by operant conditioning.

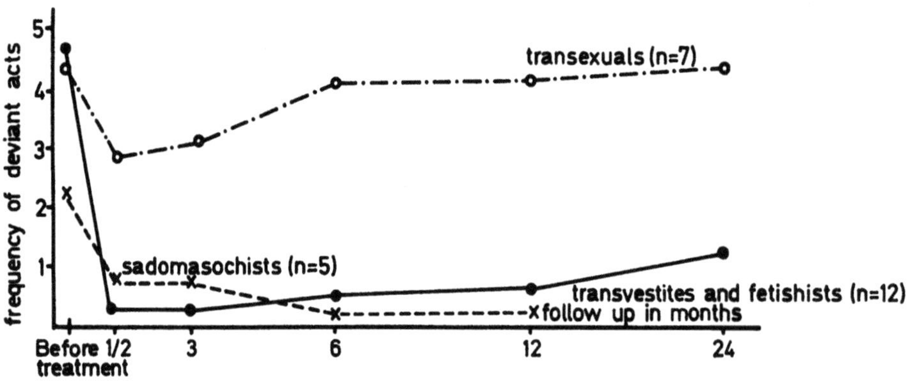

Fig. 1. Prognosis for transsexualism vs. transvestism (from MARKS et al., 1970)

References

BANCROFT, J.H.J.: Desensitization and aversion in treatment of homosexuality. M.D. dissertation, Univ. of London 1970.

FELDMAN, M.P., MacCULLOCH, M.P.: Homosexual Behaviour. New York-London: Pergamon Press 1971.

FISHER, D.: Training community agents of change for disturbed and delinquent children. Paper to 3rd Southern California Conference on Behaviour Modification. Los Angeles. October 1971.

GELDER, M.G., MARKS, I.M., WOLFF, H.H.: Desensitization and psychotherapy in the treatment of phobics states: A controlled inquiry. Brit. J. Psychiat. 113, 53-73 (1967).

HODGSON, R., RACHMAN, S., MARKS, I.M.: The treatment of obsessive-compulsive neurosis: follow-up and further findings. Behav. Res. Ther. 10, 181-189 (1972).

LADER, M.H., GELDER, M.G., MARKS, I.M.: Palmer skin-conductance measures as predictors of response to desensitization. J. psychosom. Res. 11, 283-290 (1967).
LOVAAS, O.I.: A behaviour therapy approach to the treatment of childhood schizophrenia. In: Minnesota Symposium on Child Psychiatry. Univ. of Minnesota Press 1967.
MARKS, I.M., GELDER, M., EDWARDS, J.G.: Hypnosis and desensitization for phobias: a controlled prospective trial. Brit. J. Psychiat. 114, 1263-1274 (1968).
MARKS, I.M., GELDER, M., BANCROFT, J.: Sexual deviants two years after electric aversion. Brit. J. Psychiat. 117, 193-185 (1970).
MARKS, I.M., BOULOUGOURIS, J., MARSET, P.: Flooding versus desensitization in the treatment of phobic patients: A crossover study. Brit. J. Psychiat. 119, 353-75 (1971a).
MATHEWS, A.M.: Paper to annual conference of Behavioural Engineering Association, Wexford, September 1971.
PATTERSON, G.R.: Chapter in: BERGIN, A.E., GARFIELD, S. (Eds.): Handbook of Psychotherapy and Behavior Change. New York: Wiley 1971.
ROOTH, F.G., MARKS, I.M.: Aversion, self-regulation and relaxation in treatment of persistent exhibitionism. Submitted for publication 1973.
STERN, R.S., MARKS, I.M.: Brief and prolonged flooding. In press 1973a.
STERN, R.S., MARKS, I.M.: Contract marital therapy in obsessive-compulsive neurosis. Submitted for publication 1973b.
STUART, R.B.: Operant-interpersonal therapy for marital discord. J. consult. clin. Psychol. 33, 675-682 (1969).
WATSON, J.P., GAIND, R., MARKS, I.M.: Prolonged exposure: a rapid treatment for phobias (joint article). Brit. med. J. 1971I, 13-15.
WATSON, J.P., MARKS, I.M.: Relevant and irrelevant fear in flooding - A crossover study of phobic patients. Behav. Ther. 2, No. 3, 275-293 (1971).

Subject Index

MIX
Papier aus verantwortungsvollen Quellen
Paper from responsible sources
FSC® C105338

If you have any concerns about our products,
you can contact us on
ProductSafety@springernature.com

In case Publisher is established outside the EU,
the EU authorized representative is:
Springer Nature Customer Service Center GmbH
Europaplatz 3, 69115 Heidelberg, Germany

Printed by Libri Plureos GmbH
in Hamburg, Germany